Handbook of Cannabis for Clinicians

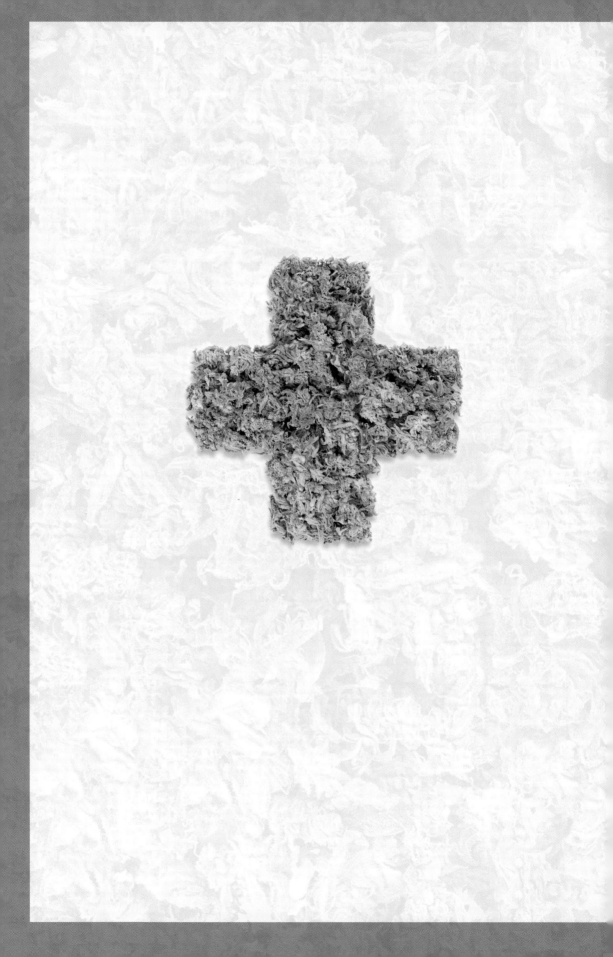

Handbook of Cannabis for Clinicians

Principles and Practice

Dustin Sulak, D.O.

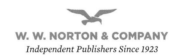

W. W. NORTON & COMPANY

Independent Publishers Since 1923

Note to Readers: Standards of clinical practice and protocol change over time, and no technique or recommendation is guaranteed to be safe or effective in all circumstances. This volume is intended as a general information resource for professionals practicing in the fields of medicine and mental health; it is not a substitute for appropriate training, peer review, and/or clinical supervision. Neither the publisher nor the author(s) can guarantee the complete accuracy, efficacy, or appropriateness of any particular recommendation in every respect. As of press time, the URLs displayed in this book link or refer to existing sites. The publisher and author are not responsible for any content that appears on third-party websites.

For information about permission to reproduce selections from this book, write to
   Permissions, W. W. Norton & Company, Inc., 500 Fifth Avenue, New York, NY 10110
For information about special discounts for bulk purchases, please contact
   W. W. Norton Special Sales at specialsales@wwnorton.com or 800-233-4830

Manufacturing by Versa Press
Book design by Daniel Lagin
Production manager: Katelyn MacKenzie

Library of Congress Cataloging-in-Publication Data

Names: Sulak, Dustin, author.
Title: Handbook of cannabis for clinicians : principles and practice / Dustin Sulak.
Description: First edition. | New York : W.W. Norton & Company, [2021] | "A Norton
   professional book." | Includes bibliographical references and index.
Identifiers: LCCN 2020034469 | ISBN 9780393714180 (cloth) |
   ISBN 9780393714197 (epub)
Subjects: LCSH: Marijuana—Therapeutic use. | Clinicians
Classification: LCC RM666.C266 S85 2021 | DDC 615.3/23648—dc23
LC record available at https://lccn.loc.gov/2020034469

W. W. Norton & Company, Inc., 500 Fifth Avenue, New York, N.Y. 10110
www.wwnorton.com

W. W. Norton & Company Ltd., 15 Carlisle Street, London W1D 3BS

1 2 3 4 5 6 7 8 9 0

This book is dedicated to all of our patients.

Contents

Part 3 Cannabis Pharmacology

Part 4 Clinical Essentials in Cannabinoid Medicine

Part 5 **Common Clinical Applications**

Foreword

It is both an honor and a pleasure to provide brief commentary on this exemplary book. While it is true that recent times have produced numerous excellent tomes on the subject of cannabis and its medical uses, Dustin Sulak has produced a detailed and scientifically accurate guide specifically geared toward the practicing physician who seeks to understand the history of cannabis in medicine, its foundations in an understanding of the endocannabinoid system that modulates human physiology, the pharmacological effects of its myriad cannabinoid and terpenoid components, their various preparations, and specific effects and contributions to combating various afflictions. Along the way in the narrative and its short discrete chapters, there are appropriate mentions of the necessary pitfalls and caveats a clinician in the trenches requires when embarking on care of patients with unfamiliar treatment modalities. Embarking on an understanding of the science of cannabis and the endocannabinoid system is clearly not for the dilettante nor for the faint of heart, but for the committed student of these disciplines, there can be few better guides than this one, which is at once lucid and practical.

Authors of scientific literature face a constant challenge in the need to present technical material in a palatable manner and must choose between a strict didactic approach versus one in which the personal touch remains clear. To my delight, and to the advantage of his readers, Dustin has peppered his text with plenty of examples of his extensive experience in applied therapeutics, not merely confined to cannabis medicine but incorporating his eclectic learning and training in the healing arts. Thus, his personality shines through the words and imparted wisdom. It has been my good fortune to know Dustin over the course of a decade, to travel with him, and to meet his wonderful extended family. I have seen him hold a huge hall of conference attendees at rapt attention, hanging on every word, and witnessed him holding court in a spontaneous impromptu yoga class of high school seniors on spring break on a Caribbean beach. I have delighted in the range and depth of his knowledge of esoteric therapeutic disciplines and obscure treatments that I encountered only after many decades of study.

Rather than wax prosaic on my own opinions on the folly of continued prohibitions on cannabis and existing roadblocks to its research, I would opt for the path of brevity here and urge the reader to press ahead to more rewarding pursuits by pushing on into this book itself. At the time of this writing, the cannabis community is mourning the passing of Lester Grinspoon, MD, one of the guiding lights of cannabis medicine. In the academic world it is often stated that we gain our knowledge by standing on the shoulders of giants. In Dustin Sulak we have another such giant, a worthy successor, at once a gifted clinician and marvelous teacher. May you be enriched by the knowledge you are about to acquire!

Ethan Russo, MD
Founder and CEO, CReDO Science
June 2020

Acknowledgments

Thank you to my patients, who have taught me the most about cannabis, intimately shared their journeys, and supported my family throughout the writing of this book.

Thank you to my beloved mentors, who gave me the confidence to follow my alternative path in medicine and who model dedication to service and teaching, open-minded yet scientific thinking, ethics, leadership, professionalism, and generosity: Rabbi Nathan Segal; Andrew Weil, MD; John McPartland, DO; Ethan Russo, MD; Jeff Hergenrather, MD; and James Jealous, DO.

Thank you to the hundreds of researchers cited in this book, the institutions that made their work possible, and the human and animal subjects who have collectively created a vast body of evidence that has guided and supported my work on the uncertain front lines of cannabis medicine. Thank you to Sci-Hub for removing barriers to scientific knowledge and making this project possible.

Thank you to my children, Arwen, Isabelle, and Samuel, for inspiring me to be my best, for understanding my dedication to this work, and for the hundreds of brief writing interruptions that filled my heart with love and my vision with beauty.

Thank you to my parents, Karen and Craig, for unconditionally supporting my work with cannabis since its beginning and comforting me in times of stress, and to my brothers and brother-in-law, Clayton, Shawn, and Brad, for joining me in this field and greatly contributing to my success.

My deepest gratitude to my wife, Danielle, for supporting this project and me at every level, including keeping me full of love and inspiration, caring for our children, caring for our clinic, understanding the subject matter and the audience, and organizing and editing the manuscript. We make an incredible team.

Thank you to the patients, parents, growers, and distributors who have risked or suffered criminal penalties by serving the health-care needs of their families and communities. Your sacrifices have helped countless others.

Thank you to cannabis, an extraordinary plant, teacher, healer, and metaphor, for taking me on this journey and empowering me to be of greater service to patients and clinicians.

Handbook of Cannabis for Clinicians

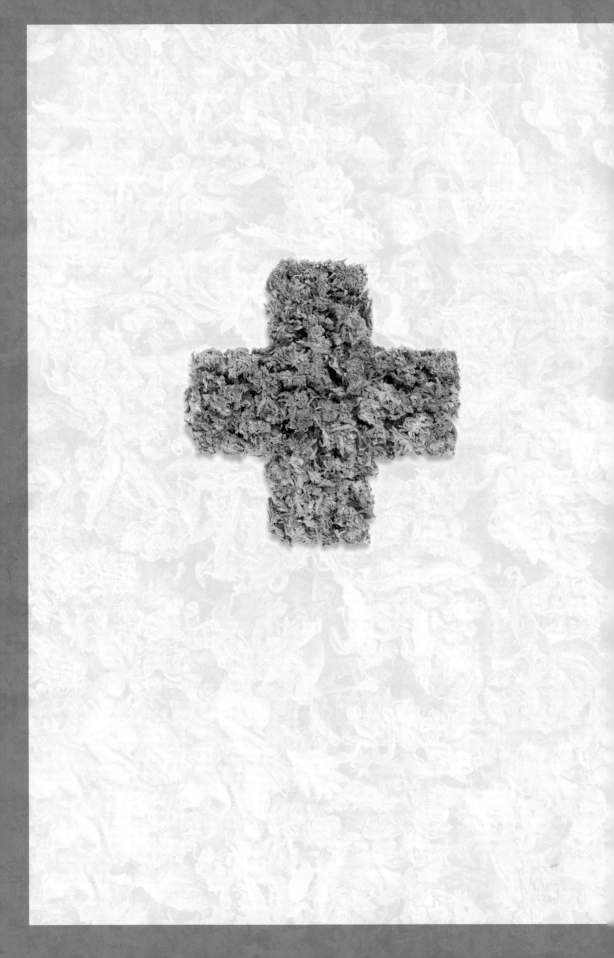

Part 1

Cannabis Is Making a Comeback in Medicine

Chapter 1

Introduction

A 54-YEAR-OLD MAN with failed back surgery syndrome returns to the office for his first 3-month follow-up visit having tapered and discontinued 60 mg of oxycodone daily, reporting less pain and better function. A 2-year-old girl with Krabbe disease, an inherited demyelinating disorder, who had spent most of her life screaming and grimacing, returns in a calm state with a slight smile on her face. A 48-year-old woman with multiple sclerosis offers to donate her walker to another patient because she does not need it anymore. An 11-year-old boy with autism stops putting his head through walls and other forms of self-injury and is now able to attend school. A 32-year-old woman with severe posttraumatic stress disorder sleeps through the night without a nightmare for the first time in over a decade.

While we may collect a few stories like this in our careers, not many clinicians see these results on a daily basis. In the last 11 years of clinical practice with cannabis, remarkable success in highly refractory patients has become the norm, not the exception. Not everyone responds to cannabis, and some that do receive only modest benefits, but after seeing what I have seen, I can hardly imagine practicing medicine without this tool. I know that I would be forced to rely on more dangerous and less effective treatments for my patients, and I would see life-changing results much less frequently.

Despite its nearly 5,000 years of recorded use as a medicine and its impressive versatility, efficacy, and safety, *Cannabis sativa* has existed outside the modern pharmacopeia since the 1940s. Primarily driven by popular demand, this botanical medicine has returned to health care, and now clinicians are seeking the essential knowledge required to identify candidates for treatment, guide dosing, maximize therapeutic benefit, and minimize harm.

Unlike most emerging medical therapies, which follow a traditional bench-to-bedside path through development, approval, and implementation in the clinical setting, the widespread public use of medical cannabis has preceded rigorous modern validation and clinical education. Medical school and residency curricula, in fact, continue to uphold the institutional bias that has challenged cannabinoid medicine for decades, often failing to even mention the plant or its mechanisms of action.

At the time of writing, clinicians and patients in the United States are challenged by a constantly evolving regulatory patchwork of state medical cannabis programs that exist despite the federal law, which continues to classify cannabis as an illegal substance with no medical use. Countries around the world are beginning to change their cannabis laws, recognizing the scientific basis and potential public health benefits of a long-overdue overhaul of the decades-old dysfunctional drug war originally exported by the United States.

In an environment of rapidly evolving cannabis policy, health-care providers are increasingly in need of readily accessible and factual information about medical cannabis, and while this book does not encompass the details of cannabis law, it provides a scientific basis that informs both clinical practice and health-care policy.

In the late 1980s and early 1990s, researchers exploring the myriad effects of Δ^9-tetrahydrocannabinol on animal physiology discovered a communication system in the body that is now known to be a widespread homeostatic controller of other physiological processes. Named the "endocannabinoid system" after the plant that led to its discovery, researchers have since published over 9,000 peer-reviewed articles that include information on this network of cell membrane receptors, enzymes, and endogenous ligands, revealing an integral component of our ability to heal from most illnesses and to maintain good health. *Therapeutics that target this system therefore have widespread potential in every bodily system and specialty field of medicine.*

Herbal *Cannabis sativa* contains hundreds of compounds that modulate endocannabinoid system activity. This distinct mechanism of action often provides efficacy where other conventional treatments fail. Cannabis, in many ways, is a therapeutic compass to the most prevalent and refractory conditions in medicine, and patients globally are turning to cannabis with or without the approval and supervision of their health-care providers.

The purpose of this book is to provide health-care professionals with an accessible and accurate reference that will empower you to have informed discussions with your patients, identify candidates for treatment, and implement cannabinoid therapies with confidence. I decided to write this book because I have been sincerely amazed by the clinical results in my practice and excited by the untapped potential to improve health and relieve suffering in millions or billions of people. As a board member of the Society of Cannabis Clinicians, I am witnessing the coalescence of a new specialty field in medicine, one that draws its members from every other specialty field and attracts progressive-thinking clinicians dedicated to their patients. In a time of rapidly growing provider dissatisfaction with the limitations of our current health-care system, cannabinoid medicine is a potent solution for patients and clinicians alike.

How to Use This Book

If you are working with a patient who may benefit from cannabis and you need a quick summary of the relevant research, potential risks and benefits, and dosing strategies, skip to Part 5: Common Clinical Applications. There you will find the basics needed for informed consent and initiation of treatment in most patients.

If you want to fine-tune dosing and delivery to improve results or mitigate adverse effects, and if you are a clinician seeing a wide range of cannabis cases, Part 4: Clinical Essentials will enable you to grasp the fundamentals of cannabis dosing that apply to many patients.

All clinicians recommending cannabis should also read the first part of Chapter 18: Adverse Effects. Those working with patients in sensitive fields like pediatrics and psychiatry must read the latter part of that chapter.

If you are open to more than a new tool and give yourself permission for a shift in paradigm, an unlearning of some of the assumptions common in conventional medicine, a deeper understanding of health and healing, and a context for your participation in a health-care revolution, start from the beginning of this book and enjoy the journey.

Chapter 2

The History of Cannabinoid Medicine

AS ONE OF THE EARLIEST plant species cultivated by humans, cannabis has an immense history—often the subject of significant debate—that is beyond the scope of this volume. Herein, I present some of the clinically-relevant history to provide context for both the medical applications and regulatory environment of cannabis.

Ancient and Premodern History

Cannabis sativa likely evolved as a distinct member of the Cannabaceae family around 27.8 million years ago, based on DNA studies.[1] The earliest robust archeological evidence of human cannabis use dates from the Copper Age (4600–3600 B.C.E. in Moldovia, Romania, and Bulgaria) and the Bronze Age (3400–3200 B.C.E. in southeastern Europe). An Iron Age steppe culture, the Scythians, likely introduced hemp cultivation to Celtic, Slavic, and Finno-Ugric cultures (700–500 B.C.E.).[2]

Humans have utilized *Cannabis sativa* in various forms preceding and throughout recorded history. Described as a ubiquitous "camp follower," cannabis accompanied the early nomads around the Old World for millennia. These nomads discovered that certain varieties were best for supplying fiber, others for edible seed, and others for their medicinal properties.[3] A single species rarely provides three or more valuable products, and while the industrial and food applications of cannabis have played a significant role in history and have much to offer our species, this chapter focuses on a concise review of the history of its medical use.

The first recorded medical use of cannabis is associated with the Emperor Shen Nong from 2700 B.C.E., though this was not transcribed until the 2nd century C.E. in the *Shen Nong Ben Cao Jing*, noting hallucinatory effects, appetite stimulation, and tonic and antisenility effects.[4] Over 30 citations demonstrate medical use in ancient Sumer and Akkad as early as 1800 B.C.E., noting utility for grief, epilepsy, neuralgia, and pediculicide.

A thorough review of medical cannabis chronology[5] reveals diverse uses over the centuries, including Egyptian use for vaginal contractions and ophthalmological conditions (1534 B.C.E.) and use in India to relieve anxiety (*Atharva Veda*, 1500 B.C.E.). Jumping forward, the Greek physician Dioscorides described the juice as a treatment for earaches in the 1st century C.E., around the same time the Roman author Pliny the Elder described the use of the herb for burns and the root for joint contractures.

In the 2nd century C.E., the Greek physician Galen described applications for earache, flatus, and chronic pain. Perhaps the oldest historical use for tumors appeared in the Egyptian *Fayyum Medical Book* from the late 2nd century C.E.

The use of cannabis as an analgesic appears throughout history, including use as a surgical anesthetic and analgesic in the 2nd century C.E. in China, for migraine and uterine pain in Persia circa 850 C.E., for neuralgia in Egypt in the 9th century C.E., for headache in Germany as described by Hildegard von Bingen in 1158 C.E., for breast pain and swelling in Italy in the 13th century, and on through premodern and modern history.

In Arabia, Avicenna, regarded as one of the most significant physicians, astronomers, thinkers, and writers of the Islamic Golden Age, described the medical use of cannabis in 1000 C.E.[6] Muslim texts mention the use of cannabis as a diuretic, digestive, and antiflatulent agent, "to clean the brain," and to soothe pain of the ears.[7] In Africa, cannabis has been used medically at least since the 15th century to treat snakebites, malaria, fever, blood poisoning, anthrax, asthma, and dysentery and to facilitate childbirth.[8] In the Americas, the use of cannabis probably began in Brazil in the 16th century, with reports of use for toothache and menstrual cramps.[9]

The pharmacology of cannabis chemovars throughout history is likely varied, and some of the reported medical applications likely involved chemovars low in D^9-tetrahydrocannabinol (THC). THC-dominant cannabis, however, was found in the Yanghai Tombs in Xinjiang, China, dating from 700 B.C.E. A Chinese description of the herb from 214 B.C.E. noted the dioecious quality of the plant and that male plants were superior for fiber, while female plants were superior for intoxication, indicating the presence of THC content.

Modern History

Cannabis was introduced to Western medicine by the Irish physician William O'Shaugh-nessy,* who learned of "gunjah" during time spent in India. He studied the literature on the plant, described various preparations, evaluated its toxicity in animals, and reported on its effect on patients with different pathologies.[10] For example, he treated three cases of tetanus with cannabis; all three patients survived the acute disorder, but one succumbed to gangrene after refusing amputation. Frequent dosing relaxed the spasmodic paroxysms and allowed nutrition and hydration until the patients recovered, sometimes weeks later.

The medical use of cannabis quickly spread throughout Europe and North America. In 1854, cannabis entered *The Dispensatory of the United States of America*, and in 1860, the first clinical conference about cannabis took place in America, organized by the Ohio State Medical Society.[11] During the rest of the 19th century, over 100 scientific articles were published in Europe and the United States about the therapeutic value of cannabis. Of note, the German physician Bernhard Fronmüller described 1,000 patients with sleep disturbance and reported cannabis produced a full cure in 53% of patients, a partial cure in 21.5%, and little or no effect in 25.5%.[12]

In the late 19th and early 20th century, numerous pharmaceutical companies marketed cannabis products, including Merck (Germany), Burroughs Wellcome (England), Bristol-Myers Squibb (United States), Parke-Davis (United States), and Eli Lilly (United States).

Physicians in the 19th century noted that cannabis is effective in sparing opiates, reducing opiate-related morbidity, and treating opiate withdrawal,[13,14] as well as in the treatment of cocaine and chloral hydrate addiction.[15]

In the first decades of the 20th century, Western medical use of cannabis significantly decreased. Some authors suggest this was due, in part, to difficulty obtaining replicable effects because of significant inconsistency of potency and efficacy of different cannabis preparations.[16]

----

* Beyond cannabis, O'Shaughnessy made another major contribution to medicine. In 1831, during a cholera outbreak in England, he analyzed the blood of patients with the condition, discovered dehydration and loss of electrolytes, and published his findings. By 1832, his work prompted the first use of intravenous saline, and the name O'Shaughnessy and the "method of saline injections" became synonymous. [Moon, J. B. (1967). Sir William Brooke O'Shaughnessy—the foundations of fluid therapy and the Indian telegraph service. *New England Journal of Medicine, 276,* 283–284.]

The Prohibition and Rediscovery of Cannabis

Several sources attribute the eventual prohibition of cannabis to the influx of Mexican immigrants to the United States after the Mexican Revolution in 1910.[17,18] The Mexicans reportedly used "marihuana" as a medicine and to relax after working in the field, especially as an alternative to alcohol, which was prohibited in 1920.

While Americans were familiar with "cannabis" because it was present in pharmacies and grown for hemp fiber, the word "marihuana" was a foreign term. So, when the media began to play on the fears that the public had about these new citizens by falsely spreading claims about the "disruptive Mexicans" with their dangerous native behaviors including marihuana use, the rest of the nation did not know that this "marihuana" was the same plant growing on farms or the source of a drug that had been in the pharmacopeia for decades.

At the federal House of Representatives hearing regarding the "Taxation of Marihuana" in May 1937, Dr. William C. Woodward, legislative counsel of the American Medical Association, strongly opposed the legislation that would eventually prohibit the sale and use of cannabis[19]:

> There is nothing in the medicinal use of Cannabis that has any relation to Cannabis addiction. I use the word "Cannabis" in preference to the word "marihuana," because Cannabis is the correct term for describing the plant and its products. The term "marihuana" is a mongrel word that has crept into this country over the Mexican border and has no general meaning, except as it relates to the use of Cannabis preparations for smoking. It is not recognized in medicine . . .
>
> I say the medicinal use of Cannabis has nothing to do with Cannabis or marihuana addiction. In all that you have heard here thus far, no mention has been made of any excessive use of the drug by any doctor or its excessive distribution by any pharmacist. And yet the burden of this bill is placed heavily on the doctors and pharmacists of the country; and I may say very heavily, most heavily, possibly of all, on the farmers of the country . . .
>
> The drug is very seldom used. That is partially because of the uncertainty of the effects of the drug. That uncertainty has heretofore been attributed to variations in the potency of the preparations as coming from particular plants; the variations in the potency of the drug as coming from particular plants undoubtedly depends on variations in the ingredients of which the resin of the plant is made up. To say, however, as has been proposed here, that the use of the drug should be prevented

by a prohibitive tax, loses sight of the fact that future investigation may show that there are substantial medical uses for Cannabis.

The Marihuana Tax Act of 1937 passed. In 1943, medical products derived from cannabis were removed from the U.S. Pharmacopeia and physicians could no longer prescribe it.

Despite its prohibition in the United States, cannabis research continued. The renowned American chemist Roger Adams isolated the active compounds in cannabis in 1940,[20] including cannabidiol and "cannabinol," which would later become known as Δ^9-tetrahydrocannabinol (THC) after its molecular structure was fully elucidated by Raphael Mechoulam in 1964.[21]

In 1944, The New York Academy of Medicine, on behalf of a commission appointed in 1939 by New York Mayor Fiorello LaGuardia, released an in-depth report that systematically refuted claims made by the U.S. Department of the Treasury that smoking cannabis results in insanity and deterioration of physical health, promotes criminal behavior, is physically addictive, and is a gateway to more dangerous drugs.[22]

In the 1950s and 1960s, the U.S. military conducted experiments using synthetic analogues of cannabinol as potential nonlethal incapacitating agents for chemical warfare.[23] Experiments into the physiological and behavioral effects of cannabis and its active components continued in the late 1960s and early 1970s, including several papers by Andrew Weil, MD, who later pioneered the field of integrative medicine.[24,25,26]

In 1969, the controversial Harvard professor Timothy Leary was arrested for the possession of cannabis. He challenged the Marihuana Tax Act on the ground that the act required self-incrimination, which violated the Fifth Amendment. The unanimous opinion of the court declared the Marihuana Tax Act unconstitutional and Leary's conviction was overturned. This apparent victory for cannabis liberation was quickly abolished.

In 1970, the Marihuana Tax Act was replaced with the Controlled Substances Act, which set up the scheduling system for illicit and licit substances. The bill was written by Attorney General John Mitchell and others, consolidating and expanding previous policies without scientific basis, pending the scientific report of the National Commission on Marihuana and Drug Abuse. Cannabis was preliminarily classified as a schedule I controlled substance: high potential for abuse, no currently accepted medical use, and lack of accepted safety for use under medical supervision.

On March 22, 1972, the chairman of the commission, Raymond P. Shafer, presented a report to Congress and the public entitled "Marihuana, A Signal of Misunderstanding," which recommends that cannabis be decriminalized for personal use, and that personal cultivation be allowed along with small transfers without profit.[27] President Nixon rejected these recommendations and cannabis has remained in schedule I status ever since, despite the lack of scientific basis and numerous legal challenges.

In 1976, a U.S. federal judge ruled in favor of Robert C. Randall, a patient with glaucoma who sued several federal agencies, arguing against criminal charges of cannabis cultivation based on his medical necessity. This ruling prompted the establishment of the Compassionate Investigational New Drug program of the U.S. Food and Drug Administration (FDA), which allowed a limited number of patients to legally use cannabis cigarettes grown at the University of Mississippi and provided by the National Institute on Drug Abuse. A total of 15 patients were granted access to cannabis via this program, which was closed in 1992. In 2002, Ethan Russo, MD, and colleagues published a study on the overall health status of four of the seven surviving patients in the program, considered the first report on the long-term effects of cannabis on patients who have used a known dosage of a standardized, heat-sterilized quality-controlled supply of cannabis. The authors noted clinical effectiveness in glaucoma, chronic musculoskeletal pain, spasm, nausea, and spasticity of multiple sclerosis, the sparing of pharmaceutical medications, mild changes in pulmonary function in two patients, and no significant sequelae in any other physiological system.[28]

Recent Progress in Cannabinoid Medicine

A decade after the FDA approved the use of herbal cannabis in select patients, dronabinol (brand name Marinol), a pharmaceutical preparation of THC, was approved in the United States in 1985 for the treatment of chemotherapy-induced nausea and vomiting.

Investigation into the physiological targets of THC led to the discovery of the cannabinoid type 1 (CB1) receptor in 1988[29] and the cannabinoid type 2 (CB2) receptor in 1993.[30]. The endogenous cannabinoid ligands anandamide[31] and 2-arachidonoylglycerol[32,33] were discovered in 1992 and 1995, respectively. Since that time, thousands of peer-reviewed articles have been published on the endocannabinoid system and the therapeutic potential of targeting its receptors and enzymes.

Psychiatrist Tod Mikuriya, MD, is considered the grandfather of the medical cannabis movement in the United States. He had been researching cannabinoid compounds since the 1960s, including a role as the leading cannabis researcher at the Center for Narcotics and Drug Abuse Studies of the National Institute of Mental Health in 1967, a position he left after realizing that the interests of the agency were biased toward the negative effects and not the medical benefits of cannabis. He was an architect of Proposition 215, the state ballot measure that made California the first U.S. state to legalize the medical use of cannabis in 1996. Practicing in the San Francisco area, Mikuriya treated over 9,000 patients with medical cannabis and developed a list of 285 ailments for which cannabis could provide therapeutic value. While such a broad therapeutic potential seemed incredible at the time, subsequent research on the endocannabinoid system supports Dr. Mikuriya's clinical findings.* In 1999, Mikuriya founded the Society of Cannabis Clinicians, a professional membership organization that continues to operate and grow in international membership.[34]

In 1999, the Institute of Medicine of the National Academy of Sciences published a comprehensive review of the scientific evidence on the potential health benefits and risks of cannabis and its constituents.[35] The accumulated data confirmed a variety of indications, particularly analgesia, antiemesis, and appetite stimulation. In general, the report emphasized the need for well-formulated, scientific research into the therapeutic effects of cannabis on patients with specific disease conditions. To this end, the report recommended that clinical trials be conducted with the goal of developing safe delivery methods. This was yet another extensive and well researched federal report refuting the schedule I status that failed to shift federal policy.

In 2003, the U.S. Department of Health and Human Services was issued a patent on "Cannabinoids as antioxidants and neuroprotectants."[36] Filed in 1999, the patent details the use of cannabis-related compounds in the treatment of "acute ischemic neurological insults," "chronic neurodegenerative diseases," and "oxidation associated diseases," including a "subset of such drugs that can be substantially free of psychoactive or psychotoxic effects, are substantially non-toxic even at very high doses, and have good tissue penetration." The hypocrisy of the federal government owning this patent while maintaining schedule I status is frequently highlighted by cannabis activists.

In 2005, nabiximols, a cannabis-derived oral spray containing roughly equal portions of THC and cannabidiol (CBD), produced by GW Pharmaceuticals, was approved in Canada for spasticity in multiple sclerosis, and with Notice of Compliance with Conditions for central neuropathic pain in multiple sclerosis and cancer pain unresponsive to optimized opioid treatment. With over 15,000 patient-years of experience,[37] nabiximols has generated the largest clinical data set on a standardized cannabis preparation. It has subsequently become available in over 25 countries with additional indications including neuropathic pain and cancer pain.

---

* The Tod Mikuriya Papers (1933–2015) were recently made available as an archival collection at the National Library of Medicine. The extensive materials include writings, correspondence, subject files, reprints, research files, business documents, clippings, photographs, audiovisual records, and memorabilia that document his professional career and medical cannabis advocacy activities. https://circulatingnow.nlm.nih.gov/2020/02/25/tod-mikuriya-papers-now-available-for-research/

Public focus on CBD exploded in 2013 after CNN aired its first cannabis documentary, *Weed*, which followed the story of a 4-year-old girl whose treatment-resistant seizures were relieved by a nonimpairing, CBD-dominant variety of cannabis, named "Charlotte's Web" after the featured patient. Soon thereafter, entrepreneurs began producing and marketing CBD products across the United States and later globally. Describing the products as "hemp," and striving for levels of THC below 0.3% by weight to comply with hemp laws, producers of oils, candies, capsules and creams claimed legality in all 50 states (which has since been refuted by the FDA[38]) and began shipping products. In recent years, demand for CBD products has grown immensely. A 2019 analysis reported 6.9% of Americans were using CBD products at that time.[39]

In 2017, the National Academies of Sciences, Engineering, and Medicine published the third comprehensive report of the U.S. government on cannabis, for the first time using the scientific term cannabis in its title, and intentionally distinguishing the data on medical use of cannabis and cannabinoid compounds from nonmedical use.[40] The report found "substantial or conclusive evidence that cannabis or cannabinoids are safe and effective" in the treatment of chronic pain in adults, chemotherapy-induced nausea and vomiting, and patient-reported spasticity related to multiple sclerosis.

In 2018, the FDA approved Epidiolex, a highly purified liquid CBD extract from GW Pharmaceuticals, for the treatment of two rare seizure disorders, Lennox-Gastaut syndrome and Dravet syndrome, in patients older than 2 years.

At the time of writing in 2019, medical cannabis has been legalized in 35 countries and in 37 states and territories of the United States. Following the enactment of medical cannabis legalization laws in the United States and globally, the widespread use of cannabis in the clinical setting has preceded gold standard clinical trial data for most conditions, though several are underway. In the meanwhile, numerous observational reports have been published, associating cannabis use with improvements in a variety of refractory conditions, decreased prescribing and dispensing of drugs for which patients use cannabis as a substitute, and low frequency of serious adverse effects.

Clinicians are increasingly realizing that both governmental regulatory and medical authorities cannot be implicitly trusted to do what is best for our patients' outcomes. As we explore the existing research on cannabis, please recall the propaganda and betrayal that deprived clinicians and our patients of a safe and effective treatment option for decades, resulting in immeasurable suffering and iatrogenic injury. This is a betrayal that needs to be intentionally addressed and prevented from recurring in other areas of medicine.

Chapter 3

Cannabinoid Medicine as a Solution to the Greatest Challenges in Health Care

DURING A PERIOD OF HISTORY with increased human life span and a shift of healthcare demands from infectious disease and trauma to chronic disease, the shortcomings of modern medicine are becoming more and more apparent. Economic forces, outdated scientific paradigms, failure to adopt evidence-based practices, clinician burnout, and other complex factors contribute to a trajectory of increased health-care spending with deteriorating outcomes. In 2016, the United States spent $10,348 per capita on health-care costs, 17.9% of its gross domestic product, a total of $3.3 trillion.[1] Despite spending more on health care than any other country, the United States consistently fails to achieve better health outcomes, ranking last or near last on dimensions of healthy lives, access to health care, efficiency, and equity, among 11 nations* compared in a 2014 report.[2] A 2013 report from the Institute of Medicine on the health of the U.S. population found the United States has worse health and premature death rates than 16 comparable high-income or "peer" countries,† in all age groups and at all income levels.[3]

For example, as of 2007, U.S. males lived 3.7 fewer years than Swiss males, and U.S. females lived 5.2 fewer years than Japanese females. For decades, the United States has experienced the highest infant mortality rate of high-income countries and also ranks poorly on other birth outcomes, such as low birth weight. American children are less likely to live to age 5 than children in other high-income countries. The U.S. death rate from ischemic heart disease is the second highest among the 17 peer countries.

---

* Australia, Canada, France, Germany, the Netherlands, New Zealand, Norway, Sweden, Switzerland, the United Kingdom, and the United States.

† Australia, Austria, Canada, Denmark, Finland, France, Germany, Italy, Japan, Norway, Portugal, Spain, Sweden, Switzerland, the Netherlands, and the United Kingdom.

Older U.S. adults report a higher prevalence of arthritis and activity limitations than their counterparts in the United Kingdom, other European countries, and Japan.[4]

The goal of a well-functioning health-care system is to ensure that people lead long, healthy, and productive lives. Sadly, 60% of U.S. adults live with one chronic disease, defined as a condition that lasts 1 year or more and requires ongoing medical attention or limits activities of daily living, and 40% of U.S. adults have two or more chronic diseases. While many chronic diseases are linked to lifestyle factors like nutrition, tobacco and alcohol use, and physical activity and may be preventable, the conventional treatment of chronic disease has numerous failures in both common and rare conditions.

Chronic pain, for example, is a common condition. In the United States, 14.4 million adults (6.4%) were classified as having the highest level of pain, category 4, with an additional 25.4 million adults (11.3%) experiencing category 3 pain. Individuals with category 3 or 4 pain were likely to have worse health status, to use more health care, and to suffer from more disability than those with less severe pain.[5] The global prevalence of chronic widespread pain is estimated to be 11.8%.[6] Amid costs of more than $150 billion annually in health care, disability, and related expenses in the United States alone[7] and the somber recognition of our devastating overuse of opioid analgesics in the management of chronic pain, the world is desperately in need of safe and cost-effective treatments. Cannabis is one such option, backed by substantial clinical evidence, with a 2017 report from the National Academies concluding that cannabis is safe and effective for the treatment of chronic pain in adults.[8]

In my clinical experience, other prevalent and rare conditions and symptoms that respond poorly to conventional treatment, including autistic spectrum disorders, epilepsy, spasticity, Tourette's syndrome, and inflammatory bowel disease, have demonstrated promising responses to cannabinoid therapies. In 2004, Dr. Ethan Russo wrote "clinical cannabis has become a therapeutic compass to what modern medicine fails to cure." [9] Why? How is it possible that one herb can offer therapeutic value in such a wide range of conditions that span every field in medicine, including neurology, psychiatry, gastroenterology, infectious disease, pain medicine, and more?

This question intrigued researchers for years prior to the discovery of the endocannabinoid system, a fundamental physiological system responsible for cellular homeostasis and the response to illness and injury, throughout the life span, in almost every tissue type, and in all vertebrates. Targeting the endocannabinoid system has therapeutic potential in almost all known human diseases,[10] but the clinical efficacy of cannabinoid medicines is the most striking in the conditions for which we lack safe and effective pharmacological options. For example, in adolescents and adults with epilepsy who have failed to respond to two antiepileptic drugs, the likelihood of becoming seizure-free on a third agent is 1%.[11] Observational data on similar patients suggests the likelihood of becoming seizure-free with cannabis is 10%, with a likelihood of >75% reduction of seizures in an additional 28% of patients.[12]

As the emerging specialty field of cannabinoid medicine grows, clinicians from a variety of disciplines are beginning to refer their most challenging patients to experts that can implement a therapeutic trial of cannabis. Patients with conditions with substantial supporting evidence, like chronic pain, as well as conditions with sparse supporting evidence, like posttraumatic stress disorder and generalized anxiety, are returning to their providers reporting success with medical cannabis, and mainstream medical providers are noticing.

Cannabis clinicians are magnets for atypical patients, refractory to conventional approaches. The work is challenging and time intensive but extraordinarily gratifying. We are often forced to rely on preclinical and limited human data to guide experimental treatments, avoid translational assumptions, emphasize risk–benefit assessments based on the available data, practice informed consent, collect observational data, and communicate with our global colleagues on the front lines of this emerging field in medicine.

Cannabinoid medicine has the potential to relieve the suffering of billions of patients for which conventional care has failed, offer cost-effective treatments, improve doctor–patient rapport, empower patients to increase participation in their own health care and even grow and produce their own medicine, and lead clinical thinking to progressive paradigms in medicine like systems biology and integrative medicine. When used correctly, cannabis is not only good medicine for our patients but also good medicine for our health care.

New patients to my practice are often given hope by the enthusiastically shared reports of follow-up patients in the waiting room. Medical residents and experienced clinicians who shadow me in my clinical training program are often filled with hope, not only for an effective new tool but also for a way of practicing medicine where we can make deep therapeutic connections with our patients and witness profound healing on a daily basis. I hope to share some of that hope with you.

Chapter 4

From the Bench to the Bedside and Vice Versa

IN ITS REINTRODUCTION to clinical practice, cannabinoid medicine has clearly taken an alternative route. Innovators, early-adopting clinicians, and researchers working with cannabis or cannabinoid-related compounds find themselves on a path toward improving patient outcomes that, like so many other features of cannabinoid medicine, is characterized by dichotomy.

Typical bench-to-bedside drug discovery, preclinical research, and phase I–III clinical trials have been the rule of medicine for decades. We clinicians often have the comfort of utilizing drugs and other treatments with known properties, informed by large data sets of placebo-controlled trials that demonstrate safety and efficacy. This process is, unfortunately, very expensive, creating a selection bias toward exploring potential treatments that are most likely to provide substantial returns on investment. It also favors monomolecular therapies that fit nicely into reductionistic experiments. While many of these drugs begin their journey as constituents of plants, fungi, and prokaryotes, pharmaceutical research has a much harder time dealing with complex botanical medicines. Despite its numerous successes, traditional bench-to-bedside drug development has failed to solve some of the greatest challenges in medicine.

Medical cannabis has turned this process on its head. Widespread clinic use of this medicine is only growing more rapidly, preceding clinical trial data supporting its use for many of its most common indications. Patients are experimenting, at best under the supervision of a medical provider or herbalist, but so often under the guidance of the internet or the dispensary attendant. Patients are simply not willing to wait, nor should they have to. Herbal cannabis has a better safety profile than most over-the-counter drugs, pain relievers, such as acetaminophen, the leading cause of acute liver failure in the U.S. In contrast, cannabis overdose is non-lethal, and 96.6% of side effects in clinical trials are non-serious. In my clinical experience, I've found that many patients have achieved satisfactory results with a little trial and error prior to medical supervision.

In an era of big data analysis, it is time for medicine to unshackle itself from its exclusive relationship with controlled clinical trials and take a look around. We can learn a lot from hundreds of thousands of patients using cannabis via observational research, and we are starting to see creative ways to collect this data from patients. The task is certainly complex, because cannabis is not a single molecule or even a single medicine. Differences in dosage and delivery route of hundreds of phytoconstituents with potential physiological activity and pleiotropic effects, combined with the inherent diversity in genetics, microbiota, lifestyle factors, and concurrent treatments in a large observational data set create quite the challenge. Luckily, cannabis seems to foster open-mindedness, creativity, and willingness to collaborate in its researchers.

Where will the bedside-to-bench and bench-to-bedside paths intersect? Perhaps in clinical practice, as it has in mine, but also in the land of network pharmacology, a novel approach to the drug discovery process that acknowledges systems biology and the complexity of chronic disease. Rather than targeting specific proteins with single molecules, network pharmacologists analyze systems to determine a set of proteins most involved in a disease state and then use chemical biology to identify molecules capable of targeting that set of proteins. This approach yields treatment that involve multiple compounds, multiple targets, and multiple physiological pathways.

Why is this better? Biological systems contain incredibly complex homeostatic and allostatic pathways with significant redundancy; most diseases are not simply caused by one single factor. This is especially true for the complex chronic diseases that plague so many of our patients. No wonder single-target monomolecular therapies so often fail to cure disease. It makes much more sense to gently nudge dozens of nodes, which is exactly what cannabis is always doing, even while we do our best to reduce it to single compounds like THC and CBD.

Using cannabinoid medicines as an example, Brodie et al.[1] described the rationale for using polypharmacology in the treatment of multifactorial diseases and developed a model for evaluating complex multitarget treatments, called the "therapeutic handshake." The model can be applied to cannabinoid medicines and can also be used to evaluate the combination of cannabinoids with other pharmaceutical and botanical agents, and may grow to include nonpharmacological interventions. The concept is ingeniously illustrated in a diagram of nabiximols (Sativex, a plant-based combination of THC and CBD) in the treatment of bone cancer pain (Figure 4.1). Twenty different molecular targets, including membrane receptors and enzymes, five tissue and pathway systems, and two well-known cannabinoids that are both multitarget agents, are arranged in the handshake model.

FIGURE 4.1

Retrospective Application of the Therapeutic Handshake Model to Nabiximols

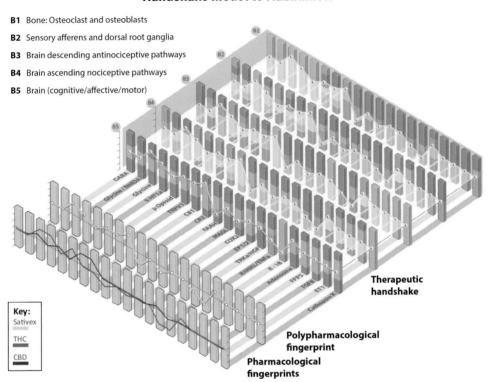

B1 Bone: Osteoclast and osteoblasts
B2 Sensory afferens and dorsal root ganglia
B3 Brain descending antinociceptive pathways
B4 Brain ascending nociceptive pathways
B5 Brain (cognitive/affective/motor)

Key:
Sativex
THC
CBD

Therapeutic handshake

Polypharmacological fingerprint

Pharmacological fingerprints

Note. Nabiximols (Sativex) is an approximately 1:1 combination of Δ^9-tetrahydrocannabinol (THC), a partial agonist for cannabinoid type 1 (CB1) receptors, and cannabidiol (CBD), a multitarget cannabinoid, as botanical extracts. Efficacy and safety of Sativex for relieving pain from bone cancer (e.g., metastatic prostate carcinoma) are predicted. Adapted from "Polypharmacology shakes hands with complex aetiopathology," by J. S. Brodie, V. Di Marzo, and G. W. Guy, 2015, *Trends in Pharmacological Sciences*, 36(12), 802–821 (https://doi.org/10.1016/j.tips.2015.08.010). Copyright 2015 by Elsevier. Reprinted with permission.

While the field of network pharmacology is still in its infancy and will require more complex models that include genetics, epigenetic factors, system perturbations induced by the modulation of primary and secondary targets, and much more data, I believe this is the future of personalized, safer, and more effective medicine.

As busy clinicians on the front lines of cannabinoid medicine, what do we do in the meanwhile? Some suggestions:

- Communicate with other clinicians in the field. Attend conferences,* join a professional society,† and participate in online forums.
- Get comfortable finding and reading the rapidly growing primary literature.‡ Recognize that institutional bias favoring research designed to show the harm of cannabis still heavily influences the literature; many papers in which the abstract seems to vilify cannabis actually contain evidence of its benefits in the findings.
- Interact with preclinical and clinical researchers; they need their study designs to be informed by what you are seeing on the front lines of clinical practice. If you read a study that fails to ask the right questions or misses opportunities to find the answers important to your clinical practice, send the author an email. The dialogues that emerge can not only be enjoyable; they can significantly impact the shape of cannabis science.
- Learn from your patients. Collect outcome data *and also* delve into the qualitative aspects of their experience. For example, if you ask if the pain is better, the response might be, "It's a little less intense." If you ask how their life is different, your cannabis-using patient will likely describe a change in the quality of pain toward less bothersome, an improvement in other symptoms you did not know they had, and an improved feeling of well-being or restored self.
- Use standardized measures in your practice. Brief subjective questionnaires can readily be added to patient intake forms. Do not worry if you lack the time to collate

---

* These are the two annual conferences I have found the most rewarding: The National Clinical Conference on Cannabis Therapeutics, organized by the nonprofit Patients Out of Time, is an excellent blend of clinicians, basic researchers, patients, activists, and legal professionals (patientsoutoftime.org). CannMed, organized by Medicinal Genomics, includes scientific presentations from the medical, horticultural, and laboratory sectors in the field (cannmedevents.com). Both usually offer continuing medical education credits.

† The Society of Cannabis Clinicians (cannabisclinicians.org) has been the home of cannabis-interested medical professionals since 1999. A nonprofit society dedicated to best practices, education, research and patient safety, it offers regular virtual meetings with expert presenters. Its online forums are a great resource for curbside consultations and collaboration opportunities.

‡ The International Association for Cannabinoid Medicines (cannabis-med.org) offers an excellent, free biweekly newsletter reviewing the most recent publications and policy changes, and their website includes a search engine of archived newsletters. In the results of a search for a full-text article, Google Scholar sometimes includes links to download. ResearchGate is another excellent online resource that facilitates communication with authors and often provides the full text of articles.

or analyze the data; it may come in handy sometime in the future when, for example, a resident contacts you looking for a research project.

- Encourage medical schools and residency programs to include endocannabinoid physiology and cannabis pharmacology in the curriculum. Offer to serve as a guest lecturer, and if you need help with material, contact me for slides.

- Expect the unexpected. Cannabis medicine is full of surprises, and though we sometimes must apply reductionistic thinking for practical purposes, when we do so, cannabis often leads us back to a world of complexity and new paradigms in medicine. Similar patients with similar conditions might respond drastically differently to the same treatment. Periodically step back and reflect to identify what questions need answering.

Sidebar: Example of Network Pharmacology

QiShenYiQi is a Chinese medicine prescription agent approved by the State Food and Drug Administration of China. Composed of *Astragalus membranaceus* (Huangqi), *Salvia miltiorrhiza* (Danshen), *Panax notoginseng* (Sanqi), and *Dalbergia odorifera* (Jiangxiang), it is widely and effectively used in China to treat cardiovascular disease, including myocardial infarction, angina, myocarditis, myocardial fibrosis, and heart failure. A network pharmacology study[2] of this multicompound treatment for multifactorial conditions demonstrates the complexity we might employ when studying cannabis. In the multicompound–multitarget–multipathway network of QiShenYiQi in the treatment of myocardial infarction, illustrated in Figure 4.2, diamonds represent compounds, circles represent target genes, and V shapes represent pathways related to cardiovascular disease. The node size of each target and pathway is proportional to the number of compounds associated with the node.

FIGURE 4.2

Multicompound–Multitarget–Multipathway Network of the Traditional Chinese Medicine QiShenYiQi

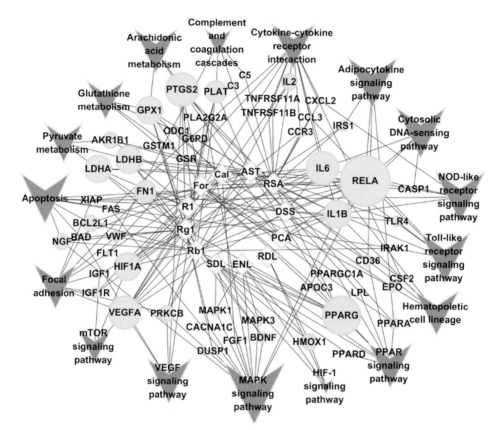

Source. From "A network pharmacology study of Chinese medicine QiShenYiQi to reveal its underlying multi-compound, multi-target, multi-pathway mode of action," by X. Li, L. Wu, W. Liu, Y. Jin, Q. Chen, L. Wang, X. Fan, Z. Li, & Y. Cheng, 2014, *PLOS ONE 9*(5), Article e95004 (https://doi.org/10.1371/journal.pone.0095004). Copyright 2014 by Li et al. Reprinted with permission.

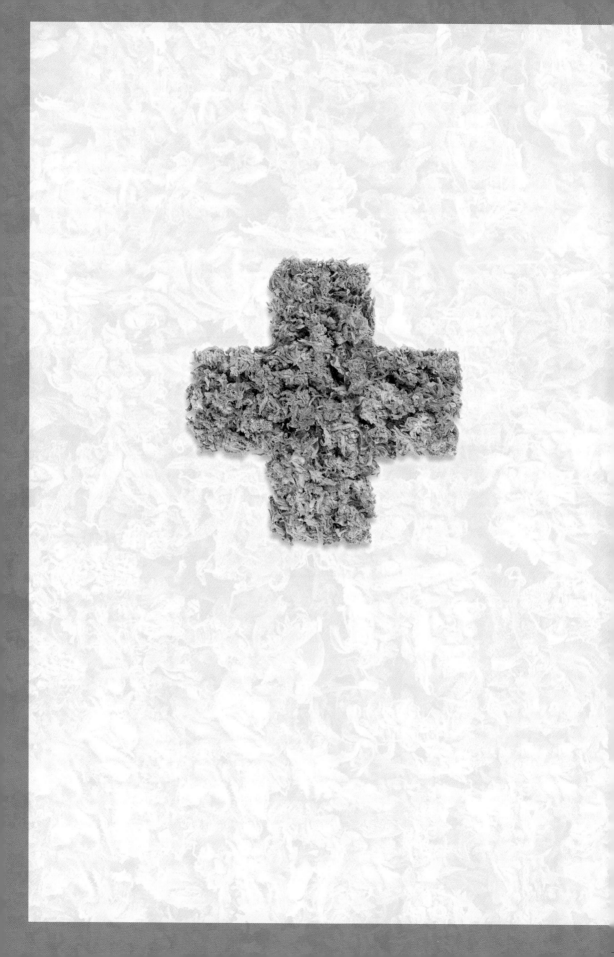

Part 2

Endocannabinoid Physiology

Chapter 5

Cannabinoid Receptors

THE CHEMICAL STRUCTURE AND DIVERSE therapeutic effects of Δ^9-tetrahydrocannabinol (THC) had been recognized for decades, and THC was even approved by the U.S. Food and Drug Administration in the form of dronabinol, before the search for the its physiological target(s) culminated in 1988, when Allyn Howlett and Bill Devane published the first evidence that a cannabinoid receptor exists in the brain.[1] The cloning of the receptor in 1990[2] provided the final evidence for the existence of a cannabinoid receptor, now called CB1, and permitted the identification of neurons expressing this receptor. At first, the CB1 receptor was thought to exist only in the central nervous system (CNS) and at low levels in the testis. In 1993, a peripherally located cannabinoid receptor was found to be present in spleen macrophages and absent in the brain; it later became known as cannabinoid receptor type 2 (CB2).[3]

CB1 receptors are abundant in the nervous system, perhaps the most abundant G protein-coupled receptors in the brain. They are primarily localized in the terminals of central and peripheral neurons, where they mediate inhibition of neurotransmitter release.[4] Beyond the nervous system, CB1 receptors are now known to exist in many other tissues, including fascia, adipose tissue, skeletal muscle, smooth muscle, liver, lungs, pancreas, kidneys, adrenal glands, heart, thymus, and tonsils.[5]

CB2 receptors are primarily expressed by immune cells, including leukocytes and splenocytes, and by osteoblasts and osteoclasts, but they are also found elsewhere, including the peripheral nervous system. Initial studies suggested that CB2 receptors were absent from the healthy brain, but it is now recognized that, during injury and inflammation, CB2 is expressed in brain cells, including microglia, astrocytes, T cells, neurons, neural progenitor cells, and endothelial cells. The presence of CB2 receptors in the healthy CNS is likely but remains somewhat controversial.[6]

In addition to the outer cellular membranes, cannabinoid receptors have been found in intracellular compartments—endoplasmic reticulum, endosomes, lysosomes, cell nuclei, and mitochondria—where they regulate ATP production and cellular respiration.[7]

As G protein-coupled receptors, CB1 and CB2 can initiate many downstream signals: ion channel coupling, inhibition and stimulation of adenylate cyclase, and coupling to the mitogen-activated protein kinase signaling pathway. The activity initiated downstream of the receptor itself often depends on the agonist, which can preferentially direct the action of the receptor toward the different functions, a process known as "functional selectivity" (also "agonist trafficking" or "ligand bias"). In other words, the same receptor may behave differently depending on whether a synthetic cannabinoid, endogenous cannabinoid, or phytocannabinoid ligand is present.[8] This level of homeostatic complexity reminds us that many discrete scientific findings tell only a small part of the story. It also reminds us to be cautious in translating findings from animal studies with synthetic cannabinoids, often full agonists, to human patients using phytocannabinoids.

Orthologs of the human CB1 receptor have been identified in primitive chordates, such as sea squirts, which suggests cannabinoid receptors evolved 600 million years ago.[9] This high level of evolutionary conservation indicates an important function. The rat and human CB1 receptors are 97% identical at the amino acid level. The CB2 receptor shows less homology between species: the human and mouse CB2 receptors share 82% amino acid identity, indicating the need for extra caution when translating rodent findings regarding CB2 to our human patients.

CB1 and CB2 receptors are distributed throughout the body and provide a cellular communication system that allows cross-talk among various cell types, are differentially expressed in conditions of health and disease, and are an integral part of the intracellular and intercellular homeostatic functions of our healing system. The CB receptors serve many functions, but are most often involved in negative feedback signaling, suppressing excessive cellular activities like neurotransmitter release or cytokine production.

Noncannabinoid Receptors Involved in the Endocannabinoid System

The endocannabinoid system (ECS) overlaps with other receptor systems. Beyond CB1 and CB2, the receptors TRPV1, GPR55, and the PPARs most notably play roles in the ECS.

TRPV1, also known as the capsaicin receptor, belongs to a family of transient receptor potential vanilloid (TRPV) channels. TRPV1 is a nonselective ion channel, permeable to mono- and divalent cations (i.e., Mg^{2+}, Ca^{2+}, Na^+). It is activated by both physical and mechanical stimuli such as high temperatures, low pH, and osmotic changes, as well as by exogenous or endogenous compounds such as capsaicin (from hot chili peppers), endocannabinoids, and phytocannabinoids. TRPV1 is mainly found in dorsal root ganglia and Aδ and C-type sensory nerve fibers, but it is also expressed in brain neurons, keratinocytes, and other cell types. [10]

GPR55 is considered an orphan receptor (a protein that has a similar structure to other identified receptors but whose endogenous ligand has not yet been identified). It is expressed throughout the brain and in the gut and has emerged as a target for modulating inflammation, endocrine function, and energy metabolism.[11,12] GPR55 is activated by THC and several endogenous compounds (anandamide, 2-arachidonoylglycerol, and N-palmitoylethanolamine).[13] It is considered by some as a third member of the cannabinoid receptor family, but this issue remains contentious because GPR55 shares little amino acid identity (~14%) and lacks the classic "cannabinoid binding pocket" present in CB1 and CB2.[14]

The 5-HT1A serotonin receptor and GPR18 (i.e., N-arachidonoylglycine receptor) are also considered by many experts to be functional components of the ECS.[15]

Peroxisome proliferator-activated receptors (PPARs) are a family of nuclear receptors that regulate gene transcription and play major regulatory roles in energy homeostasis and metabolic function. Structurally, PPARs are similar to steroid or thyroid hormone receptors, and they have three subtypes. In short, activation of PPAR-α reduces triglyceride levels and is involved in regulation of energy homeostasis; PPAR-γ causes insulin sensitization and enhances glucose metabolism; and PPAR-β/δ enhances metabolism of fatty acids.[16]

Chapter 6

Endogenous Cannabinoid Ligands: The Endocannabinoids

FOLLOWING THE DISCOVERY of the CB1 receptor, researchers postulated that it had evolved not for the sake of a plant compound but for endogenous ligands. In 1992, anandamide (named after *ananda*, the Sanskrit word for "divine joy") was the first endocannabinoid discovered,[1] and it remains the most well-studied. Two laboratories independently and simultaneously discovered 2-arachidonoylglycerol in 1995[2,3]; several similar endogenous cannabinoid compounds have subsequently been described. Though the endocannabinoids are structurally different from THC, they fit the same binding pockets on the cannabinoid receptors.

Anandamide

Anandamide (also known as *N*-arachidonoylethanolamine, AEA) acts as a partial agonist at the CB1 and CB2 receptors, similar to THC, and it may act as an antagonist in the presence of a stronger agonist. AEA is considered a full agonist at the TRPV1 receptor and is also an agonist of several members of the PPAR family of nuclear receptors.

AEA and others in the *N*-acylethanolamine class of compounds, such as *N*-palmitoylethanolamine and *N*-oleoylethanolamine, are synthesized by a variety of pathways from arachidonic acid (ω-6) precursors in the cell membrane. These compounds are catabolized by fatty acid amide hydrolase and *N*-acylethanolamine-hydrolyzing acid amidase. AEA can also serve as a substrate for cyclooxygenase 2 and for lipoxygenase and P450 enzymes that utilize arachidonic acid as a substrate.

2-Arachidonoylglycerol

2-Arachidonoylglycerol (2-AG) is the most abundant endocannabinoid in the brain and is a full agonist at the CB1 and CB2 receptors. It acts as a retrograde messenger in various types of synapses in the CNS to inhibit neurotransmitter release, and it has also been show to activate TRPV1 channels.[4] In comparison, while AEA likely functions as a relatively slow retrograde or paracrine signal in the brain, 2-AG primarily transmits a rapid, transient, point-to-point signal.[5] Also an arachidonic acid derivative, 2-AG is produced by activation of the enzymes phospholipase C and diacylglycerol lipase. It is catabolized by several enzymes, including monoacylglycerol lipase and alpha-beta hydrolase domain proteins ABHD-6, and ABHD-12, as well as cyclooxygenase 2 and some lipoxygenase subtypes.[6]

N-Palmitoylethanolamine and *N*-Oleoylethanolamine

While AEA and 2-AG are considered classic cannabinoids, based on their agonism of CB1 and CB2, a number of endogenous endocannabinoid-like compounds have been shown to influence the ECS, despite lack of direct activity at CB1 and CB2.

N-Palmitoylethanolamine (PEA) deserves special attention because it is naturally produced in many plants, as well as in cells and tissues of mammals, and has emerged as the first commercially available endocannabinoid-like nutraceutical. Surprisingly, the biosynthesis and degradation pathways of PEA in plants and humans are nearly identical. PEA has demonstrated numerous mechanisms of action, including inhibition of mast cell degranulation and agonism of PPAR-α, GPR55, and TRPV1 receptors. Clinical studies have shown that the oral administration of PEA conveys a range of benefits[7] (see Chapter 19 for more information on its clinical use).

N-Oleoylethanolamine (OEA) is a natural fatty acid amide that mainly modulates feeding and energy homeostasis by binding to PPAR-α.[8] Unlike endocannabinoids, OEA suppresses appetite and decreases food intake via several mechanisms.[9] Administration of an OEA precursor has been shown to have analgesic properties,[10] decrease inflammatory cytokines, increase awareness, improve depression, and strengthen memory in human studies.[11,12,13]

Endocannabinoid Entourage Effects

While the term "entourage effects" is commonly used to describe the potentiated interactions among the phytoconstituents of cannabis, it was originally used to describe the activity of endocannabinoids and related compounds.[14]

AEA and 2-AG are typically accompanied by an "entourage" of similar compounds with little or no activity at cannabinoid receptors, suggesting that this entourage may behave collectively as an endogenous modifier of endocannabinoid activity. The indirect actions of PEA illustrate this concept. By inhibiting expression of fatty acid amide hydrolase and stimulating expression of diacylglycerol lipase, PEA may indirectly influence activity at CB1 and CB2 receptors by impacting levels of AEA and 2-AG.[15] The entourage concept involves more complexity than just enzyme inhibition, including modulation of receptor function. For example, although PEA only slightly enhances 2-AG activation of TRPV1, it significantly increases 2-AG-induced TRPV1 desensitization, a crucial activity of TRPV1 in analgesia.[16]

Chapter 7

Endocannabinoid Enzymes and Transporters

ENDOCANNABINOIDS ARE GENERATED in one cellular compartment and move by diffusion or transport to their site of action (such as cannabinoid receptors) where they trigger a signaling cascade. To terminate the signaling, they are transported to yet another compartment where enzymes degrade the molecules.

Degradation Enzymes

Anandamide (also known as AEA), PEA, and OEA are degraded by the enzymes fatty acid amino hydrolase (FAAH) and cyclooxygenase 2 (COX-2). A third potential route of anandamide degradation is via *N*-acylethanolamine-hydrolyzing acid amidase (NAAA).[1] Like COX-2, FAAH is considered a physiological target for enzyme inhibition to slow AEA breakdown. Inhibition of FAAH may shunt anandamide metabolism to COX-2 or NAAA pathways, impacting other lipid signaling molecules and cell function independently of the cannabinoid receptors.[2]

As described previously, 2-AG is degraded by monoacylglycerol lipase (MAGL) and ABHD-6 and ABHD-12, as well as by COX-2 and some lipoxygenase subtypes.[3]

Researchers and drug developers have shown significant interest in developing agents that modulate function of the endocannabinoid system by targeting the enzymes responsible for degrading AEA and 2-AG. Several animal experiments with FAAH inhibitors have demonstrated improvements in models of pain, anxiety, and cannabis addiction. MAGL inhibitors have shown promising activities in animal models of pain and cancer.[4] Human studies are starting to emerge, demonstrating, for example, that FAAH inhibition can potentiate fear extinction and attenuate autonomic stress reactivity.[5]

In another study, a FAAH inhibitor failed to provide analgesia for osteoarthritis of the knee.[6]

Sadly, a phase I clinical trial of the FAAH inhibitor BIA 10-2474 led to the death of one volunteer and produced mild to severe neurological symptoms in four others, which made headlines in 2016. Subsequent research revealed that this compound has distinctively poor selectivity, inhibiting several other hydrolases and producing substantial alterations in human neuron lipid networks.[7] The toxicity of this agent was related to non-FAAH activity and has no bearing whatsoever on herbal cannabis.

Endocannabinoid Transport

The underlying molecular mechanisms of endocannabinoid membrane transport and cellular uptake are not completely understood. While numerous studies on AEA uptake have been performed, few data are available on the uptake of 2-AG, in part because transport assays for 2-AG uptake are hampered by its rapid degradation by both intracellular and extracellular hydrolases. Novel and more potent chemical probes to study endocannabinoid membrane transport are needed and emerging.[8]

In the meanwhile, several compounds have been identified that inhibit endocannabinoid transport. One interesting example, AM404, initially designed as an endocannabinoid membrane transport inhibitor, also activates and desensitizes the TRPV1 channel and is a metabolic product of acetaminophen in both rodents and humans. The analgesic activity of acetaminophen in rodents has been confirmed to be mediated by indirect activation of CB1 and by activation or desensitization of TRPV1,[9] though this may not be the case in humans, and with its inherent hepatotoxicity, acetaminophen is not an agent I would consider for modulation of the endocannabinoid system in my patients.

Several phytocannabinoids have been shown to inhibit endocannabinoid (eCB) transport and enzymatic degradation, as listed in Table 7.1, but perhaps not at relevant physiological concentrations: Δ^9-tetrahydrocannabinol (THC), cannabigerol (CBG), and cannabichromene (CBC) inhibit eCB transport; cannabidiol (CBD) inhibits FAAH and eCB transport; cannabidivarin (CBDV) inhibits DAGLα (biosynthesis of 2-AG) and eCB transport; cannabidiolic acid (CBDA) inhibits DAGLα and NAAA; and Δ^9-tetrahydrocannabinolic acid (THCA) inhibits DAGLα and MAGL.[10]

TABLE 7.1

Inhibition of Endocannabinoid Transport and Enzymatic Degradation by Phytocannabinoids

Phytocannabinoid		Enzyme or process inhibited
THC	Δ^9-Tetrahydrocannabinol	eCB transport
CBD	Cannabidiol	FAAH and eCB transport
CBDV	Cannabidivarin	DAGLα (biosynthesis of 2-AG) and eCB transport
CBDA	Cannabidiolic acid	DAGLα and NAAA
CBG	Cannabigerol	eCB transport
CBC	Cannabichromene	eCB transport
THCA	Δ^9-Tetrahydrocannabinolic acid	DAGLα and MAGL

Chapter 8

Endocannabinoid Signaling and Homeostatic Function

SCIENTIFIC UNDERSTANDING of endocannabinoid physiology is growing rapidly, fueled by interest in targeting the endocannabinoid system (ECS) for the treatment of several medical conditions. This book cannot cover every bodily system, and in several systems the current understanding is limited, but a tour of the ECS in various tissues demonstrates a universal homeostatic function. The ECS can bring balance to every bodily system, and I encourage each reader to study its role in the tissues relevant to your clinical areas of interest.

Nervous System

CB1 receptors are commonly expressed in the central and peripheral nervous systems and have been described as the most abundant G protein-coupled receptor in the brain,[1] but they are heterogeneously distributed. The brain regions that have the highest densities of CB1 receptors (basal ganglia, hippocampus, cerebral cortex, cerebellum, and amygdaloid nucleus) correspond with the well-known effects of THC on short-term memory, cognition, mood and emotion, motor function, and nociception. Unlike μ-opioid receptors, cannabinoid receptors are virtually absent in brain-stem cardiorespiratory centers, and thus cannabinoid receptors agonists have failed to demonstrate a lethal dose that suppresses cardiorespiratory function.[2] CB1 receptors are primarily localized in the presynaptic terminals of central and peripheral neurons, especially GABAergic but also glutamatergic, cholinergic, serotonergic, and noradrenergic neurons, where they mediate inhibition of neurotransmitter release. They are also found on astrocytes, where likewise they modulate neuronal activity.[3]

Initial studies suggested that CB2 receptors were absent from the healthy brain, but it is now recognized that CB2 is expressed during injury and inflammation in brain cells, including microglia, astrocytes, T cells, neurons, neural progenitor cells, and endothelial cells. The presence of CB2 in the healthy CNS is likely but remains somewhat controversial.[4] CB2 receptors are also expressed by peripheral nerves.

Retrograde Synaptic Transmission

Endocannabinoid signaling in the synapse differs significantly from the classic neurotransmitter model. Most neurotransmitters are stored in vesicles in the presynaptic nerve terminal, awaiting an action potential that opens Ca^{2+} channels, triggering vesicle exocytosis and neurotransmitter release into the synapse; classic neurotransmitters travel in an *anterograde* manner to the postsynaptic neuron.

Endocannabinoids are not stored in vesicles but are synthesized on demand from phospholipid precursors in the postsynaptic cell membrane. Their synthesis is triggered by activation of postsynaptic G protein-coupled receptors and increases in intracellular Ca^{2+}. The endocannabinoids are transmitted in a *retrograde* manner to CB1 receptors in the presynaptic nerve terminals (Figure 8.1). Activation of CB1 closes presynaptic

FIGURE 8.1
Endocannabinoid Signaling

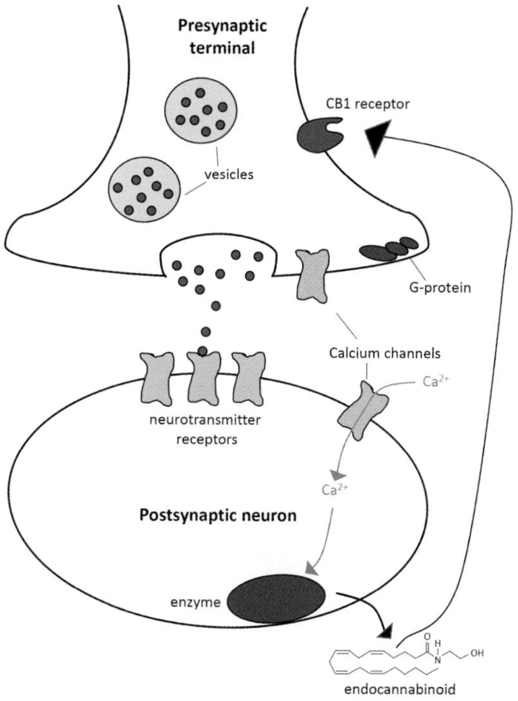

Source: Dustin Sulak

Ca^{2+} channels, preventing further release of the neurotransmitter. Thus, endocannabinoid signaling provides a negative feedback mechanism for regulating the release of neurotransmitters. After activating the CB1 receptor, the endocannabinoids are rapidly degraded by enzyme hydrolysis.[5]

Neuroplasticity

Neuroplasticity refers to the ability of the brain to develop and change throughout one's life, characterized by sprouting and pruning of synapses, changes in dendritic spine density, and changes in neurotransmitter pathways. Its outer manifestations can be readily observed in childhood development, recovery from a brain injury, learning a new skill, and even the unconscious acquisition of a new emotional response.[6] The endocannabinoid system is highly involved in neuroplasticity via multiple mechanisms.

Retrograde endocannabinoid signaling in a GABAergic synapse, which transiently suppresses the release of 4-aminobutanoic acid (an inhibitory neurotransmitter, known as GABA from its former name, gamma-aminobutyric acid), is called depolarization-induced suppression of inhibition. The same process at a glutaminergic synapse results in transient suppression of glutamate (an excitatory neurotransmitter) and is called depolarization-induced suppression of excitation. The ECS also modulates other forms of neuroplasticity including long-term depression, at both excitatory and inhibitory synapses,[7] and long-term potentiation;[8] these are two fundamental components of behavior changes.

As clinicians, we often consider short-term symptom relief valuable, and long-term efficacy even more so, but when we recall examples of healing or cure of a chronic condition, we likely note a long-lasting change in our patients' patterns of thought, behavior, and physiology. These changes are reflected in neuroplastic processes, and targeting the ECS may be one way to promote such change or healing.

Neuroprotection

Brain injuries trigger the release of harmful mediators that lead to secondary damage, including reactive oxygen species, inflammatory cytokines, and excess quantities of glutamate in the extracellular space. This leads to uncontrolled shifts in ion concentrations, cell swelling, and cell death. At the same time, the injury triggers the production of endogenous neuroprotective compounds, such as adenosine, melatonin, sex hormones, antioxidants, and endocannabinoids, to oppose the effects of the harmful mediators.

Thus, the magnitude of damage after a brain injury depends on the balance between the intrinsic degenerative and repair mechanisms of the brain.[9]

The ECS is highly involved in protecting the nervous system from injury. Anandamide (AEA) and 2-arachidonoylglycerol (2-AG) are endogenous neuroprotective substances, produced by the nervous system upon both chemical and mechanical trauma. Levels of 2-AG are significantly increased in the brain following closed head injury, and administration of 2-AG attenuates neuropathology induced by brain trauma. In contrast, chemical trauma from kainic acid rapidly raises the levels of AEA but not 2-AG. While the neuroprotective effects of endocannabinoids (eCBs) are primarily mediated through CB1 and/or CB2 receptors, evidence also demonstrates CB receptor-independent mechanisms.[10] People who use cannabis may also be more likely to survive brain injuries, as described in Chapter 29.

After an ischemic event in the brain, the tissue surrounding the infarct, described as the ischemic penumbra, is subject to reduced perfusion, waves of depolarization and glutamate excitotoxicity, pathological ion gradients, and impaired function. If perfusion and homeostatic function are not restored, the cells in the penumbra progress to permanent damage.[11] Activity of the ECS protects this vulnerable tissue via several mechanisms, including CB1-mediated dampening of glutamate excitotoxicity and hypothermia, CB2-mediated control of glial cells that results in decreased inflammatory and increased prosurvival factors, and decreased permeability of the blood–brain barrier via CB2 activation in endothelial cells.[12]

Neurogenesis

In addition to protecting the nervous system during pathological states, the ECS also regulates neurogenesis, a complex process that includes proliferation and differentiation of neural stem and progenitor cells, neuronal migration, and neuronal integration into networks of functional synapses. Neural progenitor cells express a functional ECS, including CB1 and CB2 receptors, TRPV1 channels, AEA, 2-AG, and ECS-related enzymes. The ECS is involved in the fate of these cells via both intrinsic cellular pathways (cell signaling cascades) and extrinsic cellular pathways (neurotrophins, neurotransmitters, cytokines, and hormones).[13]

CB1 and CB2 activity can induce both PI3K/Akt/mTORC and MEK/MAPK/CREB signaling pathways, which influence cell proliferation, differentiation, and survival, while also promoting integration of immature neurons into existing circuitry. In addition, ECS activation can induce transcription of brain-derived neurotrophic factor (BDNF), a signaling protein that can directly influence cell fate and neuronal plasticity. BDNF may also increase CB1 expression and endocannabinoid production, via a positive feedback loop with the ECS.

While the importance of neurogenesis in the developing brain has been widely acknowledged, neurogenesis in the adult brain was underestimated until the late 1960s and subsequently subject to skepticism until substantial research performed in the 1990s and early 2000s confirmed the presence of neurogenesis in several adult brain regions. Growing evidence implicates dysfunctional adult neurogenesis in depression and cognitive impairment, and low levels of BDNF are associated with neurodegenerative conditions such as Parkinson's disease, Alzheimer's disease, multiple sclerosis, and Huntington's disease. Cannabinoids have clear modulatory roles in adult neurogenesis through activation of both CB1 and CB2 receptors, especially in the hippocampus and the lateral ventricles.[14] These preclinical findings suggest that cannabinoid therapies may be useful in neurodegenerative conditions, not only for ameliorating symptoms but also for targeting the underlying pathophysiology and potentially for preventing these conditions.

Autonomic Nervous System

The ECS is highly involved in regulation of the autonomic nervous system, which controls innumerable physiological functions as well as our response to stress. Preclinical evidence has linked the development of stress-related disorders with dysregulation of the ECS, and several of the therapeutic effects of exogenous cannabinoids are mediated via the sympathetic and parasympathetic systems.

High densities of CB1 receptors are present in the dorsal motor nucleus of the vagus nerve and other parasympathetic centers, and CB1 signaling regulates vagal reflexes including emesis and excessive gastrointestinal (GI) motility. The antiemetic effects of THC are likely due to suppression of elevated parasympathetic activity via CB1.[15] Sympathetic nerve terminals also contain CB1 receptors that inhibit norepinephrine release.[16]

Physiological stressors (such as pain or inflammation) and psychological stressors elicit similar stress responses, including activation of the hypothalamic–pituitary–adrenocortical (HPA) axis, which releases cortisol from the adrenal cortex, and activation of the sympathetic-adrenergic system, which releases epinephrine from the adrenal medulla and norepinephrine from the sympathetic nerve terminals.

Hypothalamic–Pituitary–Adrenocortical Axis Review

Higher limbic brain regions such as the prefrontal cortex, amygdala, and hippocampus are involved in the interpretation of psychological stressors, while mid-hindbrain regions are involved in the response to physiological stressors. Both pathways converge onto the paraventricular nucleus of the hypothalamus, where they trigger the release of corticotropin-releasing hormone. Corticotropin-releasing hormone stimulates the synthesis of adrenocorticotropic hormone in the anterior pituitary, which is transported via the blood to the adrenal glands. The HPA axis is reset by glucocorticoid-mediated negative feedback, which occurs mainly at the level of the paraventricular nucleus and the pituitary gland.

Preclinical data suggests the ECS regulates activity of the HPA axis under both basal and stress-related conditions.[17] CB1 receptors, which are highly expressed in several limbic brain regions involved in HPA axis regulation, have been shown to be involved in glucocorticoid-mediated feedback of the HPA axis. CB1 receptors are expressed in the intermediate and anterior lobes of the pituitary, where they likely contribute additional modulatory effects on the HPA axis. CB1 receptors are also found in the human adrenal cortex, where their activity inhibits the production of cortisol and aldosterone.[18]

The ECS influences cardiovascular activity (including vascular tone and cardiac contractility) directly, via action on the relevant tissues, but also indirectly, via its role in the autonomic nervous system, typically conveying cardioprotection and homeostatic regulation.[19]

The ECS thus regulates the activity of both parasympathetic and sympathetic nervous systems, typically suppressing excessive activity and setting basal tone, and perhaps augmenting activity under some conditions. This universal homeostatic function in the autonomic systems makes the ECS an exciting target for treating autonomic dysfunction, a key component in most chronic disease.

Immune System

Immune cells secrete endocannabinoids and express both CB1 and CB2 receptors, though CB2 receptors in immune cells are 10–100 times more common than CB1 receptors.[20] The level of CB2 expression varies among different populations of immune cells, with B lymphocytes expressing the highest levels, followed by macrophages, monocytes, natural killer cells, and polymorphonuclear cells, in that order.[21]

The immunomodulatory activity of endocannabinoids occurs via autocrine and paracrine signaling, impacting the function of immune cells in a localized environment, and this activity is transient, due to rapid degradation. The ECS plays a role in maintaining the overall "fine tuning" of immune homeostatic balance.[22] ECS activity in lymphoid tissue may provide tonic control of immune cell activation and therefore limit spontaneous activation of immune cell function.[23]

Endocannabinoids modulate immune cells in several ways, including the following:

- T- and B-lymphocyte proliferation
- T- and B-lymphocyte apoptosis
- macrophage-mediated killing of sensitized cells
- inflammatory cytokine production
- immune cell activation by inflammatory stimuli
- chemotaxis
- inflammatory cell migration

Most immunosuppressive and anti-inflammatory effects of the ECS are mediated by CB2 receptors via inhibition of the cyclic adenosine monophosphate/protein kinase A pathway. Endocannabinoids also act at the nuclear level to enhance transcription of apoptotic genes regulated by nuclear factor κB, inhibit activated T cells via PPAR-γ, and interfere in the cell cycle via G1/S-phase arrest.[24]

The T helper cells have two main subclasses, Th1 and Th2. Th1 cells secrete interferon γ and tumor necrosis factor α and mainly protect the organism against intracellular pathogens (cell-mediated immunity). Th2 cells mainly protect against extracellular pathogens (humoral immunity). CB2 activation can induce and inhibit both Th1 and Th2 cytokines but has most often been shown to decrease Th1 cytokines and increase Th2 cytokines. Th1 cytokines are involved in the pathogenesis of a number of inflammatory disorders such as multiple sclerosis and rheumatoid arthritis. Inhibition of Th1 cytokines and the shift to a Th2-type response is considered to provide therapeutic benefit in these situations. The production of interleukin 6, a Th2 cytokine associated with malaise, fatigue, increased pain sensitivity in several chronic inflammatory conditions, is inhibited by CB2 agonism in macrophages[25] and in fibroblast-like synoviocytes derived from rheumatoid joints.[26]

The shift from Th1 to Th2 cytokines may not always be favorable, however, as Th1 cells secrete interferon γ and induce natural killer cells, an important response to cancer. In fact, almost all malignancies have been associated with suppressed Th1 activity.[27] While most preclinical studies associate CB receptor agonism with reduced neoplastic activity, likely via CB receptor-mediated proapoptotic, antiangiogenic, and antimetastatic mechanisms, some evidence demonstrates that cancers lacking CB receptor expression become more aggressive in the presence of CB2 agonists, likely due to suppression of Th1 and natural killer cell activity.[28]

Gastrointestinal System[29]

The endocannabinoid system is expressed in the gut and maintains intestinal homeostasis by modulating several functions including the immune activity, motility, sensation, and secretion.

CB1 receptors are found on both intrinsic neurons of the enteric nervous system and extrinsic (sympathetic and parasympathetic) neurons in the gut, where they modulate motility, secretion, sphincter tone, and visceral pain. CB1 signaling controls cholinergic transmission and regulates contractility, though non-cholinergic-mediated contractile responses are also suppressed by CB1 agonism. CB2 receptors are expressed by lamina propria plasma cells and activated macrophages, as well as by ganglia of the myenteric and submucosal plexus in human ileum, where they are involved in the inhibition of inflammation, visceral pain, and intestinal motility in the inflamed gut.

Regulation of gut function by endocannabinoids is complex and poorly understood. For example, 2-AG is a potent emetogen, whereas anandamide and exogenous cannabinoids exert antiemetic activity via CB1 receptors.[30]

Endocannabinoid signaling in mucosa of the jejunum is triggered by both fasting and dietary fats and is proposed to be a general hunger signal that acts at local CB1 receptors to inhibit satiation. CB1 receptors located on small intestinal enteroendocrine I cells, which produce and secrete cholecystokinin (CCK), may promote hunger while fasting and drive the intake of fat-rich foods by inhibiting the release of CCK, which normally binds CCK receptors on the sensory vagus nerve and induces satiation after a meal.

In the large intestine, the ECS likely interacts with gut microbiota and regulates epithelial barrier permeability. For example, activating CB1 in mice increased circulating levels of lipopolysaccharide, an endotoxin released from Gram-negative bacteria, through a proposed mechanism that includes decreased expression of the tight junction proteins occludin and zonula occludens 1, resulting in increased permeability. In a fascinating example of ECS homeostatic control over GI tissue function, CB1 activation can lead to both increased permeability in the large intestine (via decreased expression of tight junction proteins, potentially pathogenic) and decreased permeability (via increased expression of tight junction proteins, likely protective) of the large intestine, depending whether the CB1 agonism takes place on the luminal or basolateral side of the intestine, respectively. These findings are primarily based on ex vivo studies in which CB1 agonists can be selectively applied to the luminal or basolateral surface.[31] Thus, the route of administration of cannabis may impact these bidirectional intestinal permeability effects. Inhalation and other parenteral routes may have more of a protective effect, while enterally delivered doses of THC that reach the large intestine, or rectal administration, may increase permeability.

Increasing evidence shows that the levels of endocannabinoids and/or CB receptors are altered in the biopsy samples of patients with intestinal diseases, such as diverticulitis, celiac disease, irritable bowel syndrome, inflammatory bowel disease, and colon cancer, which suggests important roles of the endocannabinoid system in intestinal pathophysiology.[32] Dysregulation of the endocannabinoid system may contribute to the development of these conditions. Several models of GI pathological states exhibit an overexpression of enteric intestinal cannabinoid CB1 receptors, with or without increases in tissue endocannabinoid levels and turnover.[33]

Liver

CB1 receptors are expressed by hepatocytes, hepatic stellate cells, liver vascular endothelial cells, and hepatic bile duct cells.[34] CB2 receptors are expressed in Kupffer cells, the resident macrophages of the liver, in low levels. Anandamide and 2-AG are present at substantial levels, and the liver expresses the enzymes fatty acid amino hydrolase (FAAH) and monoacylglycerol lipase (MAGL). Liver injury causes a significant increase in CB2 expression by Kupffer cells and myofibroblasts; an increase in CB1 expression by hepatocytes, hepatic myofibroblasts, and endothelial cells; and increased expression of the endocannabinoids AEA and 2-AG.[35] Liver CB1 and CB2 receptor expression also follows a diurnal cycle with increased expression during the light period and decreased production in darkness.[36]

The ECS modulates liver fibrogenesis, the process of fibrotic tissue accumulation that eventually leads to cirrhosis, portal hypertension, and liver failure. CB1 activation promotes fibrosis, while CB2 activation inhibits fibrosis and liver inflammation.[37] Due to the lack of antifibrotic treatments in liver disease, CB1 antagonists and CB2 agonists are under investigation.

Preclinical evidence indicates CBD is a promising agent for treating chronic liver disease. It has been shown to reduce steatosis and fibrosis in the liver by reducing lipid accumulation, stimulating autophagy, modulating inflammation, reducing oxidative stress, and inducing the death of activated hepatic stellate cells.[38]

CB1 and CB2 are both active in liver regeneration: CB1 agonism regulates cell cycle proteins required for mitotic progression in hepatocytes, while CB2 agonism is associated with liver regeneration via activity in hepatic myofibroblasts.[39]

The ECS also modulates hepatic glucose metabolism. Under high-fat diet conditions, CB1 agonism is associated with increased lipogenesis, insulin resistance, and steatosis; CB2 agonism is associated with increased lipid accumulation, while CB2 antagonism is associated with improved insulin sensitivity.[40]

Hepatic CB1 expression has been positively correlated with higher-grade steatosis in human patients with hepatitis C.[41] Initial human clinical data associated cannabis use with worse steatosis and fibrosis in patients with hepatitis C.[42,43] Subsequent data, however, have failed to show any evidence linking cannabis use to accelerated progression of liver fibrosis or cirrhosis,[44,45,46] which suggests the earlier studies were biased by reverse causality (patients using more cannabis to relieve symptoms as liver disease progresses).

Pancreas

Human islets of Langerhans express CB1 and CB2 receptors, as well as the enzymes involved in synthesis and degradation of 2-AG. While most studies agree that CB1 is expressed in insulin-secreting beta cells, differences in experimental models result in conflicting reports about the presence of CB1 in alpha and delta cells. CB2 is likely present in somatostatin-secreting delta cells but absent in alpha and beta cells. The acinar and ductal aspects of the pancreas likely do not express an ECS.[47,48]

Endocannabinoids, predominantly 2-AG, are synthesized in the pancreas in response to glucose in a concentration-dependent manner, providing an autocrine negative feedback mechanism to avoid hypoglycemia and maintain homeostasis in insulin secretion. While CB1 signaling guards against overactivity of beta cells, in an obese state with chronic increase in circulating eCBs, excessive activation of CB1 can impede beta-cell function, promote inflammation, decrease beta-cell proliferation, and enhance beta-cell apoptosis.[49,50]

The Endocannabinoid System in Obesity and Metabolic Dysfunction

The ECS plays a key role in regulating energy homeostasis, having been shown to influence the search, intake, metabolism, and storage of calories in several preclinical and clinical evidence. ECS activation promotes consumption of palatable food, stimulates fat mass expansion and calorie preservation, and inhibits energy expenditure and thermogenesis. This system seems to have been selected by evolution to maximize intake and conservation of energy, likely to increase survival in times of scarcity. In modern society where food is plentiful, however, excessive ECS activity is a clear feature of obesity and metabolic disorders.[51]

Circulating endocannabinoid levels positively correlate with body mass index (BMI), body fat percentage, waist circumference, visceral fat mass, insulin resistance, serum triglyceride levels, and adverse cardiac events.[52,53] In one study, circulating levels of AEA and 2-AG were 35% and 52% higher, respectively, in obese women compared with lean women.[54]

Adipose tissue has higher CB1 expression than other peripheral tissues, except the stomach. The obese state, with its elevated circulating eCBs, results in decreased expression of CB1 in white adipose tissue (WAT), potentially via receptor overstimulation and downregulation, as well as decreased FAAH activity. For example, in the same cohort, adipose tissue CB1 mRNA levels were 34% lower, and FAAH levels were 59% lower, in obese subjects compared to lean subjects.[55]

The control of eCB production and degradation is clearly altered in obesity. For example, both normal-weight and obese subjects have a significant preprandial peak in AEA, which decreases after a meal in normal-weight subjects but not in obese subjects. The elevated circulating eCBs in obesity are likely produced in the gut and in WAT.

ECS dysregulation also contributes to insulin resistance. CB1 activation in the pancreas stimulates insulin secretion, while CB1 activation in the liver increases lipogenesis, inhibits insulin signaling, and inhibits insulin clearance. Insulin and leptin inhibit eCB production in WAT via both local and distant, hypothalamus-dependent mechanisms. Thus, insulin and leptin resistance, a common feature in obesity, likely leads to eCB overproduction in WAT, a feed-forward dysfunction favoring fat accumulation and further contributing to metabolic syndrome.[56]

In rodents, a high-fat diet increases plasma 2-AG and AEA levels in association with weight gain; reciprocally, FAAH deficiency (which increases AEA) promotes lipid storage and insulin resistance. Mice deficient for CB1 are resistant to obesity induced by a high-fat diet.[57] Human genetics also impact the role of the ECS in obesity[58]:

- CB1 receptor SNP rs1049353 was associated with lower BMI (17 studies), lower fat mass (five studies), and lower insulin levels (one study).
- CB1 receptor SNP rs806368 was associated with increased BMI and waist circumference (two studies).
- FAAH SNP rs324420, which results in reduced FAAH activity, was predictably associated with increased obesity (three studies).

The CB2 receptor is also involved in energy homeostasis and obesity, though its role is less well-characterized. CB2 agonists reduce food intake in lean mice and improve both body weight and obesity-associated inflammation in diet-induced obese mice; CB2 genetic ablation results in adiposity. Evidence suggests CB2 activation may induce the browning of adipose tissue.[59]

In summary, the ECS participates in feed-forward physiological dysfunction in our novel environment of excessive calorie availability. Chronic high-fat, high-calorie diets increase circulating eCBs. Increased circulating eCBs stimulate hepatic CB1, increasing insulin resistance, and downregulate adipose CB1 and FAAH, resulting in further elevation of eCBs.

Modulation of the ECS continues to provide excellent therapeutic potential in treating metabolic disorders, and related drug development is ongoing. After the clinical failure of rimonabant, a systemic CB1 antagonist, due to adverse psychiatric effects (see Chapter 15), subsequent research has focused on peripherally restricted CB1 antagonists and CB2 modulators. The phytocannabinoid Δ^9-tetrahydrocannabivarin (THCV) is one excellent candidate (see Chapter 13).

Musculoskeletal System

Fibroblasts, myofibroblasts, chondrocytes, and synoviocytes express CB1, CB2, and endocannabinoid-metabolizing enzymes. The ECS decreases inflammation in myofascial tissues and plays a role in fibroblast reorganization and remodeling.[60] Cannabinoids prevent cartilage destruction by inhibiting chondrocyte expression of cytokines and metalloproteinase enzymes.[61]

The ECS controls the utilization of energy in skeletal muscle, by reducing glucose oxidation by myofibers, and controls the extent of muscle formation, both mediated preferentially via CB1. Potential overactivity of skeletal muscle CB1 during obesity may decrease muscle insulin sensitivity and glucose metabolism and contribute to fatty acid accumulation.[62]

Bone remodeling is tightly coordinated by the ECS. Osteoblasts and osteoclasts both express CB2. AEA and 2-AG are produced locally in bone and reach concentrations similar to those in brain tissues. CB2 agonism in osteoblast precursor cells increases mitosis and expands the preosteoblastic cell pool; CB2 agonism in mature osteoblasts increases matrix mineralization. Both inhibitory and stimulatory effects of CB2 agonists on osteoclast formation have been reported under different experimental conditions; CB2 agonist have been shown to prevent ovariectomy-induced bone loss in rodents, and mice lacking CB2 display an osteoporotic phenotype.[63] Human CB2 polymorphisms have been associated with low bone mass and osteoporosis.[64]

The ECS is also involved in regulation of bone remodeling by the autonomic nervous system: norepinephrine released from sympathetic fibers inhibits bone formation and stimulates bone resorption, while parasympathetic acetylcholine decreases bone resorption. CB1 agonism in sympathetic terminals adjacent to osteoblasts inhibits norepinephrine release and decreases the tonic restraint of bone formation, as shown in Figure 8.2.[65]

FIGURE 8.2

Regulation of Bone Remodeling by the Skeletal Endocannabinoid System

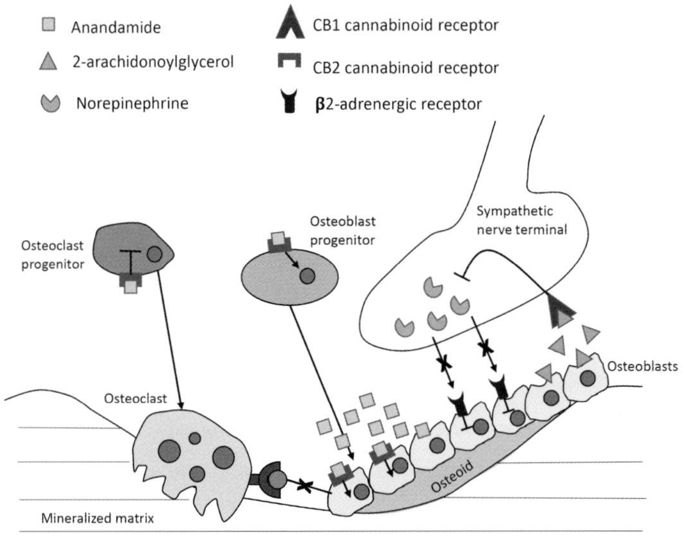

Source: Dustin Sulak

The ECS is present in the hypertrophic chondrocytes of the epiphyseal growth cartilage, which drive skeletal elongation; CB1 agonism seems to restrain bone growth related to this process.[66]

Respiratory System

Although airway epithelial cells constitute an extremely large contact surface and an important physical barrier, little research has explored the ECS in this tissue. Most research on the ECS in the lungs has focused on immunity and fibrosis. CB1 and CB2 mRNA has been found in the lungs and the bronchial tissue, with significantly higher levels of CB1. Macrophages residing in human lung express CB1 and CB2 that seem to modulate vascular remodeling in cancer and chronic inflammation.[67]

Cannabinoid receptor agonists have a bronchodilatory effect via both CB1 and CB2. The dominant autonomic innervation of the airways is parasympathetic, which induces bronchoconstriction via efferent cholinergic pathways that travel through the vagus nerve and then synapses in the parasympathetic ganglia of the airways. Prejunctional CB1 receptor activation inhibits cholinergic contraction in human bronchi.[68] The ECS also modulates airway resistance via regulation of mast cell degranulation: CB2 agonism directly reduces mast cell activity, while CB1 agonism on nerve endings innervating bronchial smooth muscle indirectly reduces their activity by reducing neural stimulation of mast cells.[69]

Endocannabinoids are a source of arachidonic acid in the lungs, which can be metabolized by immune cells into leukotrienes and prostaglandins. For example, AEA has been shown to increase permeability of airway epithelial cells in vitro via arachidonic metabolites and not CB receptor activation.[70]

While cannabis has historically been reported to act as an expectorant and antitussive,[71] it is unclear if these actions are mediated by CB receptors, though the role of CB1 receptors in respiratory secretion and smooth muscle activity may be analogous to the somewhat better characterized inhibitory actions of CB1 in gastrointestinal secretion and motility.

Renal System[72]

The ECS plays a major role in renal physiology and is involved in the pathogenesis of both acute and chronic kidney disease. While the preclinical and human data suggest trends in the function of CB1 and CB2 in the kidneys, the differing distribution and actions of CB1 and CB2 in various structures and cell subtypes results in complex signaling outcomes whose overall impact are difficult to predict.

CB1 and CB2 are found throughout the kidneys, but the receptors act via separate pathways and modulate distinct activities. CB1 is expressed in proximal convoluted tubules, distal tubules, and intercalated cells of the collecting duct in the human kidney.

Additionally, CB1 has been found in rodents in afferent and efferent arterioles, thick ascending limbs of the loop of Henle, glomerular podocytes, tubular epithelial cells, and cultured mesangial cells. CB2 has been found in podocytes, proximal tubule cells, and mesangial cells in human and rat renal cortex samples.

In the healthy kidney, 2-AG is expressed in similar levels in the cortex and medulla, while AEA levels are higher than 2-AG levels in the medulla but similar to 2-AG levels in the cortex. FAAH expression has been shown to be higher in the cortex.

The ECS regulates renal hemodynamics, handling of solutes, and handling of proteins. AEA causes vasodilation in both afferent and efferent juxtamedullary arterioles via CB1-dependent and non-CB1 mechanisms, and it stimulates nitric oxide production in the medullary thick ascending limbs, leading to an inhibition of sodium transport. CB1 activation in the podocytes and mesangial cells of the glomerulus increases urinary protein excretion. Increased activation and overexpression of CB1 was also found to enhance the expression of vascular endothelial growth factor.

In models of diabetic nephropathy, CB1 expression is upregulated in glomerular podocytes and mesangial cells while CB2 is reduced in glomerular podocyte proximal tubule cells. In rats with obesity-related nephropathy, CB2 activation can reduce albuminuria, restore podocyte protein expression, reduce monocyte infiltration, and decrease profibrotic markers. CB1 antagonism can improve renal structure and function. In models of diet-induced obesity, CB1 is upregulated and CB1 antagonism reduced weight, systolic blood pressure, plasma leptin levels, albuminuria, and plasma creatinine levels, associated with the amelioration of glomerulopathy.

In acute kidney injury (AKI), both CB1 and CB2 receptor agonists prevent tubular damage following renal ischemia/reperfusion injury, in a dose-dependent manner. The phytocannabinoid cannabidiol has also been shown to reduce renal tubular injury in rat ischemia/reperfusion injury. Inhibiting CB1 or activating CB2 can limit oxidative stress and inflammation and reduce tubular damage in kidneys of animals with cisplatin-induced AKI. Podocyte injury in AKI is associated with upregulation of CB1, AEA, and 2-AG, and AEA has been shown to exert a protective and anti-inflammatory effects on podocytes.

Integumentary System[73]

In the integumentary system, the ECS regulates cell growth, differentiation, and survival; immune and inflammatory responses; and sensory phenomena. CB1 and CB2 are expressed in suprabasal layers of the epidermis, hair follicles, and sporadic regions of the basal layer. CB1 is found in keratinocytes of the stratum spinosum and stratum granulosum, differentiated sebaceous cells, and epithelial cells of the infundibulum and inner root of hair follicles. CB2 is expressed in basal keratinocytes, undifferentiated sebaceous cells, and undifferentiated infundibular hair follicle cells. CB1 and CB2 are also seen in melanocytes, dermal fibroblasts, and myoepithelial cells of eccrine sweat glands.

CB1 and CB2 also appear in skin nerve fibers, vascular endothelium, preadipocytes, and mature adipocytes. Both cannabinoid receptors are present in the skin in mast cells, macrophages, T cells, and B cells. Various members of the transient receptor potential family are found in the skin, including TRPV1 in Langerhans cells, endothelial and vascular smooth muscle cells, sebocytes, and sweat gland epithelium.

AEA reduces keratinocyte growth and differentiation, via CB1, and induces apoptosis, via CB1 and TRPV1. In pathologies characterized by abnormally differentiated epidermis with altered barrier function, such as atopic dermatitis, early data suggests a beneficial impact of CB1 activation and a detrimental effect of CB2 activation. Conversely, in models of pathological skin fibrosis, CB1 activation appears to have a detrimental effect while CB2 activation is beneficial, similar to findings in fibrosis of the liver and other tissues. Activation of PPAR-γ can also reduce inflammation and prevent fibrosis.

In the hair follicle, CB1 activation results in decreased hair shaft elongation and induction of the catagen phase (lower portion of the follicle regresses and hair growth ends). TRPV1 activation also inhibits hair growth elongation via a distinct mechanism of action. In sebaceous glands, AEA has been shown to increase sebocyte apoptosis via CB2, and low AEA levels lead to increased lipid production. Cannabidiol has anti-acne sebostatic effects via TRPV4.

In the immune system of the skin, CB2 activity decreases mast cell degranulation, while CB1 protects against excess T-cell inflammatory response in keratinocytes and decreases mast cell infiltration into the skin. N-Palmitoylethanolamine (PEA) has demonstrated skin anti-inflammatory effects, reducing skin thickness, mast cell infiltration, and scratching behavior in a model of contact dermatitis via a mechanism involving CB2.

Embryology[74,75]

The ECS has been detected in virtually all components of the reproductive system and at virtually all stages of fertilization and development.

Human oocytes and sperm express both CB1 and CB2 receptors, which have been shown to have roles in oocyte maturation (CB1)[76], meiosis in spermatogenesis (CB2)[77], and sperm motility, acrosome function, and mitochondrial function (CB1)[78]. During pre-implantation events, CB1 is found in the oviduct and uterus from the late two-cell stage through the blastocyst stage of the embryo. The ECS has been shown to play a role in development of the preimplantation embryo, its movement through the oviduct, implantation, and placenta development. Alterations of the ECS are associated with reduced fertility and viability.

Endocannabinoids have been shown to arrest the development of two-cell embryos into blastocysts, mediated by CB1. Because AEA levels in the uterus are high, and AEA binding to CB1 receptors on blastocysts would lead to cell death, uterine AEA levels have to decrease on the day and at the site of implantation; failure to do so prevents implantation. Uterine changes required for normal gestation are facilitated by CB1 activation on the interimplantation sites of the uterine epithelium. CB1 activity is also involved in placental development: CB1 knockout mice have smaller placentas. Intriguingly, while appropriate uterine AEA levels are crucial, uterine 2-AG levels, similar to those measured in maternal milk and the developing brain, are roughly 1,000 times higher than AEA levels.

Establishment of structural components and connectivity within neuronal networks relies on several critical events, such as neuronal stem cell proliferation and differentiation, neuronal migration to target regions, and formation of synapses; all are shaped by extracellular cues provided by endocannabinoids. In chick embryos, CB1 is expressed in the earliest neurons of the CNS, followed by its appearance in the peripheral nervous system. In human brain, CB1 has been detected in the cortical plate as early as gestational week 9. CB1 is not exclusive to embryonic neurons; it has been found in the ventral forebrain, which does not produce neurons in early development, and in the mesoderm. CB2 receptors have been found in embryonic microglia.

Endocannabinoids are present in bovine and human milk, with 2-AG concentrations 100–1,000 times higher than those of AEA. CB1 receptor activation has been shown to be critically important for initiation of the suckling response.[79] Depriving neonatal rat pups of maternal contact leads to increased 2-AG in the male hippocampus, decreased CB1 expression, and increased CB2 expression.

Neoplasm

The ECS plays a fundamental role in our natural biological resistance against cancer. A large body of evidence demonstrates that cannabinoid signaling controls neoplasm via numerous and complex mechanisms of action, in vitro and in vivo. Several cancer cell lines have been shown to express CB1 and CB2 receptors; in some, the absence of either CB receptor can be associated with differing effects on the aggressiveness of the cancer.

Cannabinoid agonism is, in most studies, antitumorigenic, although a few reports have proposed tumor-promoting effects. In some types of cancer cells, such as glioma, pharmacological blockade of either CB1 or CB2 prevents cannabinoid-induced cell death with similar efficacy, and yet in other types of cancer cells (e.g., pancreatic, breast, or hepatic carcinoma cells), CB2 but not CB1 blockade inhibits the antitumor effects of cannabinoids. Why cannabinoids produce their antitumor actions through one or the other of these receptors, depending on the type of cancer cell, is poorly understood.[80]

Cannabinoids impair tumor progression at various levels. Their most prevalent effects are by inhibiting cancer cell proliferation and inducing cancer cell death by apoptosis via a CB1-mediated ceramide–caspase pathway. Autophagy, the "self-digestion" mechanism of cells, is a process that targets portions of cytoplasm, damaged organelles, and proteins for lysosomal degradation, which plays a crucial role in development and disease. Cannabinoids have been shown to induce autophagy in various cancer cell lines, with most studies showing this process is required for antiproliferative and apoptotic activities.[81] Increased tumor expression of FAAH is associated with more biological malignancy and a poor prognosis in some tumor histotypes.[82]

Cannabinoids have also been shown to impair tumor angiogenesis, by blocking the activation of the vascular endothelial growth factor pathway.[83] CB1 and/or CB2 agonists reduce the formation of distant tumor masses in animal models of metastasis, and they inhibit adhesion, migration, and invasiveness of several cancer cells in culture. This effect involves the modulation of extracellular proteases, such as matrix metalloproteinase 2.[84]

When the role of the ECS in immunomodulation is considered, it is no surprise that CB2 activation has been proposed in some reports to enhance tumorigenesis by interfering with immune tumor surveillance. Conversely, cannabinoids have also been shown to enhance immune system–mediated tumor surveillance in other contexts and to decrease migration of protumorigenic macrophages to the tumor microenvironment.[85]

Psychological distress (depression and anxiety) is associated with higher mortality rates in patients with cancer, most pronounced in those with leukemia and with colorectal, prostate, pancreatic, or esophageal cancer.[86] The interaction of our perceptual experience with the regulation of cytokine activity and immune function by the central nervous and neuroendocrine systems, known as the psycho–neuroendocrine–immune network, clearly impacts one's capacity to suppress cancer. The psycho–neuroendocrine regulation of the immune system is mainly mediated by the brain opioid and cannabinoid systems and pineal activity.[87]

Modulating the ECS in patients with cancer provides opportunity for both palliative and disease-modifying benefits, though our understanding of its complexity in neoplasm is still very limited.

Chapter 9

Influences on the Endocannabinoid System

THE FUNCTION of the endocannabinoid system (ECS) is influenced by genetics, including gender, aging and polymorphisms in genes coding for ECS receptors and enzymes (see Chapter 10 for more details), but also responds dynamically to our daily choices. A number of drugs, herbs, and lifestyle activities have been shown to exert their influence, at least in part, via the ECS.

Sex Differences

Several preclinical studies have shown gender differences in functioning of the ECS. Relative to female rodents, male rodents have higher levels of CB1 protein, mRNA, receptor density, and agonist binding.[1] In rodents, females are more sensitive than males to effects of cannabinoids on tests of antinociception, motor activity, and reinforcing efficacy.[2] Age also impacts these differences: for example, adolescent female rats were less sensitive than adult females to several pharmacological effects of THC, while male rats did not show this age-dependent difference.[3]

Estrogen has been shown to regulate CB1 expression in a brain region–dependent manner, causing both increases and decreases in CB1 density[4] and increased synthesis of anandamide (AEA) in the hypothalamus. Reciprocally, AEA regulates central gonadotropin secretion and influences sex hormone levels.[5]

Human imaging data on ECS sex differences have been mixed, with studies showing either increased or decreased CB1 availability in women. Recently, in a study of 22 healthy people from Finland, men had an average 41% higher CB1 availability than women, with a regionally specific effect larger in the posterior cingulate and retrosplenial cortices, areas thought to be involved in spatial layout.[6]

While there may be trends in gender-specific responses to the therapeutic use of cannabis, which likely vary by age and timing within the menstrual cycle, the high level of interindividual variability among patients of all genders, in my experience, precludes the utility of any clinical strategy based on a patient's gender alone.

Drug and Herb Influences

Several commonly used drugs, including NSAIDs, acetaminophen, glucocorticoids, and herbs, exert their activity, at least in part, via the endocannabinoid system.

Nonsteroidal anti-inflammatory drugs (NSAIDs) inhibit the cyclooxygenase enzymes COX-1 and COX-2 and thereby block the conversion of arachidonic acid into inflammatory prostaglandins. Ibuprofen, ketorolac, and flurbiprofen also block the hydrolysis of AEA into arachidonic acid and ethanolamine. COX-2 inhibitors have been shown to potentiate 2-arachidonoylglycerol (2-AG) release and CB1 signaling in rat hippocampal cells. In preclinical studies, some NSAIDs inhibit fatty acid amino hydrolase (FAAH) and enhance the activity of endocannabinoids (eCBs), phytocannabinoids, and synthetic cannabinoids. Combining NSAIDs with endogenous and exogenous cannabinoids produces additive or synergistic antinociceptive effects,[7] though indomethacin has been shown to decrease the subjective and physiological effects of cannabis in a small human study.[8]

The analgesic and antipyretic effects of acetaminophen are thought to occur via modulation of the ECS. Acetaminophen is metabolized into N-arachidonoylphenolamine, which is a weak agonist of CB1 and CB2, blocks the breakdown of AEA by FAAH, inhibits the AEA membrane transporter, inhibits COX-1 and COX-2, and activates TRPV1. The analgesic activity of acetaminophen in rats is blocked by CB1 or CB2 antagonists. A subeffective dose of AEA in mice became anxiolytic when it was coadministered with acetaminophen; the effect was blocked by CB1 antagonism. Some patients who consume acetaminophen report "a peculiar sense of well-being, relaxation, and tranquility" that may be related to activation of the ECS.[9,10]

Cannabinoid and glucocorticoid receptors share similar distribution in the central nervous system and other tissues, including immune cells. Preclinical rodent studies indicate that acute glucocorticoid administration enhances the activity of eCBs, while chronic exposure to glucocorticoids downregulates the CB1 expression, a scenario consistent with chronic stress.[11]

Cannabinoid and opioid receptors are also share similar distribution; acute administration of opioids has been shown to enhance the activity of endocannabinoids, while chronic administration can upregulate CB1 in some brain regions but downregulate CB1 in others.[12] The co-administration of exogenous opioids and cannabinoids produces synergistic antinociceptive effects.[13]

The anxiolytic effect of the benzodiazepine class of drugs involves CB1 signaling; a CB1 agonist and an FAAH inhibitor both synergistically enhanced the anxiolytic effects of diazepam (a benzodiazepine), while a CB1 antagonist attenuated its anxiolysis. Acute administration of diazepam to mice is accompanied by strong elevation of brain eCB levels.[14]

Alcohol influences the ECS. Acute ethanol consumption can alter eCB levels and CB1-dependent changes in neuroplasticity. Chronic consumption and binge drinking likely desensitize or downregulate CB1 and impair eCB signaling, except perhaps in areas involved in reward and motivation to self-administer alcohol.[15]

Several plants other than cannabis produce compounds that influence the ECS. β-Caryophyllene is a terpene found in cannabis, black pepper, lemon balm, cloves, and hops and in significant concentration in copaiba essential oils. As a full agonist of CB2, it provides anti-inflammatory, antifibrotic, antipruritic, and other benefits. Its oxidative product, caryophyllene oxide, has also been shown to activate CB2.[16] Echinacea, an herb widely used for immunostimulation and immunomodulation, contains alkamides that are active at CB2 and peroxisome proliferator-activated receptor γ Galangal, maca root, and cacao all contain FAAH inhibitors. Early evidence suggests that probiotic supplementation can modulate ECS function.[17] Curcumin has been shown to prevent liver fibrosis by downregulating CB1 and upregulating CB2.[18]

Nonpharmacological Influences

Several well-known, and some less common, health-promoting lifestyle interventions influence the ECS, including stress reduction, social interaction, exercise, diet, cryotherapy, fasting, manual therapies, and meditation.

Chronic stress impairs the ECS, resulting in decreased levels of AEA and 2-AG and heterogenous effects on CB1 expression. Conversely, in rats, social play increased CB1 activation in the amygdala and enhanced AEA levels in the amygdala and nucleus accumbens.[19]

Medium- to high-intensity voluntary exercise increases ECS signaling, via increased serum AEA levels, and possibly increased CB1 expression. Forced exercise, a form of stress, does not increase AEA and can decrease CB1. Anandamide levels have been shown to increase nearly 3-fold in humans after 30 min of treadmill exercise, with the subsequent magnitude of positive affect (enthusiasm, energy, and pleasurable engagement) correlated with AEA levels.[20] Thirty minutes of singing by nine women resulted in significant increases of AEA, PEA, and OEA and improved positive mood and emotions. The impact of singing on the ECS was stronger than running or dancing.[21]

Diet plays a major role in ECS function, beginning with polyunsaturated fatty acids, the precursors of endocannabinoids and related compounds. An imbalance of excessive dietary ω-6 and deficient ω-3 fatty acids is linked to several neurological and neuropsychiatric disorders.[22] A diet rich in ω-3 fatty acids, versus a "standard American diet" low in ω-3 fatty acids, reduced physical pain significantly, and pain reduction was correlated with an increase in *N*-docosahexaenoylethanolamine and 2-docosahexaenoylglycerol (the ω-3 endocannabinoids).[23] Developmental dietary ω-3 deficiency in rodents resulted in decreased eCB-dependent synaptic plasticity in the prefrontal cortex and nucleus accumbens, while a diet rich in ω-3 polyunsaturated fatty acids maintained endocannabinoid-dependent plasticity in the nucleus accumbens following a chronic social defeat stress. Consumption of ω-3 fatty acids can reduce AEA and 2-AG levels that may be causing CB1 desensitization, which is likely the case in obesity.[24]

Avoiding pesticides by consuming organic foods may protect the ECS: the pesticides chlorpyrifos and diazinon have been shown to alter ECS function. Phthalates, which are plasticizers added to food packaging and even the enteric coating of pharmaceutical pills, block CB1 as allosteric antagonists.[25]

Cold exposure and cryotherapy are ancient healing methods that have recently gained increased popularity. Cold bathing and cold-winter swimming have been associated with improvements in immune function, cardiovascular function, antioxidant activity, and metabolism;[26] with insulin sensitivity[27] and reduced inflammation and blood lipids;[28] and with activation of anti-pain centers of the brain.[29] As a powerful yet controllable stimulus of the sympathetic nervous system, cryotherapy activates brown adipose tissue (BAT) and triggers the browning of white adipose tissue (WAT) via sympathetic norepinephrine signaling at β3-adrenergic receptors in the adipocytes. The adipocytes produce eCBs as paracrine negative feedback modulators to inhibit norepinephrine release. These eCBs likely also act on the adipocytes as autocrine inhibitors of BAT activation and WAT browning, and they likely contribute to the pool of circulating eCBs.[30] A cold exposure that induces shivering thermogenesis is likely a strong enough stimulus to activate BAT and browning of WAT and to increase eCB activity; with regular cold exposure, the shivering may decrease or stop entirely, but these benefits likely persist.[31]

Wim Hof Method

I frequently recommend cryotherapy to patients with chronic pain, inflammatory conditions,[32] anxiety, or depression, with impressive results, and I personally use this modality to support my own health. For those interested, I recommend the Wim Hof method, a clinically studied technique that includes a breathing exercise that effectively prepares one for the cold exposure. The breathing temporarily produces hypocapnia, respiratory alkalosis, hypoxia, and high levels of adrenaline,[33] a powerful combination of hormetic stressors that likely activate the ECS. You can visit wimhofmethod.com for more information and a free app that teaches the technique.

Like cryotherapy, various fasting techniques have also gained widespread attention and scientific validation as tools to combat insulin resistance, inflammation, and associated sequelae.[34] The ECS is intimately involved in regulation of hunger, satiety, and energy utilization, and while the interactions are complex, data suggest that fasting can both trigger increased production of eCBs[35] and restore balance to the ECS in scenarios consistent with obesity and metabolic syndrome.[36]

Manual therapies like osteopathic manipulation and massage have demonstrated early findings that suggest ECS involvement in analgesia and other benefits.[37] Electroacupuncture has also been shown to impact the ECS both in the periphery and centrally.[38,39]

Finally, meditation may convey benefits partially mediated through the ECS. Anecdotally, many practitioners report meditation, yoga, and deep breathing exercises impart mild cannabimimetic effects and can both potentiate and be potentiated by the use of cannabis. One clinical study found the analgesic effects of meditation were not dependent on opioid signaling; in fact, analgesia improved with naloxone treatment 5 min prior to a pain stimulus. The authors proposed that the ECS may be involved in the analgesic effects of meditation.[40]

Chapter 10

Endocannabinoid System Dysfunction

CONSIDERING THE CRITICAL ROLE of the endocannabinoid system in homeostasis, one might presume that ECS dysfunction would predispose an individual to pathological states. Ethan Russo presented the theory of clinical endocannabinoid deficiency in 2001, and increasing evidence has emerged to support the concept that endocannabinoid deficiency is a component of certain disorders, such as chronic migraine, irritable bowel syndrome, endometriosis, and fibromyalgia. All are characterized by hypersensitivity or hyperalgesia, lack of diagnostic laboratory findings, and high rates of comorbidity with each other. Chronic migraineurs, for example, have been shown to have lower levels of AEA than controls in the cerebrospinal fluid.[1] Women with endometriosis have lower levels of CB1 receptors in endometrial tissue; reduced ECS function has been suggested to lead to growth of endometriosis tissue and a more severe pain.[2] Children with autistic spectrum disorder had lower levels of AEA, PEA, and OEA than their neurotypical controls.[3] Alterations in ECS tone have been reported in patients with inflammatory bowel disease[4] and irritable bowel syndrome.[5]

While human evidence for clinical endocannabinoid deficiency is still in its infancy, and confounded by the numerous influences on circulating eCB levels, preclinical evidence continues to support this theory.[6] Rodents that lack DAGL have 2-AG deficiency and are used to model low stress resilience and behavioral alterations analogous to mood disorders, such as increased anxiety, impaired reward sensitivity, compromised fear extinction, and alterations in structural plasticity.[7] Authors have proposed ECS dysfunction as a factor in postconcussive headache on the basis of preclinical data.[8]

When optimal ECS function to support health and prevent disease is considered, it is important to note that either deficiency, as described above, or excess of circulating endocannabinoids, as in obesity and metabolic syndrome, could weaken the homeostatic capacity of the ECS.

Our genetics play a clear role in ECS function. A surprisingly large body of evidence associates a variety of clinical outcomes with polymorphisms in the ECS genes, such as those coding for the CB1 and CB2 receptors and for the enzyme FAAH. A partial list of outcomes includes schizophrenia subtypes,[9] alcohol dependence,[10] body mass index,[11] central obesity,[12] ADHD and PTSD,[13] happiness,[14] serum lipid profiles,[15] and risk of cyclic vomiting syndrome.[16]

An interesting case was reported in which a 66-year-old woman required no postoperative analgesia after a normally painful orthopedic hand surgery (trapeziectomy). Further investigations revealed a lifelong history of painless injuries, such as frequent cuts and burns, which were observed to heal quickly. She was found to have a microdeletion in a FAAH pseudogene and high levels of anandamide.[17]

Cannabinoid hyperemesis syndrome (CHS) may be another example of ECS dysregulation, in this case triggered by exogenous cannabinoids. Characterized by cyclic, intense episodes of nausea and vomiting, and frequent hot bathing as the only means of short-term relief, CHS occurs in individuals after long-term, high-dose cannabis use, and the onset of CHS is typically years after initiation of cannabis use. While the pathophysiology has yet to be elucidated, it may involve abnormal HPA axis and sympathetic activation, compromised regulation by the ECS, and genetic susceptibility[18] (see Chapter 18 for more information).

Our ECS function changes as we age. While both rodent and human studies provide some conflicting results regarding levels of CB1 expression, there is consistent evidence of reduced CB1 function in both species and of reduced 2-AG levels in rodents. Authors have proposed a link between ECS changes and reduced amplitude of circadian activity in aging, and they have highlighted the preclinical evidence that suggests the ECS can be targeted to address age-related conditions like disturbed sleep and cognitive decline.[19] Perhaps by supporting optimal ECS function with health-promoting activities, as described in Chapter 9, and appropriate use of exogenous ECS modulators, we can help prevent age-related disease.

Chapter 11

Osteopathic Perspectives on the Endocannabinoid System

OSTEOPATHY IS A MEDICAL SCIENCE keenly interested in the anatomy and physiology of health and the mechanisms of healing. Doctors of osteopathy use manual therapies and other treatments to support the patient's homeostatic capacity, and they spend hundreds of hours developing the ability to palpate subtle alterations in anatomy and physiology and to sense the innate self-correcting therapeutic activities present in states of both health and disease.

Our understanding of the ECS is ever growing, one small puzzle piece at a time, and is far from complete. As researchers and clinicians work to assemble these pieces into a picture that can serve humanity, I believe this information provides us with more than new drug targets or an explanation of the results we have seen with one useful herb.

Endocannabinoid physiology can lead us into paradigms of systems biology, where we accept our inability to understand every discrete cause and effect and instead recognize that every living system is subject to negentropic organizing forces that counteract entropy throughout its life span. In osteopathy we ask, from where these forces emerge, how do they work, and how can we support them? We quietly put our hands on a patient and feel the physiology of homeostasis at work. The sensory experiences that result leave us better prepared to understand the science of healing.

Several principles of osteopathy are exemplified by our current picture of the ECS and may help orient readers, interested in working with the ECS for the benefit of their patients, to a health-care approach based primarily on supporting health rather than fighting disease.

Preference for Endogenous Medicines

Andrew Taylor Still, the founder of osteopathy, hypothesized that osteopathic techniques stimulated the production and release of endogenous compounds that promoted homeostasis and healing. In 1897 he wrote, "Man should study and use the drugs compounded in his own body." [1]

In 2005, osteopath and cannabinoid researcher John McPartland tested endocannabinoid levels before and after osteopathic manipulative treatment. Average anandamide levels more than doubled following treatment.[2] This may explain the psychotropic changes that often accompany osteopathic treatment, such as anxiolysis and euphoria. Other activities that likely enhance the production of cannabinoids from our inner pharmacy, such as exercise, singing, fasting, and meditation, produce comparable psychotropic and healing effects.

When a patient's inner pharmacy is unable to adequately supply cannabinoid medicines, as in the case of ECS deficiency or dysfunction, we may consider the potential benefit of phytocannabinoids, like THC; exogenous supplementation of endocannabinoids or endocannabinoid-like compounds, such as PEA; and the utility of nonpharmacological ECS modulators, including manual medicine and exercise.

Forces of Development Are Forces of Healing

Osteopathic pioneer James Jealous stated, "The formative and regenerative forces that organize embryological development are present throughout our life span [. . .]. In other words, the forces of embryogenesis become the forces of healing after birth."[3]

As described previously, the ECS regulates numerous activities of embryonic development, especially in the nervous system, and is intimately involved in postnatal neurogenesis, neuroplasticity, and recovery from neurological injury throughout the life span. The ECS is an embryological force available for healing in the adult. By interfacing with the ECS in our therapeutic approaches, intentionally or not, perhaps we are more likely to promote a healing process capable of regenerating tissue and repatterning function, rather than simply ameliorating patients' symptoms.

Unity of Body, Mind, and Spirit

The ECS, present throughout the CNS and peripheral tissues, provides a system of communication that integrates our triune aspects, as well as spanning the function of the psycho–neuroendocrine–immune axis. Cannabinoid ligands, such as THC, and non-drug methods, likely characterized by increased ECS activity, can promote spiritual experiences, emotional shifts, and physical effects. While we may use language to describe these as distinct occurrences, they are often experienced as a singular process.

Disengagement from Compensatory Patterns

Anatomical and physiological dysfunctions are often compensated for via redundant and alternative pathways in an effort to maintain function. While these compensatory activities are helpful in the short term, their accumulation can limit resilience and capacity to adapt to an ever-changing external environment.

During an osteopathic treatment, we often disengage from compensatory patterns, most easily observed in the autonomic and musculoskeletal systems. A sense of wholeness in the patient ensues, characterized by more homogenous tissue texture, increased translation of respiratory motions through peripheral tissues, and augmentation of innate therapeutic activity. This state of wholeness, frequently referred to as the patient's "neutral", is not unique to osteopathic treatments; the Eastern healing practices of yoga and qigong also promote this state as an important step in healing. Essentially, new patterns of thought, behavior, and physiology more congruent with our current position in life are more likely to emerge if we first disengage from old compensatory patterns.

The ECS is most active as a negative feedback system, suppressing excessive physiological activity throughout other bodily systems, liberating physiology from allostatic load, and restoring our capacity for homeostasis and adaptation. I suspect that the ECS is heavily involved in the processes of defacilitation, disengagement, and return to neutral.

Coherence in a Complex Polyrhythmic System

The human being is a complex polyrhythmic system of biological oscillations, involving tissue and fluid movement, intracellular and intercellular signaling activity, chemical and ionic gradients, and more. The periods of these rhythms range from the life span to the circadian rhythm to the vibration of the microtubules. We observe increased coherence, or harmony, among these oscillations in states of wellness and increased interference, or discord, in states of illness. The ECS influences our health through modulation of our biorhythms, as McPartland eloquently explains:[4]

> The endocannabinoid system alters every biological oscillator or pacemaker cell investigated to date, beginning with somite formation in the embryo.[. . .]
> Human consciousness represents the rhythmic entrainment of synchronously

firing neurons. In five regions of the human brain, such neurons are particularly enriched with CB1:

- The **hippocampus** is a source of theta and gamma band oscillations and is the neural substrate responsible for declarative memory.
- **Striatal tissues** contribute to the "beat frequency" model of time perception.
- The **cerebellum** plays a role in rhythm production and self-paced-behaviors, and cannabis accelerates the cerebellar clock.
- The **suprachiasmatic nucleus** is responsible for controlling circadian rhythms.
- The **pineal gland** produces melatonin and 2-AG in a circadian rhythm driven by the suprachiasmatic nucleus and regulated in part by CB2 in animal studies.

Imagine the function of our nervous system as interactions of rapidly oscillating networks of nerve transmission and neurotransmitter signaling. The cadence of these oscillations is defined, in part, by the pause, characterized by the strength of the postsynaptic endocannabinoid signal and the sensitivity of the presynaptic endocannabinoid receptor. In the CNS and beyond, the ECS helps set the tempo of our biology.

Axonal Transport

Seventy years prior to the discovery of axonal transport, A. T. Still described a "nutritive" function of nerves that transported essential components of health from the CNS to the peripheral tissues.[5] He attributed the cause of disease to "partial or complete failure of the nerves to properly conduct the fluids of life,"[6] and his approach to treatment frequently describes correcting the "compression, stretching, angulation, and torsion" on nerves that block this nutritive supply and disrupt peripheral physiology.

As previously described, many of the anti-inflammatory, antinociceptive, autonomic regulating, and other homeostatic effects of the ECS require the presence of CB1 receptors in the terminals of peripheral nerves. The CB1 protein is produced in the body of the nerve and subsequently transported, sometimes great distances, to the nerve terminal by axoplasmic flow. A rodent study enables us to visualize the interruption of axonal transport of CB1 to the periphery, perhaps analogous to myofascial and other structural nerve compressions in our patients. After ligation of the sciatic nerve with a suture loop, CB1 receptors are seen accumulating proximal to the ligation and failing to make their way to the nerve terminal (Figure 11.1).[7] In the words of McPartland, "By obstructing axoplasmic flow and cellular trafficking of CB1, the pathophysiology of somatic dysfunction perpetuates itself."[8]

FIGURE 11.1

Cannabinoid Receptors in Sciatic Nerves

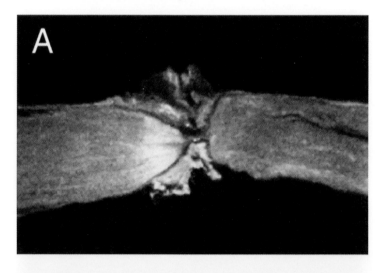

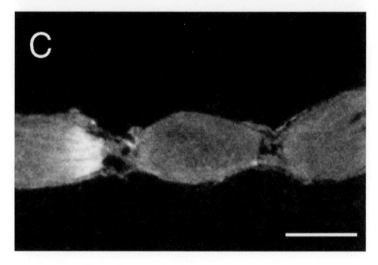

Note. Cannabinoid binding sites accumulate proximal to a tight ligation of the sciatic nerve, demonstrating the flow of cannabinoid receptors to the periphery. Dark-field photomicrographs show damming of cannabinoid receptor binding sites proximal, as opposed to distal, to a single tight ligation (A) or the more proximal of two individual ligatures (C) applied to the sciatic nerve. From "Cannabinoid receptors undergo axonal flow in sensory nerves," by A. G. Hohmann and M. Herkenham, 1999, *Neuroscience, 92*(4), pp. 1171–1175 (https://doi.org/10.1016/S0306 -4522(99)00220-1). Copyright 1999 by Elsevier. Reprinted with permission.

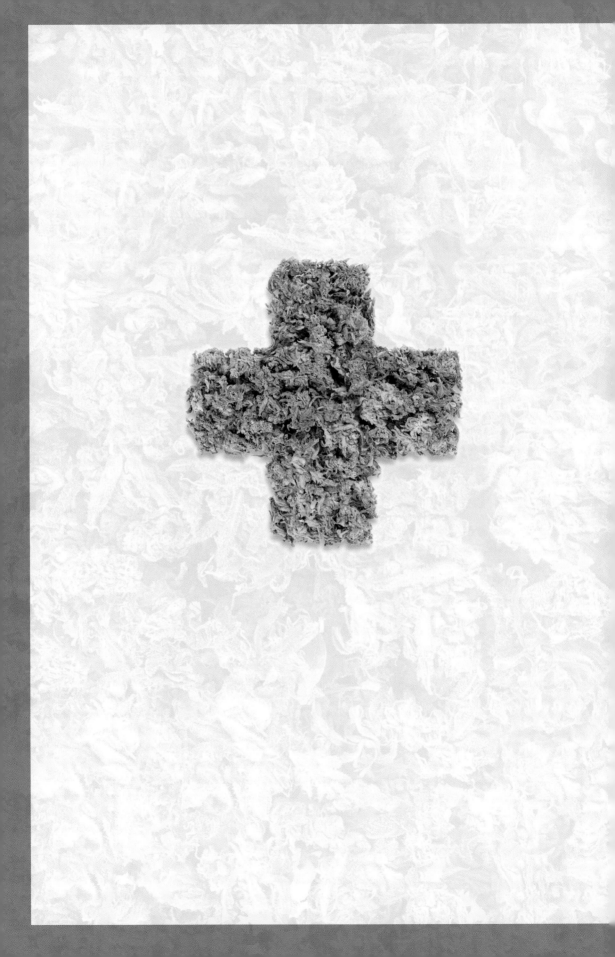

Part 3

Cannabis Pharmacology

Chapter 12

Clinically Relevant Botany

CANNABIS SATIVA, of the family Cannabaceae, is an annual, dioecious plant, producing separate male and female plants. It is thought to have evolved approximately 28 million years ago on the basis of molecular clock studies.[1] Its closest relative is *Humulus*, which produces a female flower known as hops, widely used as a flavor and aroma ingredient in beer.

Most of the medicinal compounds in cannabis are produced in trichomes, glandular protuberances that grow on the leaves and flowers, and to a lesser extent in bracts and stems, of the female plants. The trichomes produce a resin rich in phytocannabinoids, thought to provide defense and interaction with herbivores and pests, and terpenoids, which provide a strong aroma, repel insects, and potentially suppress growth of surrounding vegetation. The resin also has antibiotic and antifungal properties and protects against water loss, and the antioxidant activity of the phytocannabinoids likely protects the reproductive structures from ultraviolet radiation and oxidative damage.[2]

The female plants produce inflorescences, or clusters of flowers, which continue to grow until they are wind-pollinated. When the male plants are culled before they release their pollen, female flowers continue to grow in size and increase in potency, often referred to as *sinsemilla* (without seeds). Most cannabis grown for medicine is unfertilized, with flowers containing up to 30% phytocannabinoids and 4% terpenes by weight and trichomes containing up to 60% phytocannabinoids and 10% terpenes.[3]

The cannabis plant synthesizes phytocannabinoid acids, such as Δ^9-tetrahydrocannabinolic acid (THCA). These acids are converted into neutral cannabinoids, such as Δ^9-tetrahydrocannabinol (THC), upon exposure to heat and time through a process called decarboxylation (dissociation of the carboxylic acid group). Raw, cured cannabis flowers often contain 5–10% of the phytocannabinoids in the neutral form.

Medical varieties of cannabis are often divided into three categories based on cannabinoid content: type I is THC-predominant, type II contains both THC and cannabidiol (CBD), and type III is CBD-predominant. While sometimes referred to as "strains," a term technically reserved for microbes, the varieties of cannabis selected for their biochemical attributes are increasingly called "chemovars."[4] The term "cultivar" is also sometimes used, though some plant taxonomy experts argue this term should be reserved for officially registered varieties.

Most cannabis flowers are prepared for smoking by trimming the lower potency leaves surrounding the higher potency inflorescence and then "curing" to allow the flower to undergo further biochemical changes and reach ideal dryness for smoke quality and taste. The trimmed material may contain up to 15% cannabinoids by weight and is often processed into cannabis concentrates and/or medical products.

Various methods of concentrating the active constituents of cannabis have been employed over millennia. For example, rubbing the flower over fine screens causes the trichomes, which appear like tiny crystals, to fall off into a powder called *kief*. Other mechanical methods can be used to concentrate the resin into *hash*. More recently, hydrocarbons, supercritical CO_2, and distillation techniques have been used to produce cannabis concentrates with cannabinoid potency up to 90% by weight. These newer forms of cannabis concentrates are mostly smoked by nonmedical users and are identified with names that describe their physical properties, such as *shatter* or *wax*. Concentrates can be infused into oils, tinctured in ethanol, or processed in other manners to make medicinal preparations.

Until recently, "hemp" varieties of cannabis were grown for nonmedical crops, including fiber, hurd (the center of the stalk), and seed. Most countries have regulations that limit the THC content (e.g., 0.3% by weight) of dietary hemp products, such as seed and seed oil. Due to the exploding popularity of CBD, cannabis breeders have developed type III, CBD-rich flowers with ultra-low THC content, in an effort to qualify as a hemp product. Because CBD is typically a more lucrative product than fiber or seed, many hemp farmers are choosing to grow "hemp" varieties whose morphology appears no different than traditional "drug-type" cannabis varieties. The morphology of "fiber-type" cannabis, traditionally referred to as hemp, is quite distinct, with much longer stalks, less branching, and smaller inflorescences.

The chemical composition, and thus medicinal properties, of cannabis flowers can be influenced by their environment, with increased cannabinoid production associated with low humidity, sparse rainfall, increased ultraviolet radiation, soil nutrients including magnesium and iron, and parasites. The soil microbiome has also been shown to influence the production of medicinal compounds by the plant, and certain bacterial communities show cultivar specificity.[5] The same cannabis variety grown outdoors or indoors, in soil or hydroponically, or in different regions will likely produce medicine with somewhat different pharmacological properties.

Beyond innocuous soil microbes, cannabis flowers can contain potentially pathogenic microbes. Using molecular amplification and sequencing, researchers have demonstrated the presence of several toxigenic fungi in dispensary-derived cannabis samples, including toxigenic *Penicillium* species (*P. paxilli*, *P. citrinum*, *P. commune*, *P. chrysogenum*, and *P. corylophilum*) and *Aspergillus* species (*A. terreus*, *A. niger*, *A. flavus*, and *A. versicolor*). Interestingly, several of these microbes were not detected by use of traditional culture-based platforms from food safety testing that are also used in the cannabis industry.[6] Several cases of pulmonary aspergillosis in immunocompromised patients associated with cannabis inhalation have been reported, and methods of sterilization have been developed[7] (see Chapter 18 for more information).

Cannabis root preparations have been described in the medical literature for millennia, primarily indicated for the treatment of joint pain, burns, and tumors. Devoid of phytocannabinoids, the roots contain the triterpenoids friedelin and epifriedelanol, alkaloids, sterols, and other minor compounds, including choline.[8] Very little modern research has explored the therapeutic properties of cannabis roots.

Cannabis botanical terminology is fraught with inaccuracy and controversy, especially regarding the terms "sativa," commonly used to describe taller varieties with thin fan leaves and more euphoric psychological effects, and "indica," commonly used to describe shorter, bushy varieties with more sedating effects. Though widely used, the terms are both inaccurate and inadequate for describing qualities relevant to medical use. In a recent review, John McPartland stated that "Categorizing Cannabis as either 'Sativa' and 'Indica' has become an exercise in futility. Ubiquitous interbreeding and hybridization renders their distinction meaningless."[9] Ethan Russo agreed, choosing to "eschew the irreconcilable taxonomic debate as an unnecessary distraction, and rather emphasize that only biochemical and pharmacological distinctions between Cannabis accessions are relevant."[10]

Nevertheless, patients often face product choices with indica, sativa, or hybrid as the only indication of pharmacological profile. In general, indica products may be best for sleep, pain, and spasticity; sativa products may be best for daytime nonsedating use and antidepressant effects but may be more likely to exacerbate anxiety; and hybrid products may be the most versatile.

Chapter 13

Phytocannabinoid Pharmacology

FIVE HUNDRED THIRTY-EIGHT natural compounds have been identified in cannabis, with over 120 identified as "phytocannabinoids" on the basis of a chemical structure shared with Δ^9-tetrahydrocannabinol.[1] Despite the name, very few of the phytocannabinoids have been shown to have activity at cannabinoid type 1 and type 2 (CB1 and CB2) receptors. For many, we know little to nothing about their pharmacological effects and only refer to them based on chemical nomenclature. Early research has identified that some of these lesser-studied cannabinoids, typically found in trace quantities, can have synergistic pharmacological effects with their more well-known counterparts.[2] Often referred to as the "entourage effect," a term borrowed from endocannabinoid physiology research, phytoconstituent synergy is the rule in cannabis-derived medicines, contributing to the diversity of therapeutic effects and potential clinical applications and demanding a more systems-based approach to therapeutics.

This chapter details the pharmacology of the nine cannabinoids most clinically relevant and most commonly available to patients. Unless otherwise noted, the information herein references excellent reviews from Roger Pertwee (2014)[3] and Russo and Marcu (2017).[4]

Δ⁹-Tetrahydrocannabinol

FIGURE 13.1

Δ⁹-Tetrahydrocannabinol (THC) Chemical 2D Structure

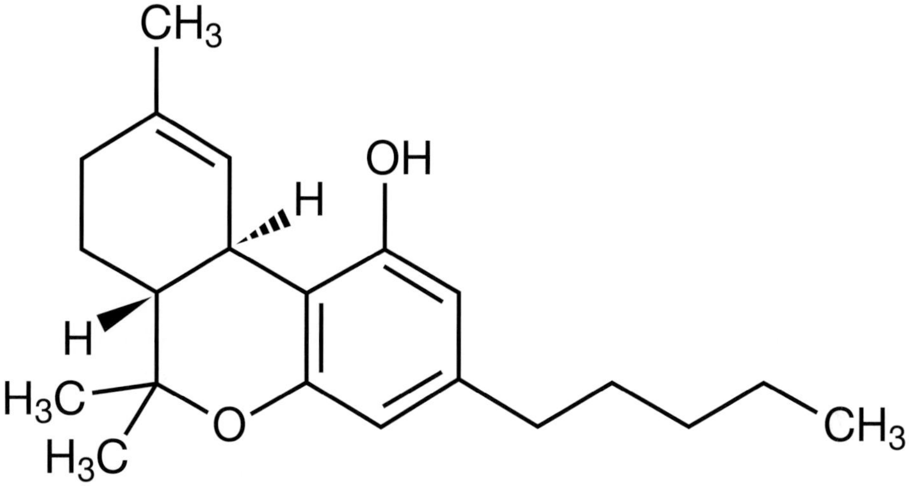

Δ⁹-Tetrahydrocannabinol (THC, Figure 13.1) mimics the endocannabinoids anandamide (*N*-arachidonoylethanolamine, AEA) and 2-arachidonoylglycerol (2-AG) by acting as a partial agonist at the CB1 and CB2 receptors. As a partial agonist, THC is an ideal agent for activating but not overstimulating the endocannabinoid system (ECS), and it can also act as an antagonist or inverse agonist under certain conditions, especially at CB2 or in the presence of stronger agonists. Due to the distribution and nature of the cannabinoid receptors, THC demonstrates myriad pharmacological effects, including the following:

- analgesic
- antipruritic
- antispasmodic
- antiemetic
- antioxidant
- anti-inflammatory
- anxiolytic
- bronchodilatory
- neuroprotective
- psychoactive

Beyond CB1 and CB2, THC has been shown, mostly in vitro, to affect a variety of other receptor targets, but the clinical relevance of these actions is unknown. For example, THC has been shown to activate GPR18, GPR55, PPAR-γ nuclear receptor, TRPA1, TRPV2, TRPV3, and TRPV4 and to inhibit 5-HT3A, TRPM8, and GPR55.

THC has additionally been shown to influence numerous enzymes and transporters at low concentrations in vitro: it enhances phospholipases, which may catalyze the release of arachidonic acid from membrane phospholipids; it inhibits the uptake of adenosine and serotonin, increasing the uptake of norepinephrine; and it may stimulate or inhibit the reuptake of dopamine.

Δ^8-THC is a stable metabolite of Δ^9-THC that occurs in small quantities in the plant but can be produced by acid isomerization of Δ^9-THC.[5] Though the pharmacology of Δ^8-THC has received little investigation compared to Δ^9-THC, it has been shown to similarly act upon the CB1 receptor, to induce ataxia in dogs and cannabis-like psychopharmacological effects in humans and rhesus monkeys, though with less potency than Δ^9-THC.

Δ^9-Tetrahydrocannabinolic Acid

FIGURE 13.2

Δ^9-Tetrahydrocannabinolic Acid (THCA) Chemical 2D Structure

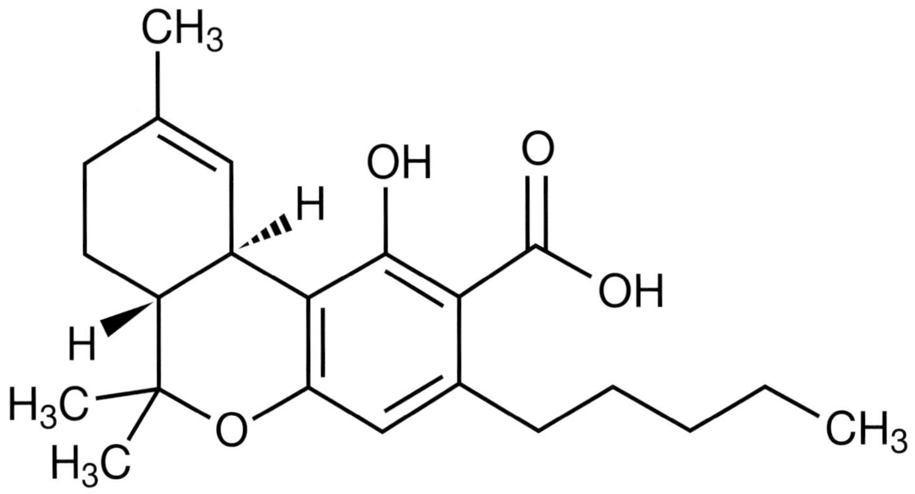

Though Δ^9-tetrahydrocannabinolic acid (THCA, Figure 13.2) is the direct natural precursor of THC, the two compounds exhibit distinct pharmacology. Primarily, THCA has little to no activity at CB1 and CB2 receptors[6] and does not cause a cannabimimetic effect in rhesus monkeys (≤5 mg/kg), mice (≤20 mg/kg), or dogs (≤7 mg/kg).[7]

In vitro, THCA has been shown to exert immunomodulatory, anti-inflammatory, neuroprotective, and antineoplastic effects, including suppression of tumor necrosis factor α release, preventing nerve damage from 1-methyl-4-phenylpyridinium in a model of Parkinson's disease, scavenging free radicals, and inhibiting prostate carcinoma (androgen-receptor-positive and -negative) and breast carcinoma (triple-negative and HER2-negative) cell lines.[8] In vitro and ex vivo models of inflammatory bowel disease have demonstrated anti-inflammatory effects of THCA without the biphasic pro-inflammatory effects seen with CBD.[9]

In vivo, THCA has been shown to exert antiemetic effects at 10 times the potency of THC.[10] In a mouse model, THCA was shown to have poor penetration of the blood–brain barrier, likely due to its more hydrophilic nature,[11] though clinically I have observed THCA exerting anticonvulsant effects at remarkably low doses.[12] One explanation may be the increased permeability of the blood–brain barrier noted in epilepsy and other neurological disorders.[13] An older preclinical assay did find anticonvulsant effects of THCA at high doses (200 mg/kg),[14] though recently it has been shown that even pure standards of THCA contain at least small amounts of THC, a potential confounder.[15]

Ethnobotanical and anecdotal reports of the healing properties of cannabis tea are likely attributed to THCA, the most abundant constituent due to the increased water solubility related to the carboxyl group.[16] Its hydrophilicity also impacts absorption and distribution; human pharmacokinetic data demonstrates high oral bioavailability of THCA in oil and decoction, with 30 and 50 times more absorption than THC, respectively.[17]

Cannabidiol

FIGURE 13.3

Cannabidiol (CBD) Chemical 2D Structure

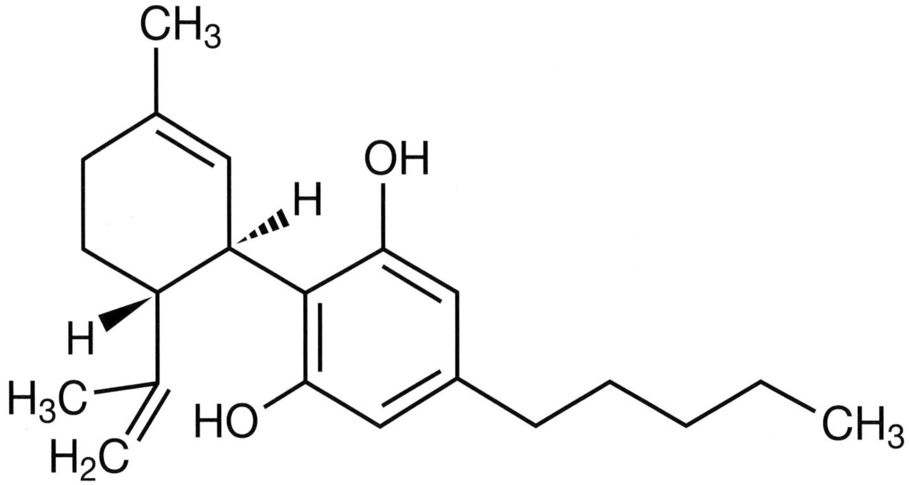

Over 65 distinct pharmacologic targets for cannabidiol (CBD, Figure 13.3) have been identified on the basis of in vitro studies, including receptors, ion channels, enzymes, and transporters.[18] While the activity at many of these targets requires concentrations that are unlikely to occur in vivo, CBD is strongly pleiotropic, yet it is remarkably safe and well-tolerated. In pre-clinical and/or clinical studies, CBD has demonstrated the following physiologic effects:

- anticonvulsive
- anti-inflammatory
- analgesic
- antioxidant
- antifibrotic
- anxiolytic
- antipsychotic
- procognitive
- neuroprotective

Cannabinoid Type 1 and Type 2 Receptors

CBD acts as a negative allosteric modulator of the CB1 receptor: it binds to a site on the receptor distinct from agonists like AEA, 2-AG, and THC, decreasing but not abolishing the activity level of the receptor when stimulated by CB1 agonists.[19,20] This is the likely mechanism by which CBD is able to mitigate the adverse effects of THC when coadministered. The impact of CBD on CB2 is less well characterized, but it likely also acts as an allosteric modulator.[21]

Beyond modulating signal intensity at the cannabinoid receptors, CBD also likely regulates the functional selectivity of the receptors (see Chapter 5), especially in regard to the activity of AEA.[22] While the activity of CBD at CB1 and CB2 receptors is thought to be less relevant in the treatment of neurological disorders,[23] preclinical data suggests cannabinoid receptor involvement in the impact of CBD on behavioral disorders, such as its ability to disrupt the consolidation of fear memories[24] and to inhibit sucrose self-administration.[25]

Serotonin Receptors

CBD stimulates the serotonin 5-HT1A receptor,[26] possibly a common mechanism for reducing anxiety,[27,28] reducing the damage of brain ischemia,[29] reducing nausea,[30] and improving cognition in hepatic encephalopathy.[31] The 5-HT1A receptor is the most widespread serotonin receptor in the central nervous system and is involved in the activity of several antianxiety and antidepressant medications. 5-HT1A activation is also associated with improved cognition, decreased aggression, increased sociability, decreased impulsivity, inhibition of drug-seeking behavior, and facilitation of sex drive and arousal.

Adenosine Receptors

Adenosine receptors have several functions in the body, including regulation of heart function, inflammation, and dopamine and glutamate release in the brain. The adenosine receptor is well-known as a target of caffeine, which inhibits the A1 and A2 receptors and provides a stimulating effect. Studies have shown that CBD likely stimulates the adenosine A1 receptor, perhaps indirectly by inhibiting the uptake of adenosine. This mechanism has been shown to prevent irregular heart rhythm in a rodent model of heart attack.[32] CBD also likely stimulates the adenosine A2 receptor, leading to anti-inflammatory[33] and potentially neuroprotective[34] effects. Activating these receptors typically produces sedation, so this is likely not the mechanism by which CBD increases alertness, which is more likely related to 5-HT1A activation.

Glycine Receptor

Glycine receptors mediate neuropathic pain and inflammation. CBD and its analog dehydroxyl-CBD have been shown to suppress neuropathic pain in rats with spinal nerve injury by targeting the α3 glycine receptor[35] and to reduce chronic inflammatory pain caused by noxious heat stimulation by targeting the α1 glycine receptor.[36] Glycine signaling is also involved in spasticity,[37] and glycine receptor activity may contribute to the antispasmodic effects of CBD.

Dopamine Receptors

CBD has been shown to act as a partial agonist at the dopamine D2 receptor, explaining its antipsychotic effects at high doses in humans. The inhibition follows similar biphasic trends as the dopamine partial agonist antipsychotic drug aripiprazole.[38]

GPR55

CBD antagonizes GPR55, resulting in anti-inflammatory effects[39] and decreased migration of neutrophils.[40] CBD has also been shown to reduce neuronal excitability via GPR55 antagonism, likely one of its antiepileptic mechanisms of action.[41]

Ion Channels

CBD is also an agonist at transient receptor potential vanilloid type 1 (TRPV1), likely a mechanism of analgesic, anti-inflammatory, and antiepileptic effects and potentially contributing to its antipsychotic effects.[42] Unlike capsaicin, the classic TRPV1 agonist commonly used in topical preparations for arthritis, CBD does not cause a burning sensation in the mouth or on the skin. The ability of CBD to stimulate and desensitize TRPV1 may contribute to its commonly observed bell-shaped or biphasic dose–response effects.[43]

Voltage-dependent anion-selective channel 1 (VDAC1), also known as mitochondrial porin, is an ion channel most often located on the outer membrane of mitochondria, although it has been reported to be present on cell plasma membranes as well. VDAC1 plays a complex and important role in a variety of cell functions such as cellular energy rationing, calcium homeostasis, apoptosis, and protection against oxidative stress. The activity of CBD on VDAC1 and mitochondrial calcium likely contributes to its neuropro- tective[44] and antineoplastic[45] effects.

Transporters and Enzymes

CBD has been shown to inhibit the uptake of several neurotransmitters, including nor- epinephrine, dopamine, serotonin, GABA (4-aminobutanoic acid, formerly known as gamma-aminobutyric acid), and anandamide. Thirty-two specific enzymes have been identified that CBD acts upon, many with unknown significance. Several are in the cyto- chrome P450 family (see the Drug Interactions section in Chapter 18). CBD weakly inhib- its fatty acid amide hydrolase (FAAH), but its ability to increase anandamide levels is more likely due to the inhibition of anandamide transport. CBD has not been found to have significant effects on cyclooxygenase (COX-1 or COX-2) activity.[46]

Cannabidiolic Acid

FIGURE 13.4

Cannabidiolic Acid (CBDA) Chemical 2D Structure

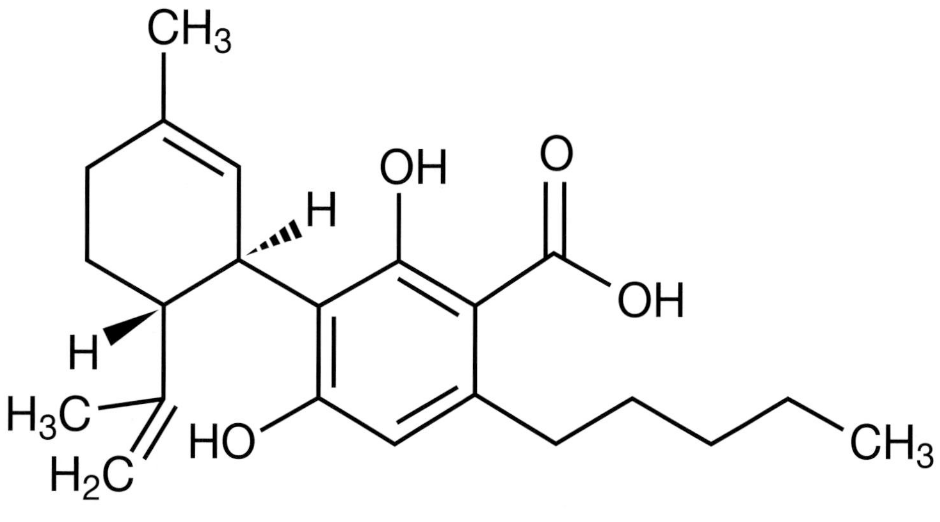

Cannabidiolic acid (CBDA, Figure 13.4) is a promising therapeutic agent due to its over-lapping pharmacological properties with CBD but superior bioavailability and efficacy at lower doses. For example, both CBD and CBDA are antiemetics via activation of the 5-HT1A serotonin receptor in rodent models of nausea, but while CBD demonstrated antiemetic effects at 5 mg/kg ip, CBDA was effective at 0.0005 mg/kg ip.[47] Further-more, the dose–response curve for the antiemetic effect of CBDA was not biphasic, as has been reported for CBD, with potentiation of vomiting at 20–40 mg/kg. Similarly, in a rodent model of carrageenan-induced hyperalgesia, orally administered CBD was effec-tive at preventing hyperalgesia at 10 mg/kg, while oral CBDA was effective at 0.1 mg/kg.[48] In a rodent model of the seizure disorder Dravet syndrome, CBD reduced seizures at 100 mg/kg, while CBDA was effective at 10 mg/kg.[49]

CBDA has been shown to act on the following physiological targets:

- indirect agonist of the 5-HT1A serotonin receptor, responsible for its antiemetic and anxiolytic effects[50,51]
- agonist at the TRPV1 receptor (EC50 = 19.7 ± 3.9 µM),[52] responsible for its antihy-peralgesic effects[53]
- agonist at TRPA1 (EC50 = 12.0 ± 8.8 µM),[54] a receptor involved in pain, sensory sig-naling, and cerebral vasodilation[55,56]
- antagonist at TRPM8 (IC50 = 1.6 ± 0.4 µM),[57] also known as the cold and menthol receptor 1, also implicated in the inflammatory response of bronchial epithelial cells to both cold temperature and cigarette smoke[58]
- inhibition of tumor necrosis factor α release at low concentrations (1 mg/ml) in human U937 cells stimulated with lipopolysaccharide[59]
- inhibition of the COX-2 enzyme (IC50 = 2 µM) in one model, at approximately $^1/_{10}$ the potency of diclofenac,[60] and inhibition of COX-1 (IC50 = 470 µM) in another model[61]
- downregulation of c-Fos, one component of the activator protein 1 dimer complex, a transcription factor for positive regulation of the COX-2 gene[62]
- decreased expression of matrix metallopeptidase 9[63]

Regarding COX-2 inhibition, it remains to be seen whether this effect occurs in vivo and whether CBDA produces the side effects common with other COX-2 inhibitors. CBDA has been shown to inhibit breast cancer cell migration in vitro via mechanisms including downregulation of COX-2, matrix metallopeptidase 9, transforming growth factor β, and parathyroid hormone-related protein.[64,65]

CBDA has not been found to act upon CB1 or CB2, either directly or as an allosteric modulator like CBD. While the pharmacological strategy of combining CBD with THC is often helpful for mitigating adverse effects of THC, some data suggest CBD can, to some extent, also inhibit the therapeutic effects of THC, such as analgesia.[66] Combining CBDA with THC can convey additive or synergistic benefits, as demonstrated in a rodent study of nociception and inflammation,[67] without diminishing the power of THC, a strategy that might be useful in patients who are not overly sensitive to the adverse effects of THC.

In humans, the oral bioavailability of CBDA is higher than that of CBD in decoction and oil by 5- and 11-fold, respectively.[68] Overall, early results with CBDA indicate promising therapeutic attributes that warrant more investigation.

Cannabinol

FIGURE 13.5
Cannabinol (CBN) Chemical 2D Structure

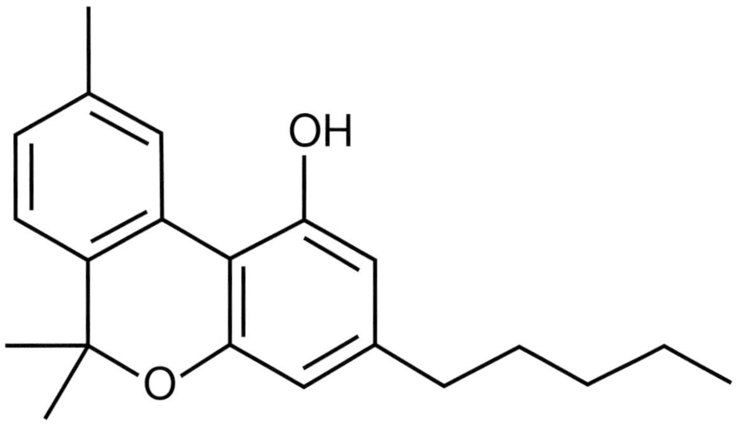

Oxidation of THC produces cannabinol (CBN, Figure 13.5), which has activity similar to that of THC as a CB1 and CB2 partial agonist but with only ¼ the potency of THC and with somewhat higher affinity for CB2 than CB1. Animal and human experiments have demonstrated sedative, anticonvulsant, anti-inflammatory, and antibiotic properties, including activity against methicillin-resistant *Staphylococcus aureus* (MRSA). The 11-OH-CBN metabolite is more potent at CB1 and CB2 than the parent molecule, so CBN taken by mouth may produce effects with similar potency to THC.

The CBN content of cannabis products is directly related to storage conditions: time, temperature, and exposure to ultraviolet light. One study found that 41% of the THC in cannabis plant material had converted to CBN after 4 years of storage at 20–22°C.[69] In tropical and equatorial regions where cannabis is dried in the sun, CBN content is likely to be higher. Commercially, some cannabis products designed to promote sleep intentionally contain higher levels of CBN, though I have not observed a clear trend of improved efficacy and have had a few reports of paradoxical effects, with higher levels of CBN associated with wakefulness or disturbed sleep. During the oxidation of THC to CBN, several other phytoconstituents likely also undergo oxidative changes, which may serve as confounding factors.

Cannabigerolic Acid and Cannabigerol

FIGURE 13.6

Cannabigerolic Acid (CBGA) Chemical 2D Structure

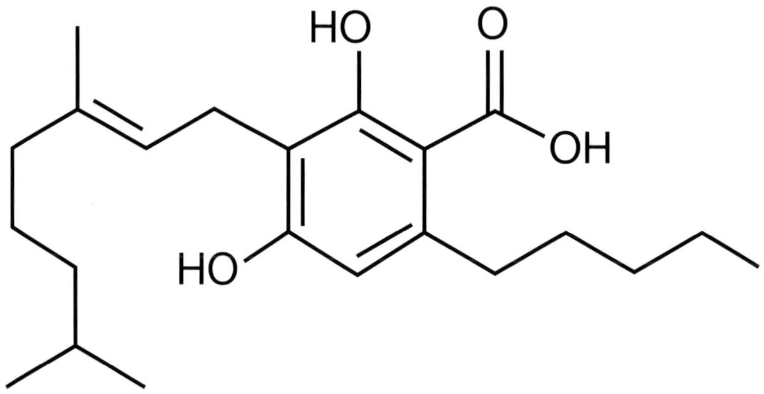

FIGURE 13.7

Cannabigerol (CBG) Chemical 2D Structure

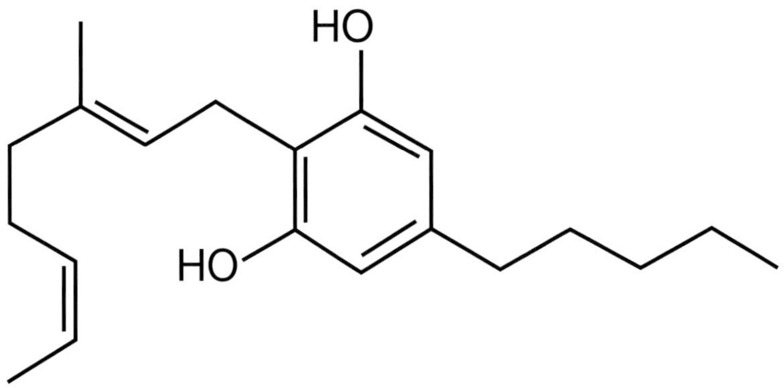

Cannabigerolic acid (CBGA, Figure 13.6) is the original phytocannabinoid biosynthesized in the plant from olivetolic acid and geranyl pyrophosphate; it is later converted into the other cannabinoid acids via enzymatic processes. While most chemovars contain very low quantities of CBGA and cannabigerol (CBG), some varieties have been bred to lack the enzymes responsible for this conversion. Currently, varieties of CBGA/CBG-predominant cannabis with ≤0.3% THC content have become commercially available for production as hemp. Compared to CBD, little research has explored the physiological effects of CBG, and even less has focused on CBGA.

CBG (Figure 13.7) has low activity at the CB receptors, but it stimulates TRPV1, TRPV2, TRPA1, TRPV3, TRPV4, and α2 adrenoceptor. The latter is likely related to its analgesic effects, which were reported to be stronger than THC in one experiment, and to its mild antihypertensive effects. CBG potently antagonizes TRPV8, suggesting therapeutic potential in prostate cancer, bladder pain, and detrusor muscle overactivity.

CBG inhibits the uptake of anandamide, serotonin, norepinephrine, and GABA. In vitro experiments have found that that CBG can oppose the activation of both CB1 and 5-HT1A receptors with significant potency, respectively suggesting potential for mitigating the adverse effects of THC and for antidepressant effects as demonstrated in rodent models. CBG inhibits keratinocyte proliferation, suggesting utility in dermatology.

CBG also demonstrates significant antineoplastic activity in basic research models; antibacterial effects, including activity against MRSA; and modest antifungal activity. Both CBG and CBGA have been shown to be dual PPAR-α/γ agonists in vitro, with therapeutic potential in regulating lipid metabolism.[70]

Cannabichromene

FIGURE 13.8

Cannabichromene (CBC) Chemical 2D Structure

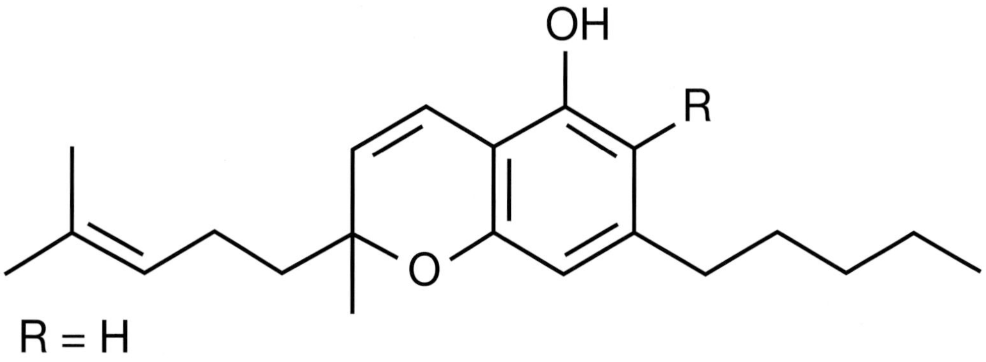

R = H

Cannabichromene (CBC, Figure 13.8) is one of the more abundant cannabinoids after THC and CBD, but it still occurs with relatively low potencies in most chemovars. Some varieties have been selectively bred to contain the recessive genes needed for significant CBC content. While CBC does not have any significant activity at CB1, it has been shown to have its own antinociceptive effects and to potentiate the antinociceptive effects of THC in rodent models. CBC can stimulate and desensitize TRPA1 channels, stimulate TRPV4 and TRPV3 channels, desensitize TRPV2 and TRPV4 channels, and, at a lower potency, stimulate TRPV1 channels. CBC can inhibit both the cellular uptake of anandamide and the metabolism of 2-AG by monoacylglycerol lipase. It has been shown to reduce inflammation in rodent models by inhibiting macrophage and monoacylglycerol lipase activity.

Δ⁹-Tetrahydrocannabivarin

FIGURE 13.9

Δ⁹-Tetrahydrocannabivarin (THCV) Chemical 2D Structure

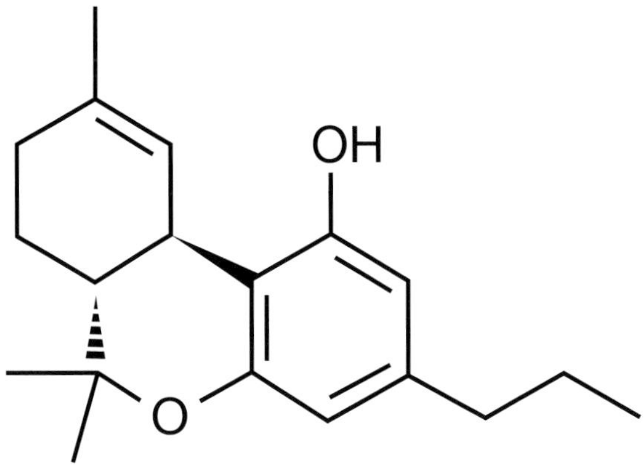

While the aforementioned better-studied cannabinoids contain a five-carbon pentyl group in their tails, the varin cannabinoids have a three-carbon propyl group. Δ⁹-Tetrahydrocannabivarin (THCV, Figure 13.9), quickly gaining interest for its therapeutic potential, is typically found in low concentrations, but selectively bred chemovars have been shown to contain up to 16% THCV by weight.

THCV acts as a CB1 antagonist at lower doses and a CB1 agonist at higher doses. It has been shown to produce weight loss, decreased body fat and serum leptin concentrations, and increased energy expenditure in obese mice. Importantly, the in vivo effects of

THCV are distinct from those of the CB1 antagonist rimonabant, and it is unlikely to cause similar psychiatric and somatic adverse effects. In a randomized, placebo-controlled trial, THCV 5mg administered orally twice daily for 13 weeks decreased fasting glucose by 12.6 mg/dL ($p < 0.05$), increased adiponectin ($p < 0.01$), and improved beta-cell function with only mild to moderate adverse events. Interestingly, the benefits of THCV were lost when it was combined with CBD.[71]

In a placebo-controlled crossover study of 10 male cannabis users, THCV (10 mg) or placebo was administered orally for 5 days, followed by intravenous administration of THC (1 mg) on day 5. The THCV was well tolerated and subjectively indistinguishable from placebo but was mildly anxiogenic. THCV inhibited some of the well-known effects of THC: increased heart rate, intensity of subjective effects, and THC-induced memory impairment.[72]

THCV also binds to CB2 with high affinity and acts as a partial agonist, with the typical mixed agonist–antagonist properties of a partial agonist, inducing signs of agonism when CB2 is highly expressed and antagonism when CB2 is expression is lower. THCV can antagonize CB1 at the same doses that have been shown to activate CB2. THCV has also demonstrated preclinical evidence of anticonvulsant activity.

Cannabidivarin

FIGURE 13.10
Cannabidivarin (CBDV) Chemical 2D Structure

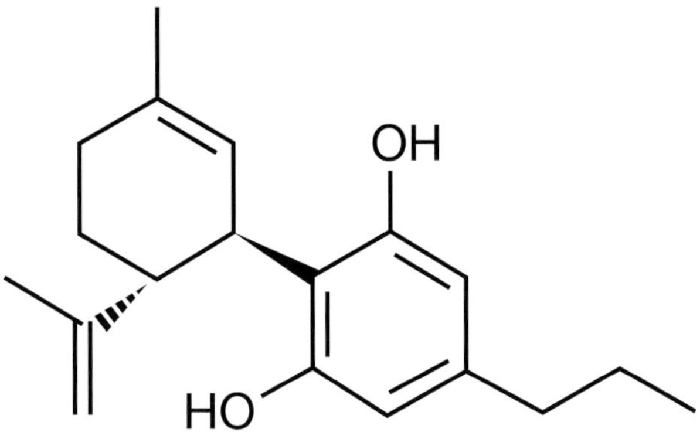

Cannabidivarin (CBDV, Figure 13.10), the propyl variant of CBD, has also been reported to show significant anticonvulsant properties, particularly in partial-onset seizures, as well as antiemetic effects. The pharmacology of CBDV is poorly understood, but it seems to interact with several TRP channels, to inhibit anandamide degradation via diacylglycerol lipase and *N*-acylethanolamine-hydrolyzing acid amidase, and to inhibit the cellular uptake of anandamide.

Phytocannabinoid Pharmacokinetics

Unless otherwise noted, the information in this section is referenced in two excellent reviews: Pertwee (2014)[73] and Lucas et al. (2018).[74] For more on the clinical utility of various routes of administration, see Chapter 16.

The pharmacokinetics of THC have been the best elucidated but likely apply to the other phytocannabinoids. After absorption via the lungs, gastrointestinal tract, or skin, the cannabinoids are concentrated in extracellular fluid, where they can bind to albumin or lipoproteins, be stored in adipose tissue, and concentrate in hair, saliva, and sweat. The cannabinoids are metabolized by hepatic microsomal and nonmicrosomal processes, as well as by nonhepatic processes, and excreted in the bile and urine.

Absorption

When inhaled, cannabinoids are rapidly absorbed and exhibit pharmacokinetics similar to those for intravenous administration, reaching peak plasma concentrations within 3–10 min that are much higher than the maximum concentrations from oral ingestion. The bioavailability after inhalation ranges from 10% to 35%, attributable to variability in inhalational techniques and equipment. When cannabis is smoked, 23%–30% of the THC may be lost to pyrolysis and another 40–50% to noninhaled and exhaled smoke. The pharmacokinetics of cannabinoids via flower vaporization are similar to those for smoking, though my patients often report a slightly slower onset of effects.

Oromucosal preparations may undergo rapid absorption via the oral mucosa, producing plasma drug concentrations higher relative to enterally absorbed cannabinoids but lower relative to inhaled cannabinoids. This route avoids some first-pass metabolism, though typically part of the dose is swallowed and absorbed enterally.

An oral solution of THC (50% ethanol and 5.5% propylene glycol) administered in the fed state was absorbed much faster than a capsule (THC and sesame oil), with mean time to the first measurable concentration 0.15 hr versus 2.02 hr, respectively. The oral solution also had less interindividual variability in plasma levels during early absorption, and taking the oral solution with food increased its bioavailability by 2.1-fold.[75]

Nabiximols, an oromucosal spray containing THC and CBD with ~50% ethanol, may have less oromucosal bioavailability than expected, since one pharmacokinetic study showed no statistically significant difference in first-pass metabolism and total bioavailability at lower doses, and only minor differences at high doses, when compared to oral THC capsules.[76] The formulation of the product and the administration technique (holding in mouth vs. swallowing) may impact the actual amount of oromucosal absorption.

Enteral bioavailability of THC is as low as 6%, with *Tmax* at 2–6 hr after ingestion; many patients complain of erratic onset when taking THC in capsule or edible form. The bioavailability of a 5-mg THC capsule was increased by 2.4-fold when taken with food, but the time to maximum plasma concentration was delayed from 1.7 hr when fasting to 5.6 hr with food.[77] A phase I trial of high oral doses of CBD described *Tmax* at 4–5 hr, with CBD reaching a steady state after approximately 2 days of moderate accumulation (1.8–2.6-fold), with half-life estimates at 10–17 hr, a profile that supports twice-daily oral dosing. The bioavailability of CBD was over 4 times higher when taken with a high-fat meal compared to fasting.[78]

The rectal bioavailability of THC has been studied, as this is a potentially useful delivery route for avoiding first-pass metabolism and the need to swallow (desirable for antiemetic effects). The suppository composition can impact absorption, with THC hemisuccinate demonstrating 2.4 times higher bioavailability than capsules.[79] From the clinical experience of my colleagues and myself, and especially considering numerous reports of little to no psychoactive effects of high doses of THC delivered rectally, I suspect that most patients using cannabis suppositories are failing to absorb the cannabinoids and simply making expensive excrement.

The transdermal route, appealing for similar reasons, likely requires permeation enhancement because the hydrophobic nature of cannabinoids limits diffusion across the aqueous layer of the skin. Several of the terpenes found in cannabis have been shown to act as permeation enhancers.[80] In vitro studies with human skin have determined the permeability of CBD to be 10-fold higher than that of THC, consistent with CBD being relatively less lipophilic.[81] See Chapter 16 for more information on the use of topical cannabis products.

Distribution

Cannabinoids rapidly distribute into well-vascularized organs (such as lung, heart, brain, and liver), and later into less vascularized tissue. With repeated use, cannabinoids can accumulate in adipose tissues, where they can be released later and result in notable pharmacological activity several weeks postadministration. Despite higher oral bioavailability demonstrated in humans, a recent rodent study showed that the acidic cannabinoids have poor blood–brain barrier permeability, both likely related to their increased hydrophilicity due to the carboxyl group.[82]

THC rapidly crosses the placenta, though concentrations found in human umbilical cord blood were 3–6 times lower than in maternal blood. THC also concentrates into breast milk, with exclusively lactating infants exposed to approximately 2.5% of the mother's dose per kilogram of body weight.[83] For more information on cannabinoids in pregnancy and lactation, see Chapter 18.

Metabolism

The metabolism of THC, much better characterized than that of other phytocannabinoids, is predominantly hepatic, via cytochrome P450 isozymes CYP2C9, CYP2C19, and CYP3A4. THC is mainly metabolized to 11-hydroxy-THC (11-OH-THC) and 11-nor-9-carboxy-THC (THC-COOH), which undergoes glucuronidation and is subsequently excreted. Metabolism also occurs in extrahepatic tissues that express cytochrome P450, including the small intestine and brain. Rising plasma THC-COOH concentrations tend to surpass those of THC 30–45 min after smoking and 1 hr after oral ingestion. There is no significant difference in metabolism between men and women. The 11-OH-THC metabolite has similar activity to THC and is psychoactive, while THC-COOH is an inactive metabolite that can persist for days or weeks. Patients typically report differences in subjective effects between various routes of administration of THC, which may be explained by the somewhat differing activity of THC and 11-OH-THC. The plasma concentrations of THC and its metabolites after smoking and oral ingestion are illustrated in Figures 13.11 and 13.12.

CBD is also hepatically metabolized, primarily by cytochrome P450 isozymes CYP2C19 and CYP3A4 (as well as CYP1A1, CYP1A2, CYP2C9, and CYP2D6). Little is known about the primary metabolites, which are 7-COOH-CBD, 7-OH-CBD, and 6-OH-CBD, in order of abundance after oral dosing. 7-OH-CBD, but not 7-COOH-CBD, demonstrated anticonvulsant activity in mice. A molecular modeling study, however, found similarities between 7-COOH-CBD and $\Delta^{2(E)}$-valproic acid, a nonteratogenic bioactive metabolite of the commonly used antiepileptic drug valproic acid.[84]

Elimination

After a single dose of THC, 80%–90% is excreted within 5 days, with more than 65% via the feces and 25% via urine. A significantly longer half-life is seen in regular users, likely due to slow redistribution from deep compartments such as fatty tissues. The average half-life of CBD was found to be 31 hr after inhalation and 2–5 days after oral administration.

FIGURE 13.11

Mean Plasma Concentrations of THC and Its Metabolites After Smoking a Cannabis Cigarette Containing THC (34 mg)

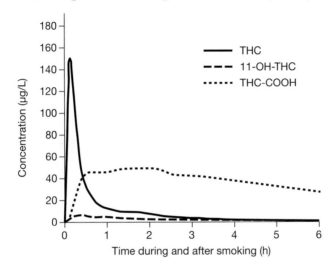

Note. From Dustin Sulak. Data from "Blood cannabinoids. I. Absorption of THC and formation of 11-OH-THC and THC-COOH during and after smoking marijuana." by M. A. Huestis, J. E. Henningfield, and E. J. Cone, 1992, *Journal of Analytical Toxicology, 16*(5), pp. 276–282 (https://doi.org/10.1093/jat/16.5.276). Copyright © 1992 Oxford University Press.

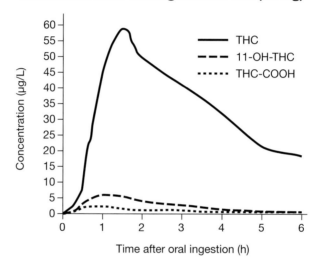

FIGURE 13.12

Mean Plasma Concentrations of THC and Its Metabolites After Oral Ingestion of THC (15 mg)

Note. From Dustin Sulak. Data from "Metabolic studies of delta-9-tetrahydrocannabinol in cancer patients," by S. Frytak, C. G. Moertel, and J. Rubin, 1984, *Cancer Treatment Reports, 68*(12), pp. 1427–1431. Copyright © 1984 by National Institutes of Health.

Chapter 14

Other Phytoconstituents in the Cannabis Entourage

CANNABIS PRODUCES HUNDREDS of non-cannabinoid compounds, many of which have potential therapeutic properties. Among them, the terpenoids, flavonoids, and seed constituents are the best characterized and likely the most clinically relevant.

Terpenes and Terpenoids

Unless otherwise noted, the information in this section references the material reviewed in Russo and Marcu (2017).[1]

Terpenoids are aromatic compounds produced in the flowers, fruit, leaf, and sap of plants for protection from predation, attraction of pollinators, and other ecological roles. Formed of five-carbon isoprene units, terpenes contain only carbon and hydrogen, while terpenoids also contain oxygen. For simplicity, I will henceforth use the term terpene to describe this entire class. Monoterpenes (e.g., limonene and pinene) contain 10 carbons and are the most volatile, sesquiterpenes (e.g., β-caryophyllene) contain 15 carbons, diterpenes (e.g., phytol) contain 20 carbons, and triterpenes (e.g., friedelin, found in cannabis roots) contain 30 carbons.

Terpenes are responsible for the distinct and strong odor of cannabis, with concentrations totaling 4% of weight or higher in certain chemovars. Despite their lower concentration than cannabinoids, they are highly bioavailable via inhalation (especially the monoterpenes) and have proven to be potent: small amounts in ambient air have been shown to increase or decrease activity levels in rodents, even when the observed serum levels are low or negligible. The terpenes discussed in detail here are "generally recognized as safe" by the U.S. Food and Drug Administration (FDA) and/or are approved as food additives by the Flavor and Extract Manufacturers' Association.

Though it is not proven, terpenes are widely considered to modulate the effects of THC and to be a major contributor to the "entourage" and distinct subjective effects of various chemovars. Cannabis users report selecting chemovars on the basis of their aromas, often described as earthy, sweet, piney, citrus, skunky, or spicy, and believe they can predict different therapeutic properties on the basis of these aromas. One study found that untrained panelists are able to consistently discriminate flower aroma from different cannabis chemovars and that odor impacts perception of product quality.[2] The same terpenes found in cannabis are found elsewhere in the plant kingdom, and the essential oils of other plants may begin to inform the therapeutic properties of some cannabis terpenes. For example, lemon essential oil has been shown to produce antidepressant effects and has been used in aromatherapy for this purpose; similarly, cannabis consumers sometimes expect chemovars with strong citrus aromas to be best for improving mood.

Terpenes have been shown to improve THC pharmacokinetics by increasing vasodilatation of alveolar capillaries (which permits more absorption of THC by the lungs) and by increasing blood–brain barrier permeability.[3] Several terpenes found in cannabis (e.g., myrcene, limonene, and linalool) have demonstrated their anticonvulsant activity in rodent models at high doses.[4]

β-Myrcene

β-Myrcene, a monoterpene also found abundantly in hops, is the most prevalent terpene in modern cannabis chemovars and is likely responsible for the sedative effects. Hops, a close relative of cannabis, has long been used by herbalists for treating anxiety and sleep disturbance. β-Myrcene has demonstrated a number of effects in preclinical studies:

- anti-inflammatory activity via prostaglandin E2
- anticarcinogenic activity against aflatoxin in the liver
- long-lasting analgesia involving α2 adrenoceptors and μ-opioid receptors
- muscle relaxation and sedative effect
- prevention of peptic ulcers with increased mucus production, decreased levels of superoxide dismutase, and increased levels of glutathione
- prevention of ischemic or reperfusion oxidative injury

D-Limonene

D-Limonene is a cyclic monoterpene found in citrus rinds with high bioavailability (70% absorption after human pulmonary administration), rapid metabolism, accumulation in adipose tissues and the brain, and low toxicity with an estimated human lethal dose of 0.5–5 g/kg. Preclinical studies have found the following effects:

- strong anxiolysis mediated via 5-HT1A receptors, boosting serotonin levels in pre-frontal cortex and dopamine in hippocampus
- increased mouse motility by 35.25% after inhalation and decreased activity after caffeine by 33.19%
- prominent antibiotic effects versus *S. aureus* and *Pseudomonas aeruginosa*; inhibition of biofilm formation of *Streptococcus pyogenes* SF370 and *Streptococcus mutans*
- induction of apoptosis in breast and colon cancer cells
- agonist activity at A2A adenosine receptors
- reduced hyperalgesia
- increased mitochondrial biogenesis
- induction of adipocyte browning

In human clinical studies, depressed patients exposed to citrus scent experienced normalization of depression scores, allowing discontinuation of antidepressants in 9 of 12 hospitalized patients, and stimulated immune function (CD4/8 ratio normalization).[5]

D-Limonene was utilized in high doses in phase II randomized controlled trials of breast cancer, with good tolerability but unimpressive efficacy. A more recent study in women with preoperative breast cancer found a daily oral intake of 2 g of D-limonene produced a mean concentration of 41.3 µg/g in biopsy breast tissue and reduced cyclin D1 expression, which could lead to cell cycle arrest and decreased cancer proliferation.

α- and β-Pinene

The monoterpene α-pinene, the most widely distributed terpene in nature, has 60% bio-availability via inhalation and rapid metabolism. Preclinical studies (unless otherwise noted) indicate the following pharmacological effects:

- anti-inflammatory activity via prostaglandin E1
- antibiotic activity against MRSA and other resistant bacteria; antibiofilm activity in MRSA, *Cryptococcus neoformans*, and *Candida albicans*; potentiation of

ciprofloxacin, erythromycin, and triclosan against the gastroenteric pathogen *Campylobacter jejuni*.

- acetylcholinesterase inhibition, which could potentially mitigate short-term memory deficits induced by THC (The documented mental health–promoting effects of "shinrin-yoku" or "forest bathing" are often attributed to pinene inhalation.)
- bronchodilation in humans at low exposure levels
- increased mouse motility after inhalation
- in vitro antineoplastic effects against hepatoma and non-small-cell lung carcinoma

β-Pinene is typically found with its structural isomer α-pinene and has demonstrated similar antimicrobial properties. Less is known about its other physiological effects.

Linalool

Linalool is a monoterpenoid present in lavender, coriander, rose, basil, and other botanicals and can be found in high levels in certain cannabis chemovars. Pharmacological properties include the following effects:

- anxiolytic and sedative
- antidepressant
- anticonvulsant and antiglutamatergic, promotion of axonal regeneration
- anti-inflammatory: attenuated production of tumor necrosis factor α and interleukin 6 in vitro and in vivo and attenuated cigarette smoke–induced lung inflammation via decreased production of tumor necrosis factor α, interleukins 6, β, and 8, and monocyte chemoattractant protein 1 in mice, both via inhibitory action in the nuclear factor κB pathway; also inhibits COX-2 and activates the Nrf2/HO-1 signaling pathway[6]
- antineoplastic effects in vitro against numerous cancer cell lines, via cell cycle arrest and proapoptotic activity, as well as activation of T-helper cells[7]
- antihyperlipidemic[8]
- antibacterial and antifungal[9]
- local anesthesia comparable to procaine and menthol

β-Caryophyllene and β-Caryophyllene Oxide

β-Caryophyllene (BCP) is a sesquiterpene commonly found in plants and food products (FDA-approved food additive), including clove and black pepper, and abundantly present in cannabis. It is the major constituent of copaiba oil, an oleoresin extracted from plants of the genus *Copaifera,* which is an important anti-inflammatory herbal medicine of the Brazilian Amazon that is globally commercialized. β-Caryophyllene accounts for approximately 40% of the oil extracted from *Copaifera reticulata,* the most abundant species in the Brazilian Amazon.[10] In addition to the study of BCP as an individual compound, copaiba oil has also accumulated a large body of evidence demonstrating anti-inflammatory, antimicrobial, antineoplastic, and other effects.[11]

BCP is most notably a selective and strong full agonist at the CB2 receptor, as well as an agonist of the PPAR-γ receptor. These targets, and their cross-talk, are likely responsible for the antinociceptive, anti-inflammatory, and other benefits demonstrated in numerous animal models against the following conditions:[12]

- inflammatory arthritis
- nervous system diseases (Parkinson's disease, Alzheimer's disease, multiple sclerosis, amyotrophic lateral sclerosis, stroke)
- atherosclerosis
- cancer (colon, breast, and pancreatic cancers, lymphoma, melanoma, and glioma)
- *Streptococcus* infections
- osteoporosis
- seizures
- depression
- hepatic injury associated with oxidative stress, inflammation, and steatosis[13]
- doxorubicin-induced chronic cardiotoxicity[14]
- reduction of ethanol consumption and preference in rodents[15]

In human patients with *Helicobacter pylori* infection, BCP (126 mg/day) was superior to placebo for reducing nausea and epigastric pain but did not eradicate the infection.[16] The myriad physiological effects and therapeutic potential of BCP should be no surprise, considering the widespread distribution and function of the CB2 receptor. BCP is nontoxic in rodents, with an LD50 greater than 5,000 mg/kg, but it inhibits various cytochrome P450 isoforms, especially CYP3A4.[17]

β-Caryophyllene oxide (BCPO), found in high concentrations in lemon balm and eucalyptus, is an oxidative product of BCP that was traditionally used for cannabis identification by drug-sniffing dogs; it also has antifungal efficacy in a model of clinical onychomycosis and anti–platelet aggregation properties.[18] Though in vitro studies had failed to show CB2 activity of BCPO, a recent experiment demonstrated BCPO to have

10 times the potency of BCP in reducing the ethanol consumption and preference of rodents, reversed by a CB2 antagonist.[19] Thus, BCPO is also likely a strong CB2 agonist, perhaps stronger than BCP.

Humulene

Humulene, a sesquiterpene also known as α-caryophyllene, is found abundantly in the essential oil of hops. While little is known about its pharmacology, a few studies have demonstrated antineoplastic properties in vitro against breast[20] and colon cancer cells[21] and in vitro and in vivo activity against hepatocellular carcinoma.[22]

Terpinolene

Terpinolene is a monoterpene found predominantly in parsnips and many pine species. Its presence in cannabis is said to be characteristic of "sativa" varieties. The following effects have been reported:

- sedative effect in mice, though humans have reported stimulating effects with terpinolene-rich chemovars
- antifungal and larvicidal activity
- antineoplastic activity at high concentrations

β-Ocimene

β-Ocimene is one of the most common monoterpenes found in nature, prominently found in basil. While it has seldomly been investigated in isolation, essential oils with high ocimene content have demonstrated anticonvulsant, antifungal, antiviral,[23] and pest resistance properties.

Nerolidol

Nerolidol, also found in citrus peels, is a sesquiterpene with sedative properties. It has also been shown to reduce colon adenoma formation in vivo, enhance skin penetration of 5-fluorouracil, and inhibit the growth of dermophytes.

Friedelin

Cannabis roots contain no phytocannabinoids or mono- or sesquiterpenes, but they do produce triterpenoids, which as a general class of compounds have displayed a wide spectrum of anti-inflammatory, antipyretic, and anticarcinogenic effects with low toxicity. Friedelin is the most prominent triterpenoid in cannabis roots and has demonstrated the following properties:

- anti-inflammatory effects in carrageenan-induced hind paw edema of adult Wistar albino rats; results of friedelin (40 mg/kg) were comparable to those of indomethacin (10 mg/kg)
- hepatoprotective effects in a carbon tetrachloride model of liver injury in rats; results of friedelin (40 mg/kg) were comparable to those of silymarin extract from *Silybum marianum* (milk thistle; 25 mg/kg) and produced highly significant increases in superoxide dismutase, catalase, and glutathione peroxidase levels
- protection against ethanol-induced gastric ulceration in rats at 35 mg/kg, comparable to the effects of omeprazole
- antipyretic effects comparable to acetaminophen

Flavonoids

Cannabis produces approximately 20 flavonoids (aromatic, polycyclic phenols), including quercetin, apigenin, and cannaflavin A. The leaves contain approximately 1% total flavonoids. Flavonoids may be absorbed via cannabis smoke, but this is unlikely via flower vaporization since they do not vaporize at temperatures below combustion.[24]

Cannflavin A (CFA) is unique to cannabis; in addition to the aerial parts, certain varieties of sprouted hemp seeds can produce it.[25] CFA has been shown to inhibit prostaglandin E2 30 times more powerfully than aspirin and to have anti-inflammatory potency intermediate between that of aspirin and dexamethasone without COX-1 or COX-2 inhibition.[26] Recently, CFA demonstrated hormetic effects on amyloid β–mediated neurotoxicity in vitro, with concentrations of 1–10 μM increasing cell viability by 40% but higher concentrations (>10–100 μM) causing neurotoxicity.[27]

An unnatural isomer of cannflavin B, FBL-03G, was shown to have activity against pancreatic cancer in vitro (increased apoptosis in combination with radiotherapy) and in vivo (delayed metastatic tumor progression and increased survival).[28]

Cannabis Seed Constituents

Cannabis seeds are considered one of the most nutritionally complete foods on earth, containing 25% protein as edestin and albumin, both highly digestible and storable, with all the essential amino acids, including high levels of arginine. The seeds also contain 30% oil, rich in polyunsaturated fatty acids including essential fatty acids in a 2:1-3:1 ω-6:ω-3 ratio, which is often considered ideal for human health, plus γ-linolenic acid.[29]

Chapter 15

Synthetic Cannabinoids and Endocannabinoid System Modulators

NABILONE IS A SYNTHETIC ANALOGUE of Δ^9-tetrahydrocannabinol (THC), with a ketone substituted for a methyl group in the third carbon ring, with similar activity to THC as a partial agonist at CB1 and CB2 receptors. It is approved in the United States and Canada for the treatment of chemotherapy-induced nausea and vomiting, and it is commonly used in Canada off-label for treating pain and posttraumatic stress disorder. Nabilone, available in 1-mg capsules, has higher oral bioavailability and clearer dose linearity than THC.[1]

Hundreds of synthetic cannabinoids have been developed as research tools to explore the endocannabinoid system (ECS). In the early 2000s, clandestine laboratories began producing and spraying synthetic cannabinoids on plant material resembling herbal cannabis, marketed as legal cannabis alternatives with names like "Spice" and "K2" and labeled "not for human consumption." While many of these compounds are now considered schedule 1 drugs by the U.S. Drug Enforcement Administration, structurally diverse cannabimimetic compounds continue to emerge. Their popularity is attributed to intense psychoactive effects, lack of detectability in routine urine drug tests, and availability in head shops and on the internet.[2]

Many of the synthetic cannabinoids have potencies 2–100 times higher than that of THC, producing similar physiological and psychoactive effects but with greater intensity, resulting in medical and psychiatric emergencies. Human adverse effects include nausea and vomiting, shortness of breath or depressed breathing, hypertension, tachycardia, chest pain, muscle twitches, acute renal failure, anxiety, agitation, psychosis, suicidal ideation, and cognitive impairment. [3] Coagulopathy, intracranial hemorrhage, immune thrombocytopenia, ischemic stroke, and seizures have also been reported.[4,5] Cross-sectional studies have shown that synthetic cannabinoid users have lower performance on cognitive tasks and elevated symptomatology (such as paranoia) compared to both natural cannabis users and nonusers.[6]

The damage caused by the illicit use of synthetic cannabinoids highlights the therapeutic importance of partial agonists of the CB1 receptor, the danger of high-potency full agonists, and the risk of toxicity related to non-CB receptor targets of these novel compounds. Sadly, it also demonstrates the futility and public health repercussions of cannabis prohibition.

Rimonabant, a CB1 receptor inverse agonist (functional antagonist), developed in 1994 for preclinical ECS research and originally named SR141716A, suppressed appetite and weight gain in animal models and, in four major clinical trials, was consistently found to produce a placebo-subtracted weight loss of 4–5 kg. Although never approved in the United States due to the awareness of its neuropsychiatric side effects, rimonabant (Acomplia) was licensed in Europe as an anti-obesity agent by the European Medicines Agency in June 2006. By October 2008, increasing reports of serious psychiatric problems (e.g., anxiety, depression, and suicide) led to suspension of marketing authorizations by the European Medicines Agency. This decision in turn rapidly led to the termination of several CB1 receptor antagonist–based anti-obesity drug development programs.[7] The history of rimonabant reminds us of the crucial function of the CB1 receptor in human health and warns against heavy-handed blockade of the ECS.

A number of ECS-modulating drugs are currently being investigated for a wide range of potential indications, including peripherally restricted CB1 agonists and antagonists, selective CB2 agonists, inhibitors of endocannabinoid metabolism/transport, positive allosteric modulators of CB receptors, and more. Thus far, synthetic drugs have failed to modulate the ECS with comparable safety and efficacy to botanical preparations of cannabis. Perhaps, in the future of cannabinoid medicine, the therapeutic value of monomolecular agents will remain limited in comparison to complex botanical preparations, though I suspect that some of the agents currently under investigation, or their analogs, will eventually make their way through clinical trials and drug approval.

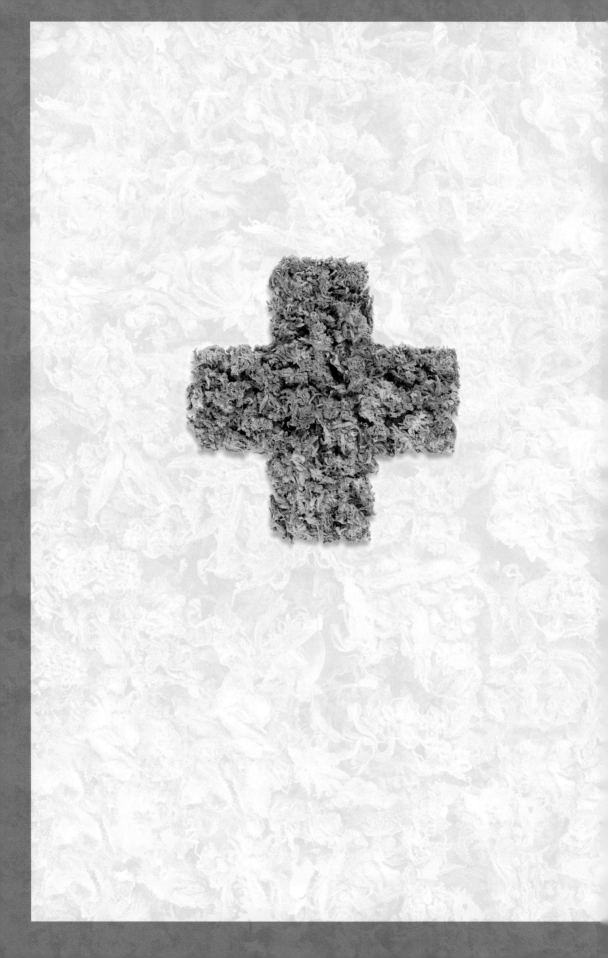

Part 4

Clinical Essentials in Cannabinoid Medicine

Chapter 16

Cannabis Preparations and Delivery Methods

IN ADDITION TO THE COUNTLESS CHEMOVARS and their varied pharmacology, numerous options for preparing and administrating cannabis produce distinct effects. Understanding the properties, strengths and weaknesses of the various preparations and delivery methods allow clinicians and their patients to customize treatment plans and improve outcomes.

Dried Flower

Raw, dried cannabis flower can be used for inhalation, tea, or decoction or can simply be eaten or swallowed like a capsule.

Inhalation

Cannabis flower can be inhaled via pipe, cigarette (i.e., joint), or flower vaporizer. Inhaling cannabis flower can be an effective delivery method for patients who infrequently require a rapid onset of effects to treat episodic conditions or breakthrough symptoms. For example, some patients find that if they inhale cannabis smoke at the earliest sign of a migraine or cyclic vomiting syndrome episode they are able to abort it, but if they wait too long the cannabis is less effective. It is also useful for patients who are unable to tolerate oral administration (i.e. vomiting) or the delay in onset with oral administration (i.e. severe flashbacks in PTSD).

Long-term, heavy cannabis smokers are more likely to develop respiratory symptoms like bronchitis with symptoms of productive cough, but unlike tobacco smokers, they do not develop chronic obstructive pulmonary disease, irreversible airway damage, or recurrent infections.[1] Acutely, inhaled cannabis causes bronchodilation. Infrequent low-dose smoking (*e.g.*, ≤4 grams per week) is unlikely to significantly harm the respiratory tract. If the cannabis is to be smoked, I recommend using a pipe made of glass, ceramic, or stone, to avoid potentially inhaling components of paint, varnish, or metals. A longer pipe will allow the smoke to cool somewhat before reaching the airway, potentially decreasing respiratory irritation.

Some patients prefer the use of a water pipe (i.e., bubbler or bong) in which the cannabis smoke bubbles through water before it is inhaled. This can cool the smoke, making it less irritating and enabling the smoker to consumer larger volumes of smoke in a single inhalation. Many believe that the water also filters harmful compounds and makes the smoke safer. This may not be the case, as some data indicate that the water removes more cannabinoids than tar, resulting in a worse ratio of therapeutic to toxic compounds after the water filtration.[2] I typically recommend against the use of water filtration, though some infrequent users find it is the most effective method for delivering a high-dose, single inhalation without causing them to cough, a side effect that can be hard for those with migraine onset or acute nausea. I also recommend against smoking joints for therapeutic purposes because patients typically take more inhalations than they need when they see the visual prompt of a joint that is still smoldering. I frequently see patients who have developed tolerance to Δ^9-tetrahydrocannabinol (THC) and loss of therapeutic effects due to smoking joints.

A flower vaporizer is a device that heats the cannabis flower to a temperature in the range 175–205°C (350–400°F), causing the resin from the flower to vaporize without combusting the remaining plant material. Though there may be small amounts of combustion products in the inhaled material, it is significantly less than cannabis smoke. Thus, the flower vaporizer is the safest method of inhaling cannabis and can be more cost-effective than smoking, which can pyrolyze ~30% of the cannabinoids prior to inhalation. Likely due to the lower temperature and reduced respiratory irritation, patients often report a somewhat slower onset when vaporizing versus smoking, and most vaporizers take 1–2 min to reach the desired temperature, so vaporizing may not be as effective for patients who require very rapid action.

Flower vaporization has been used and studied for over 20 years, with early studies demonstrating comparable pulmonal uptake of THC[3] with drastic reductions in products of combustion.[4] Survey data show that cannabis users who vaporize report fewer respiratory symptoms than those who smoke, especially those who use larger amounts.[5] Though they are similar, I believe the pharmacodynamic effects of smoking and vaporizing are slightly different, as numerous patients have described distinctions in the therapeutic effects from the same dose of the same chemovar via the two inhalation methods.

One potential explanation is the likelihood that vaporized cannabis does not deliver flavonoids, which do not vaporize at temperatures below combustion.[6]

It can be difficult to precisely discuss the dosage of inhaled cannabis, especially because the inhalation technique can drastically impact the delivered dose. I typically recommend my patients take 1–2 inhalations, wait 10 min, and repeat if needed. I document the inhalation device used, how many inhalations they take per session, the frequency of sessions per day or week, and the weekly amount of cannabis flower they smoke. I consider less than 3.5 g (⅛ oz) per week a low dose, up to 14 g (½ oz) per week a moderate dose, and greater than 14 g per week a high dose of inhaled cannabis flower. Suggestions for converting inhaled doses of cannabis to equivalent oral doses are described in Chapter 19, Off-Label Use of Prescription Cannabinoids.

Cannabis Tea, Decoction, and Raw Consumption

Traditional use of cannabis tea has been documented in Jamaica for treating marasmus, infantile diarrhea, teething, and as an all-purpose remedy,[7] and in Morocco cannabis tea combined with mint tea has been used for intestinal worms.[8]

Most dried cannabis flower contains >90% cannabinoid acids and <10% neutral cannabinoids. For patients who benefit from consuming the acidic cannabinoids, which are more hydrophilic, tea (steeping in hot water) or decoction (simmering while covered) can be an ideal delivery method. Because the acidic cannabinoids are well-tolerated and rarely cause adverse effects, the dosing often does not need to be precise. In one study, adding 1 g of cannabis flower to 1 L of boiling water and simmering for 15 min resulted in a solution containing 43 mg of Δ^9-tetrahydrocannabinolic acid (THCA) and 10 mg of THC per liter. The THC reaches saturation around 0.01 mg/ml and then precipitates out, typically adhering to the container; thus, the THC potency of the final solution is limited. Very little decarboxylation of THCA into THC occurs in boiling water for 15 min. Refrigeration or storage of cannabis tea results in loss of potency via precipitation, but the addition of coffee creamer or cyclodextrin was shown to prevent this loss.[9]

A more recent study prepared a decoction by boiling 500 mg of flower in 500 ml of water for 15 min. The flower contained 5–8% THC (including THCA) and 7–12% cannabidiol (CBD) (including cannabidiolic acid [CBDA]), and a 200-ml portion of the final decoction contained 2.22 ± 0.66 mg of THCA, 1.85 ± 1.6 mg of THC, 8.82 ± 2.02 mg of CBDA, and 1.93 ± 1.17 mg of CBD. Pharmacokinetic data from human consumption of the decoction found that CBDA was absorbed ~5 times more than CBD, and THCA was absorbed ~50 times more than THC.[10]

A single-arm clinical trial assessed the effects of long-term use of a cannabis decoction in 338 patients with chronic pain. The recipe involved boiling 200 ml of water, adding 30 ml of milk and a tea bag containing 28 mg of cannabis flower (19% THC/THCA by weight), and simmering for 20 min. Unfortunately, the cannabinoid content of the final preparation was not analyzed. Patients took a range of 1–8 servings per day after titration and were followed for 12 months. Pain, disability, anxiety, and depression scores all improved, most notably from the baseline measurement to the 3-month follow-up, with modest improvements thereafter. Somnolence and confusion were the most common adverse effects that led to stopping the treatment, likely related to THC and not THCA.[11] I suspect the fat content of the milk increased the THC content of the final product.

For patients that might do well with lower but less precise doses of neutral cannabinoids in combination with acidic cannabinoids, I frequently recommend cannabis tea or simply adding a pea-sized portion of cannabis flower to whatever hot beverage they typically consume. For those who are sensitive to the adverse effects of THC, this can be an effective strategy since patients rarely complain of psychoactive side effects from cannabis tea. The most common positive responses observed in my practice are in patients with arthritis, with benefits typically appearing 2 weeks after starting consistent use twice daily.

As an alternative to taking the time to prepare cannabis tea, some patients who wish to try daily dosing with acidic cannabinoids do well with simply eating a pea-sized raw cannabis flower or taking it like a pill twice daily. If the flower has not been exposed to high temperatures, the THC content of a small piece of cannabis flower will be low and unlikely to cause adverse effects.

Indica or Sativa?

The terms indica and sativa are frequently inaccurate and inadequate for describing qualities relevant to medical use (see Chapter 12 for more details). Common chemovar or "strain" names are also often unreliable, with significant variability in chemical profile and genetics among various growers and distributers. The best way to identify potentially effective flower chemovars for a patient's specific symptom is for the patient to consult a knowledgeable customer service agent who can identify the best-selling products for patients with various complaints. Patients can purchase small quantities of a few potential chemovars and test them to find the best options. Periodically rotating chemovars can be helpful.

Oils and Tinctures

I have found liquid preparations of cannabis to be the most useful and versatile delivery method. The liquids can be held in the mouth for several minutes to promote oromucosal absorption, with the remaining medicine swallowed and delivered enterally. Many patients report onset within 10 min and duration of 4–8 hr; most do well with dosing three times a day. The liquid preparations are also easy to titrate and therefore especially useful for those new to cannabis. Drops of cannabis tincture or oil can be applied directly under the tongue or first placed into a spoon. An oral syringe also works well for precision dosing and for those with fine motor challenges using a dropper.

A tincture is technically an ethanolic extract of an herbal medicine, though many in the medical cannabis field (erroneously) refer to any liquid preparation as a "tincture." Ethanol is an excellent solvent for extracting the phytoconstituents of cannabis and typically produces a high-quality medicine, plus it is a simple process amenable to home and artisanal production. Unfortunately, the ethanol can irritate the oral mucosa, depending on its concentration, and many patients do not tolerate the experience. Those who do often report faster onset with tinctures compared to oil-based liquids. The tolerability can be improved by first adding the tincture to a small amount of water before consumption.

Most liquid preparations of cannabis available commercially are oil-based and sold in a dropper or spray bottle. A carrier oil, such as olive oil or medium-chain triglyceride coconut oil, is typically infused with a cannabis concentrate and diluted to a desirable potency. Cannabis flowers can be directly infused into oil via gentle heating and stirring for several hours, but the direct infusions are usually weaker—they typically do not reach potencies above 10 mg of cannabinoids/ml of oil.

The oromucosal bioavailability of infused cannabis oils may be dependent on the terpene content, as several terpenes are known permeation enhancers. Some patients report rapid onset of infused oils in 10 min or less, while others describe onset after 1 hr or more, consistent with enteral absorption. Several patients have reported that mechanical agitation from brushing one's teeth prior to holding a liquid cannabis preparation in the mouth speeds onset. A pharmacokinetic study of dronabinol oral solution (5 mg/ml THC with 50% ethanol and 5.5% propylene glycol) demonstrated the presence of THC in the blood on average ~10 min after administration. All of the subjects receiving the oral solution, but only 16.8% of those receiving dronabinol capsules, had THC in the blood at 15 min. THC oral solution and THC capsules had roughly equal bioavailability, but the oral solution had significantly less interindividual variability.[12]

Troches, dissolvable tablets, dissolving films, and other innovative delivery methods are emerging to take advantage of oromucosal absorption and improve upon the convenience and palatability of tinctures and infused oils, but the liquid preparations are likely the best for incremental titration, often essential for patients new to cannabis.

Capsules and Edibles

Cannabis capsules are a convenient delivery method for patients with chronic conditions who require long-duration baseline treatment and do not require rapid onset. Capsules may contain cannabis concentrates or simply ground flower that has been decarboxylated (if desired). The enterally absorbed cannabinoids will undergo significant first-pass metabolism, which many patients report changes the subjective effects with significant interindividual variability. Some find oral delivery of THC, when compared with inhalation, more or less psychoactive, more or less analgesic, more or less of a muscle relaxant, and sedating versus stimulating. These differences may be related to increased blood levels of the active metabolite 11-OH-THC, or they may be related to other pharmacokinetic differences.

Enteral absorption of cannabis often produces erratic onset and bioavailability, even in the same individual at the same dose. Patients report more rapid onset (in as little as 30 min) with stronger psychoactive effects on some days and delayed onset (up to 3 hr) with more mild effects on other days. These differences may be influenced by the numerous factors affecting gastrointestinal (GI) motility and secretion, including meal timing, food choices and fat content, anxiety, stress, pain, sleep, and overall autonomic function. Taking a 5-mg THC capsule with food increased the bioavailability by 2.4-fold but delayed the Tmax from 1.7 hr (fasting) to 5.6 hr.[13] The oral bioavailability of CBD was over 4 times higher when taken with a high-fat meal compared to fasting.[14]

I have also infrequently encountered patients who experience little to no effect from even hundreds of milligrams of orally delivered THC, though they are able to benefit from low to moderate doses of inhaled THC; for some, oral bioavailability seems extremely low.

I most frequently use cannabis capsules to improve sleep maintenance, and I titrate the dose to promote restorative sleep without causing morning grogginess. Patients must be cautioned to mitigate fall risks and prepare for potential psychomotor effects in the middle of the night. For more information on using cannabis for sleep, see Chapter 22.

Cannabis can also be added to food products, commonly called "edibles," and more often used for nontherapeutic purposes. Cannabis edibles are the single most common cause of THC overdose for several reasons:

- repeat dosing prior to delayed onset, based on an assumption of low potency and absence of effects

- heterogenous distribution of cannabinoids in the recipe, rendering some servings stronger than others
- psychoactivity and appetite stimulation from the initial dose leading to excessive consumption thereafter
- accidental ingestion by those who are unaware of the cannabis content

In general, I dissuade my patients from preparing or using cannabis edibles to prevent these mistakes, though there are certain clinical scenarios in which edibles are preferred, such as overcoming issues with palatability, especially in pediatrics, autism, and dementia cases. For patients with GI conditions, recipes high in soluble fiber may provide extended release effects and/or deliver the cannabinoids more directly to the intestine.

Cannabis Concentrates

The trichomes and/or resin of cannabis can be concentrated by a variety of methods. Solventless, mechanical methods such as sifting on a fine screen to make *kief* (collected trichomes) or *hash* (collected resin of various purities) can achieve a cannabinoid potency up to 50% by weight and typically include a broad spectrum of phytoconstituents. Hash and kief are typically smoked or vaporized directly or first mixed with cannabis flower, and they can also be used in oil infusions and other recipes. Another solventless technique using pressure and heat produces *rosin*; it may provide a phytoconstituent profile similar to hash or kief, and closely resembling that of the original flower, but at a higher potency.

While ethanol is an excellent extraction solvent for cannabis, the use of rotary evaporation or slow cookers to evaporate the ethanol and concentrate the cannabinoids typically results in loss of volatile terpenes. These tarlike oleoresins go by many names, including *hash oil*, *full extract cannabis oil* (FECO), *Rick Simpson oil** (RSO), and even the extraordinarily misleading *hemp oil*; they are viscous, sticky, and difficult to work with and are typically stored in a syringe. The usual route of administration is to place a rice-grain-sized amount in contact with the buccal mucosa, via capsules, or added to recipes. The concentrates are typically 50–80% decarboxylated cannabinoids by weight, and even a tiny portion can result in overdose. Due to the inaccuracy inherent in measuring these substances, I typically recommend dilution into a carrier oil, using a warm magnetic stir plate for even mixing, prior to consumption.

---

* Rick Simpson is a celebrated Canadian cannabis activist who popularized the use of cannabis concentrate to treat cancer and other chronic conditions; he recommended using naphtha or isopropyl alcohol, solvents with potential toxicity.

Other hydrocarbons are frequently used to concentrate cannabis, including butane and propane, producing oleoresins with a more honeylike or waxlike consistency. Frequently called *butane honey oil* (BHO), these concentrates are typically used for inhalation. Supercritical and subcritical CO_2 methods are commonly used to extract cannabis commercially; these methods are appealing for their lack of toxic solvents but have also been shown to alter the terpene composition.[15] Some extractors strive to capture the volatile terpenes as they escape, with condensation techniques, and later reintroduce them to the concentrate. CO_2 concentrates can be used for inhalation, infused into oils, and added to other products. A variety of postprocessing techniques, including distillation, can increase the potency, reduce the terpene content, and alter the physical properties of hydrocarbon and CO_2 extracts, with the resulting compounds often named after their appearance (such as shatter, wax, or diamonds). Such concentrates may have >90% THC content by weight.

The inhalation of various concentrates has become known as *dabbing*, a process in which a small portion of the concentrate (dab) is applied to a glass or metal "nail" that has been heated with a butane torch, often to 600 °C (1100 °F) or higher, and subsequently inhaled by use of a variety of devices that often include water filtration. Electric devices are also used for dabbing. This delivery method provides a rapid onset of a very high dose of THC that seldom has therapeutic value. Though I have seen dabbing, in certain patients, provide rapid analgesia superior to any other delivery method, users typically experience strong psychoactive and cardiovascular effects (including orthostasis, resulting in falls and injury), rapidly build tolerance (so that the THC loses efficacy), and require stronger, more frequent doses. Furthermore, dabbing presents additional risks: analysis of extracts used for dabbing has revealed the presence of significant levels of pesticides and residual solvents[16]; the high temperatures can cause terpenes to degrade into methacrolein, benzene, and other toxins[17]; and cases of acute hypersensitivity pneumonitis[18] and acute respiratory distress syndrome[19] have been reported.

Parallel with the increase in dabbing, electronic cigarettes (i.e., vape pens) have become increasingly adopted by users of both therapeutic and nontherapeutic cannabis. These devices, typically containing a diluted cannabis concentrate, pose a number of health concerns. First, the diluent may be propylene glycol, poly(ethylene glycol), glycerol (aka vegetable glycerin), medium-chain triglyceride oil, or plant-derived terpenes. Though safe for oral consumption, these compounds have not been proven safe for inhalation, and they have been shown to produce acetaldehyde, acrolein, and formaldehyde when exposed to high temperatures.[20] The term "vape" is a misnomer because, unlike flower vaporization, these devices typically reach combustion temperatures. Second, the starting material typically used to produce the contents of vape pen cartridges is typically low-quality trim at best and may be contaminated with pesticides, mold, and mycotoxins at worst. Finally, the hardware in the vape pens often contains heavy metals that leach into the solution and are present in the inhaled material, though often at low levels that may not necessarily be harmful.[21] There has been one report of pneumonia secondary to cobalt poisoning from a cannabis vape pen.[22]

At the time of writing (February 2020), 2,807 cases of e-cigarette or vaping product use–associated lung injury (EVALI) hospitalizations have been reported to the U.S. Centers for Disease Control, including 68 deaths. Around 82% of the cases involved THC-containing products, though some cases have been associated with only nicotine e-cigarette use.[23] No single compound or ingredient has been implicated, and the etiology may be multifactorial, though the use of vitamin E acetate as a diluent is likely involved.

It may be possible to vaporize cannabis extracts without harm. Some products use pure cannabis extract with no diluents, probably the safest form. Temperature-controlled vape devices, free from heavy metals and other contaminants, are emerging for medical use due to popular demand. Vaporized extracts are more convenient and discreet than flower vaporizers and could potentially deliver a standardized dose. I look forward to innovation in products and extraction methods and to the scientific investigation that is needed before these products are considered safe for patient use.

Topical and Transdermal Preparations

Cannabis salves, balms, lotions, and creams are very popular with my patients, who commonly report relief from neuropathy, arthritis, muscle spasms, tender points, pruritis, and inflammatory dermatological conditions. Topical delivery is generally well-tolerated and rarely produces adverse effects; in patients with localized pain (e.g., monoarthropathy) and few comorbid symptoms, I often start with a trial of topical cannabis. Interestingly, patients sometimes prefer preparations of THC, CBD, or mixed THC/CBD for treating pain, and I have yet to identify characteristics that may predict a beneficial response to a particular formulation, except that THC-dominant preparations seem to work best for pruritis.

Little preclinical and very little human clinical research has examined the use of topical cannabinoids for pain or skin conditions. Topical WIN 55,212-2, a synthetic CB1/CB2 agonist, in a solution of dimethyl sulfoxide was shown to decrease nociception[24] and to enhance the antinociceptive effects of topical morphine in mice.[25] Topical THC (1.5 mg/ml), applied 30 min before and 24 and 48 hr after a contact allergic challenge, was shown to attenuate inflammation in mice by decreasing keratinocyte-derived pro-inflammatory mediators via a CB1/CB2-independent mechanism.[26] Another study found that rat skin had 13-fold more permeability to Δ^8-THC than human skin,[27] suggesting that preclinical data may not translate well.

In human studies, three cases of epidermolysis bullosa responding to topical CBD oil with faster wound healing, less blistering, and amelioration of pain have been reported.[28] A retrospective study of 20 patients with psoriasis, atopic dermatitis, and/or resulting scars who applied topical CBD ointment (also containing other herbs) twice daily for 3 months demonstrated improvement in skin parameters (hydration, transepidermal water loss, elasticity, and photographic assessment) and in patient-reported symptom severity and quality of life.[29] Three cases of pyoderma gangrenosum experienced clinically significant analgesia and reduced opioid use with topical cannabis oil containing 5–7 mg/ml THC + 6–9 mg/ml CBD.[30] A double-blind trial in patients with temporomandibular disorders found significant improvements in pain and masseter activity after application of 1.46% CBD oil over the masseters twice a day for 14 days.[31] And in one small open-label study, topical N-palmitoylethanolamine significantly reduced pain and pruritis in patients with acute, but not chronic, postherpetic neuralgia.[32]

Several cannabis-containing patches and other products intended for transdermal systemic absorption have been marketed, though I have been unable to find any published preclinical or clinical pharmacokinetic studies validating the claims related to specific products. One rat study using a monoarthritic knee joint model showed that a 1% CBD gel applied to the shaved back of the animal resulted in systemic absorption and significantly reduced joint swelling and pain-related behavior.[33] In an open-label safety trial, a CBD gel was also shown to be well tolerated and produced clinically meaningful reductions in anxiety and behavioral symptoms in children and adolescents with fragile X syndrome.[34] This suggests transdermal systemic delivery may be feasible, but more data are needed to confirm this.

Anecdotes of patients using cannabis for precancerous and cancerous skin lesions, typically with direct application of undiluted concentrates, are common both in my practice and on the internet, though I have only directly observed before-and-after responses in a few patients. Historical medical texts also report efficacy in skin tumors.[35] Preclinically, topical synthetic cannabinoids were able to inhibit tumor growth in the two-stage mouse skin carcinogenesis model.[36] Several case reports of skin cancers responding to topical cannabis treatment, with photographic evidence, were reported in a non-peer-reviewed compendium of cases.[37] For some patients, topical cannabis concentrates may be a safe and cost-effective solution for precancerous and cancerous skin lesions, and a short trial may be practical prior to more aggressive treatment. When doing so, I recommend against continuing use unless there is a clear initial response, because at such a high potency the cannabis concentrate could potentially impair local antitumor immune function. If there is a clear response, patients often describe a cyclical process of healing and sloughing.

Patients who use topical THC often ask if it is possible for them to experience psychoactive effects or fail drug tests; little scientific evidence can help answer this question. I rarely hear reports of psychoactive side effects associated with topical cannabis use, though at least two patients have reported psychoactive effects after applying an ethanolic cannabis concentrate topically. One study failed to find THC in the blood and urine of three volunteers after they applied cannabis salves every 2–4 hr for 3 days,[38] but the salves were extraordinarily low potency (0.01% THC by weight) and not representative of those commonly used by my patients.

I suspect the formulation of topical cannabis products strongly impacts their efficacy. Many of the products my patients find most effective have cannabinoid potencies in the 1–2% range and contain other herbs and essential oils such as arnica, lavender, and menthol. Topical cannabis has a lot to offer patients, and more research is clearly needed to identify optimal formulations and appropriate indications.

Summary of Delivery Methods

The majority of medical cannabis patients use more than one delivery method. In a survey study of 1,321 cannabis-using patients with chronic pain, 93.4% used two or more administration routes and 72.5% used three or more.[39] Why? By *dose layering* (utilizing multiple products and delivery methods), clinicians can custom-tailor patients' treatment regimens for best results.

The rationale is analogous to the common practice of using multiple medications to address different symptoms, except in this case one herb is used in a variety of formats. For example, a patient with chronic pain, periodic daily exacerbations, and comorbid anxiety and sleep disturbance might be prescribed a daily extended-release opioid analgesic, an instant-release opioid for breakthrough pain, a sleep aid, and an anxiolytic. A similar patient could be treated with longer-acting oromucosal or enteral cannabis products, with higher levels of CBD during the day and higher levels of THC before bed, plus inhaled cannabis for breakthrough symptoms, with certain chemovars selected for breakthrough pain and other chemovars for breakthrough anxiety. I encourage you to familiarize yourself with the strengths and weaknesses of the various cannabis delivery methods (summarized in Table 16.1) and remember that cannabis dose layering is the norm rather than the exception.

TABLE 16.1

Comparison of Routes of Administration

Delivery route	Strength	Weakness	Clinical utility
Inhaled	• Rapid onset • Easy dose titration • Non-invasive parenteral, ideal for anti-emesis • Long safety record for vaporized flower	• Shorter duration of action • Narrow therapeutic window • Respiratory irritation • More cardiovascular side effects • Higher abuse potential • Risk of pulmonary adverse effects from inhaled concentrates, vape pens, and heavy smoking	• Abrupt onset and episodic conditions (e.g., migraine, panic attack, flashbacks, cyclic vomiting episode) • Breakthrough symptoms • Sleep onset
Oromucosal	• Intermediate onset • Easy dose titration using dropper, oral syringe, or spray	• Palatability • May have variable onset and effect if swallowed vs held in mouth	• Broadly applicable • Good for cannabis-naïve patients • Baseline treatment
Enteral	• Convenient (capsules) • Longer duration of action • Edibles can improve palatability over liquid preparations for sensitive patients.	• Slow onset • Erratic onset and bioavailability • First-pass metabolism may result in higher psychoactivity • Edibles most common to be used inappropriately and to cause adverse effects	• Baseline treatment • Sleep maintenance • Direct treatment of GI pathology
Topical	• Non-psychoactive at typical doses • Anti-pruritic • Analgesic • Anti-inflammatory • Muscle-relaxant	• Sparse research to guide formulation of constituents and potency	• Localized pain (arthritis, neuropathy) • Skin conditions • Trigger points
Suppository	• Rectal: potentially (though not likely) higher bioavailability and faster onset than oral with less psychoactive effects (avoids first-pass metabolism) • Vaginal: may be helpful in treating vulvodynia, dyspareunia	• Inconvenient for most patients • Formulation determines bioavailability • Most suppository use results in little to no absorption and a waste of medicine • THC may worsen vulvovaginal candidiasis[40]	• Rectal and vaginal pruritis, pain • Inability to tolerate other routes of delivery • End of life care

Chapter 17

Cannabis Dosing

CANNABIS IS UNLIKE any other medicine I've encountered due to its wide range of effective dosages, impressive safety profile, broad physiological mechanisms of action, and versatility in treating a wide range of symptoms and diseases. I've found that using the correct dose of cannabis is the single most important factor in minimizing potential harms and maximizing potential benefits.

Unlike most medications, cannabis cannot be prescribed at a certain quantity and frequency based on body weight, age, and medical condition. Due to the complexity of the endocannabinoid system and interindividual variability, as well as the wide range of cannabis chemovars and formulations, patients typically require an individualized dosing plan that includes titration and self-awareness. With an understanding of the dosing range of cannabis, dose–response effects, therapeutic window, and phytoconstituent synergy, you can provide your patients with an individualized plan to achieve maximal benefit and minimal harm.

Broad Safe and Effective Dosing Range

When I started seeing medical cannabis users in my practice, I was surprised to find that some patients were using a very low dose (e.g., one inhalation), while other patients required much higher doses (e.g., an entire large joint or a potent edible) to achieve therapeutic benefits. Over the years, I have seen this range grow even wider, with some patients safely and effectively using ultrahigh doses and others using ultralow doses.

While I typically calculate dosing per body weight for pediatric patients only, the oral dosing range I have observed in my practice, including patients of all ages, extends from 0.01 to 50 mg·kg^{-1}·day^{-1} total cannabinoids. Interestingly, human use in this range is reported in the peer-reviewed literature, with Δ^9-tetrahydrocannabinol (THC) reported to be effective for pediatric spasticity at doses as low as 0.08 mg·kg^{-1}·day^{-1},[1] and safety trials conducted on cannabidiol (CBD) for seizures at doses up to 50 mg·kg^{-1}·day^{-1}.[2]

Despite this 5,000-fold dosing range, even the highest clinically observed doses are well below the acute toxic dose found in primates, with single doses of THC up to 9,000 mg/kg in rhesus monkeys proving nonlethal and producing no histopathological changes;[3] daily doses up to 250 mg/kg were nonlethal over 28 days.[4]

The 0.01 and 50 mg·kg^{-1}·day^{-1} responders are clearly outliers in my practice, with most patients experiencing efficacy and tolerability in the 0.1–2 mg·kg^{-1}·day^{-1} range of total cannabinoids. A general rule for cannabis dosing and titration is to start low, go slow, and do not be afraid to go all the way. Some patients do very well with high doses.

Multiphasic and Bidirectional Dose–Response Effects

Within the broad safe dosing range, cannabinoids are notorious for producing multiphasic and bidirectional dose–response effects.* If a certain dose of a cannabinoid causes a particular effect, one cannot assume that a higher dose will produce a stronger effect or that a lower dose will cause a weaker effect. Patients and clinicians are often surprised to find that reducing the dose of cannabis can increase therapeutic effects, and that different doses of cannabis could produce opposite effects in the same individual.

A straightforward example of multiphasic and bidirectional dose–response effects can be seen in the activity of rats exposed to various doses of THC (Figure 17.1). A triphasic effect was demonstrated: low doses of THC (0.2 mg/kg) suppressed locomotor activity, higher doses (1–2 mg/kg) dose-dependently stimulated movement greater than baseline, until catalepsy emerged at even higher doses (>2.5 mg/kg), accompanied by decreases in activity. Interestingly, the suppression of activity at 0.2 mg/kg was more profound than at 5 mg/kg.[5]

---

* A multiphasic dose–response effect indicates that the magnitude of effect undergoes different phases of direct and indirect relationship with increasing dose. Bidirectional dose–response effects are opposite effects from different doses of the same agent.

FIGURE 17.1

Dose–Response Curve Showing Effects of Systemic Administration of THC on Horizontal Activity in Rats

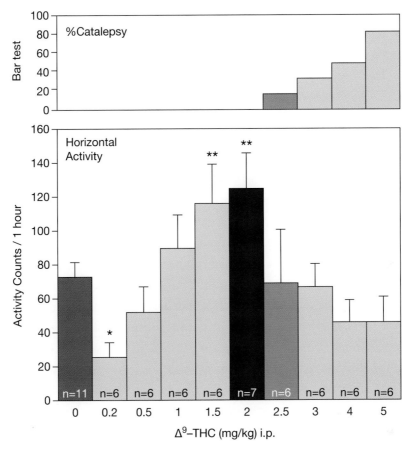

Note. *significantly different from the rest of the groups except those receiving 4 or 5 mg/kg, p<0.05; **significantly different from the rest of the groups except the one receiving 1mg/kg, p<0.05

Adapted from "Activational role of cannabinoids on movement," by M. C. Sañudo-Peña, J. Romero, G. E. Seale, J. J. Fernandez-Ruiz, and J. M. Walker, 2000, *European Journal of Pharmacology*, *391*(3), pp. 269–274 (https://doi.org/10.1016/S0014-2999(00)00044-3). Copyright © 2000 by Elsevier. Reprinted with permission.

Cerebral metabolism in rodents has also been shown to exhibit a biphasic dose–response relationship to THC: very low doses increased cerebral metabolism, measured by 2-deoxyglucose uptake, while higher doses of THC decreased cerebral metabolism. Limbic regions, particularly the hippocampus, were more sensitive to THC, suggesting a selective regional action of THC at lower doses.[6] This highlights the complexity of cannabinoid-related biphasic dose–response patterns, with varying responses in one organ or responses in different tissues potentially shifting phase at different doses.

THC is well-known for its biphasic and bidirectional effects on anxiety in animals and humans. Several studies have shown that acute administration of low doses of THC and CB1 agonists can reduce anxiety behaviors in a variety of animal models, while higher doses or administration under stressful environmental conditions can increase anxiety behaviors and neuroendocrine responses to acute stress. Promoting relaxation and reducing tension are some of the most commonly reported benefits in cannabis users; paradoxically, the most consistently documented adverse effects of cannabis intoxication are anxiety and panic-like reactions. The complex biphasic dose–response curve of cannabinoids on anxiety appears to undergo a leftward shift under stressful environmental conditions, may undergo a rightward shift under socially permissive situations, and could also be shifted by personality factors or comorbid anxiety disorders.[7]

Biphasic psychological effects are common in domains other than anxiety. For example, in human subjects with some history of cannabis use, oral THC was shown to dampen negative emotional responses without impairing performance at 7.5 mg but increased negative affect and impaired performance at 12.5 mg.[8] This suggests that mood benefits of THC can be achieved with doses lower than those causing impairment.

CBD has also been shown to exhibit biphasic effects on anxiety in several animal models and two human clinical experiments. In one study, using a simulated public speaking test model of anxiety in 57 healthy male volunteers, pretreatment with 300 mg of CBD resulted in significant reductions in anxiety compared to placebo, while doses of 150 and 600 mg were not effective.[9] Another study evaluated 60 healthy subjects of both sexes in a real-life public speaking test; 300 mg of CBD, but neither 100 nor 900 mg, reduced anxiety in the postspeech phase.[10]

Similar to its effects in models of anxiety, CBD has also demonstrated biphasic dose–response relationships in animal models of depression,[11,12] compulsive behavior,[13] and pain.[14] This reminds us that the optimal dose of CBD likely depends on the condition and the individual, and it highlights the importance of testing different doses in experimental studies as well as in the clinic.

THC and CBD can have biphasic effects on pain, demonstrated in a placebo-controlled study of opioid-treated cancer patients with poorly controlled chronic pain treated with nabiximols (THC/CBD oromucosal spray) at three doses or placebo (Figure 17.2). The low-dose group, receiving 4 sprays/day (20.8 mg of THC + CBD), had an overall 26% reduction in pain, while the medium-dose group (10 sprays/day) had 19% reduction and the high-dose group (16 sprays/day) was no different than placebo, ~14% reduction.[15]

FIGURE 17.2

Analysis of Change from Baseline
in Average Pain Score

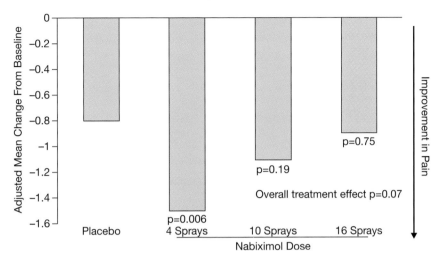

Note. From "Nabiximols for opioid-treated cancer patients with poorly-controlled chronic pain: A randomized, placebo-controlled, graded-dose trial," by R. K. Portenoy, E. D. Ganae-Motan, S. Allende, R. Yanagihara, L. Shaiova, S. Weinstein, R. McQuade, S. Wright, and M. T. Fallon, 2012, *The Journal of Pain, 13*(5), pp. 438–449 (https://doi.org/10.1016/j.jpain.2012.01.003). Copyright 2012 by American Pain Society. Reprinted with permission.

THC can have bidirectional effects on pain depending on dose, experience with cannabis, and the nature of the pain. For example, THC has been known to increase the intensity of acute pain, especially at higher doses and in the cannabis-naïve,[16,17] though THC is well-known to ameliorate chronic pain.

As mentioned above, bidirectional effects are not always dose-dependent but are related to factors inherent in set (external environmental conditions) and setting (internal mindset and expectations of the participant): the same dose of THC in the same individual may cause anxiolytic effects in a serene environment or anxiogenic effects in a stressful environment; anxious individuals may be more likely to experience anxiolytic effects, while nonanxious individuals may be more likely to experience anxiogenic effects.[18] Different chemovars at the same dose have also been reported to produce bidirectional effects; patients often prefer certain chemovars for daytime use, due to awakening effects, and others for evening use, due to sedating effects.

Perhaps the clearest example of bidirectional effects of cannabinoids is the acute effects of a THC overdose, which produces a symptom constellation characterized by many of the same symptoms often ameliorated by appropriately dosed THC: anorexia, nausea, vomiting, diarrhea, anxiety or panic, dyskinesia, spasticity, and pain.

Why do we see so many multiphasic and bidirectional dose–response effects in cannabinoid medicine? There are likely several reasons, including tolerance building via receptor downregulation, complex heterogenous effects on the endocannabinoid system and the other physiological systems it modulates, and interindividual variability, including the influence of set and setting.

Ultralow Doses

On the basis of surprising clinical observations, I have been keenly interested in the ultralow-dose range of cannabinoids, and I suspect that more research in this area will yield additional therapeutic applications, including health promotion and disease prevention.

Ultralow doses of cannabinoids have been shown to be physiologically active in several preclinical models. A single intraperitoneal (ip) injection of 0.002 mg/kg THC to mice induced long-lasting activation of protective signaling molecules in the brain, including the transcription factor CREB and brain-derived neurotrophic factor (BDNF), and provided protection against a variety of neuronal insults.[19] Incredibly, another study found that the same single dose induced mild but long-term cognitive deficits in young mice that lasted for at least 5 months.[20] Yet another study showed that the same ultralow single dose in female older mice improved performance in six different behavioral assays of memory and learning, with 24-month-old treated mice scoring similarly to naïve 2-month-old mice; remarkably, the beneficial effect lasted for at least 7 weeks.[21] This suggests a bidirectional effect of ultra-low-dose THC based on one's age and baseline physiological activity.

Other preclinical studies have reported that ip injection of 0.002 mg/kg THC reduced damage and preserved cardiac function when administered to mice 2 hr before myocardial infarction[22] and also reduced apoptotic, oxidative, and inflammatory injury in mice with hepatic ischemia and reperfusion.[23] Keep in mind that 0.002 mg/kg is extraordinarily low for mice, with an allometrically scaled dose in humans around 0.00016 mg/kg or 0.16 μg/kg.

I have also observed acidic cannabinoids at ultralow doses to be effective in my practice, supported by preclinical literature. In a rat model of nausea, Δ^9-tetrahydrocannabinolic acid demonstrated antiemetic effects at 0.05 mg/kg, $\frac{1}{10}$ the minimal effective dose of THC.[24] Subsequent work on cannabidiolic acid (CBDA) found an effective dose as low as 0.5 μg/kg, approximately 2,000 times lower than that of CBD (1–5 mg/kg).[25] Interestingly, the dose–response curve for the antiemetic effect of CBDA was not biphasic in the ranges tested, as has been reported for CBD, which potentiated vomiting at 20–40 mg/kg.[26]

Ultra-low-dose synergistic effects have also been described among the cannabinoids. For example, in a rodent model of hyperalgesia and inflammation, doses of THC (100 µg/kg, orally) or CBDA (0.1 µg/kg, orally) that were ineffective alone effectively reduced symptoms when combined.[27] Cannabis users are frequently exposed to dozens of minor cannabinoids in this dosing range, perhaps contributing to chemovar-specific entourage effects.

Hormesis, a dose–response phenomenon characterized by low-dose stimulation and high-dose inhibition, explains some of these surprising results and is far from unique to cannabinoids. A simple example of hormesis is the ability of ultralow doses of disinfectants to stimulate the growth of *Candida*, while higher doses inhibit growth and even higher doses are fungicidal. A number of mechanisms have been described, commonly involving the activation of protective and regenerative cellular pathways upon low-dose exposure. An understanding of the paradigm of hormesis, recently reviewed in relation to the effects of THC on memory and cognition,[28] is important for the cannabis clinician.

Therapeutic Window for Δ^9-Tetrahydrocannabinol

The therapeutic window, which is the range between the effective dose and a dose that causes intolerable adverse effects, can be most narrow in cannabis-naïve patients, who are more likely to experience adverse effects. This can be managed with appropriate dosing strategies.

Compared to the cannabis-naïve patient, frequent users have shown blunted responses to the psychotomimetic, perception-altering, cognition-impairing, anxiogenic, and cortisol-modulating effects of THC but not to the euphoric effects.[29] This heterogenous tolerance-building to various effects may be due to cannabinoid receptor downregulation and desensitization occurring at varying rates and magnitudes in different brain regions. For example, CB1 downregulation upon exposure to THC occurs faster in the hippocampus, an area that contributes to the effects of THC on memory, than in the basal ganglia, an area that contributes to the euphoric effects of THC.[30]

In general, the therapeutic effects of THC, especially those produced by lower doses, are more resistant to tolerance development than adverse effects or effects produced by higher doses. For example, rodents build tolerance to high-dose behavioral effects of THC faster than moderate-dose hypothermic effects, and they are slowest to build tolerance to low-dose analgesic effects.[31]

Thus, when titrated appropriately, THC has the ability to widen its own therapeutic window, a strategy that can be intentionally utilized with patients who have not recently or ever been exposed to THC. Cannabis-naïve patients tend to have a narrow therapeutic window at first but are typically able to tolerate higher and more therapeutic doses with fewer adverse effects after a period of regular administration, which in my experience ranges from a few days to 2 weeks.

Strategically, I start my cannabis-naïve patients on a subtherapeutic dose of THC that is unlikely to produce any noticeable effects, titrate up to the minimum dose needed to produce mild effects, hold at that dose for 3 days, and then resume slow titration. I believe the therapeutic window widens during the 3-day pause at the minimal noticeable dose, increasing the likelihood of success with subsequent titration. In those who can more patiently wait for satisfactory results, I typically titrate every 3–5 days, which accomplishes a similar goal.

Δ⁹-Tetrahydrocannabinol and Cannabidiol Synergy

Among the synergistic effects of cannabis constituents, the interaction of THC and CBD is the most well-studied. Preclinical and clinical literature demonstrate that adding CBD can help mitigate many of the adverse effects of THC, such as intoxication, sedation, and tachycardia, while potentiating many of the benefits of THC, such as analgesia and antiemesis. While the reduction in adverse effects is likely related to the activity of CBD as a negative allosteric modulator of the CB1 receptor, pharmacodynamic interactions and pharmacokinetic interactions (such as decreased 11-hydroxylation of THC) that are not mediated by cannabinoid receptors likely also play a role.[32]

Though CBD certainly offers therapeutic effects on its own, its most useful clinical property may be its role as an adjunct to THC, widening the therapeutic window of THC while providing additional benefits. The large body of clinical trial evidence and long history of effective clinical use of nabiximols THC/CBD oromucosal spray support this strategy.

For example, in a clinical trial of 177 patients with chronic cancer-related pain not adequately responding to chronic opioid treatment, subjects were randomized into groups receiving a THC-dominant oromucosal spray, a combined THC/CBD spray, or a placebo spray and allowed to titrate the dose within basic guidelines over the course of a week with minimal dosing adjustments thereafter. By the end of 2 weeks, the THC group took an average of ~10 sprays/day, for a total of ~27 mg of THC daily, while the combined THC/CBD group took ~11.5 sprays/day, for a total of ~31 mg of THC and ~29 mg of CBD daily. The two groups experienced similar rates of adverse effects, despite the slightly higher dose of THC in the combined THC/CBD group, but the THC/CBD recipients were nearly twice as likely to experience a ≥30% reduction in pain scores compared to the THC-only group (43% vs. 23%, respectively).[33] In this study, the combination of THC and CBD resulted in improved tolerance of a higher total cannabinoid dose with improved benefits.

Clinicians with access to products containing a variety of THC:CBD ratios are able to adjust the dosing based on patient goals, personal preference, and clinical response. For example, those with a history of being highly sensitive to adverse effects from THC may want to start with a THC:CBD ratio in the range 1:10–1:5, whereas others may do well on a nabiximols-like formula in the range of 1:1.

From a practical standpoint, it is important to note that for many patients a lower THC:CBD ratio results in the need for a higher total daily dose of cannabinoids, which typically results in a more expensive treatment. For example, a patient with pain may experience relief at THC (5 mg) that is comparable but less well tolerated than the relief experienced with THC (4 mg) + CBD (8 mg), but the latter treatment may cost more than twice as much, based on the total number of milligrams needed per dose.

Though it is widely reported that CBD mitigates euphoria and psychoactive adverse effects of THC while enhancing its benefits, some contrary data have been reported. In one study of 31 healthy cannabis users, treatment with 200, 400, or 800 mg of oral CBD 90 min prior to inhalation of THC-dominant cannabis did not change ratings of feeling "high," an experience typically desired by nonmedical users but avoided in medical users.[34] Older studies report that CBD changes the type of psychological reaction induced by THC in infrequent cannabis smokers, reducing their anxiety and thereby rendering THC more enjoyable.[35] Thus, CBD may heterogeneously mitigate the adverse effects of THC, especially in regard to psychoactivity, and this likely varies significantly among individuals and delivery methods.

Furthermore, some evidence exists that CBD may pharmacodynamically inhibit the analgesic effects of THC. In a small study on women with fibromyalgia that compared three chemovars of vaporized cannabis (type 1, THC-dominant; type 2, mixed THC and CBD; and type 3, CBD-dominant) with placebo, pharmacokinetic data suggested that CBD inhalation increased THC plasma concentrations but diminished THC-induced analgesic effects, indicative of synergistic pharmacokinetic but antagonistic pharmacodynamic interactions.[36] Since the analgesic effects of THC are mainly CB1-mediated and CBD somewhat antagonizes this signaling, it should not be surprising that CBD can decrease the power of therapeutic effects of THC in addition to its adverse effects.

Adverse and Beneficial Psychoactive Effects

The psychoactive effects of cannabis, primarily related to CB1 agonism, are often reported as adverse effects. Patients may feel somnolence, time distortion, impaired short-term memory, confusion, anxiety, and perceptual disturbances that can interfere with function and may be dangerous when combined with driving and other activities. When the goal of treatment is typically to improve patients' function while reducing their symptoms, THC-related intoxication and impairment are undesirable.

Often grouped with other psychoactive properties of cannabis, euphoria is also frequently considered an adverse effect, the sixth most commonly reported based on one meta-analysis.[37] Euphoria is defined as "a feeling of great happiness or well-being."[38] An older definition from The Century Dictionary, which I find especially applicable to cannabis, is "the state of feeling well, especially when occurring in a diseased person."

Is it undesirable for our diseased patients to feel well? In most situations, euphoria should be considered a valuable side benefit, and clinical strategies to maximize the euphoric properties of cannabis are appropriate in many cases. In fact, hundreds of my patients have reported this feeling of well-being as the primary therapeutic effect of cannabis, with reduction in symptoms noted as less profound and less important to their clinical course.

An Israeli qualitative study of 19 patients, ages 28–79 years, using cannabis to treat chronic pain illustrates this concept. All the interviewees described the experience of chronic pain in terms of "losing one's self" and "losing one's life," and many used the word "normal" to describe their lives after beginning to use cannabis. They talked about how cannabis allowed them to sleep, focus, and function and, through this, to attain a sense of normality in their lives once again. Interviewees generally reported that cannabis changed their pain to a different and more tolerable form and more often distanced the pain rather than reducing it. They frequently described a return to normality or "restored self," a term proposed by the authors: for example, "I can smoke and feel normal," "I behave much more normal than before. It is simply easier," and "I was a shadow of my former self, and now I am a normal human being again."[39]

I also frequently hear these phrases in my clinic—perhaps the most common is, "cannabis has given me my life back." Importantly, in the qualitative data mentioned above, regaining oneself was not described as a passive process facilitated solely by the use of medical cannabis; the interviewees consistently described a state in which they became more proactive in reclaiming their lives. I also observe this in my patients, many of whom become more inspired and engaged in meaningful and therapeutic activities after they start using cannabis. After observing this trend for a couple of years in my most successful patients, I began promoting it to all my patients by first suggesting they explore the psychoactive effects of cannabis as an adjunct to meditation, prayer, reflection, and exercise.

Beyond restored self, my patients report a variety of psychological benefits attributed to the psychoactive effects of cannabis, many of which are experienced or learned during the acute effects but often persist long after the drug effects resolve:

- greater acceptance of symptoms and illness
- increased self-awareness and insight into one's situation
- enhanced capacity for mindfulness and decreased emotional reactivity
- ability to view oneself from a different vantage point
- increased ability to find creative solutions to problems
- increased mental, emotional, and physical flexibility and capacity for change
- increased desire to interact socially and help others
- sense of connection to God, nature, or the universe

Furthermore, many patients with pain describe a process of unbundling, or increasing their ability to recognize and modulate the various aspects of their condition, illustrated in Figure 17.3:

FIGURE 17.3
Unbundling of Chronic Pain Perception and Behavior

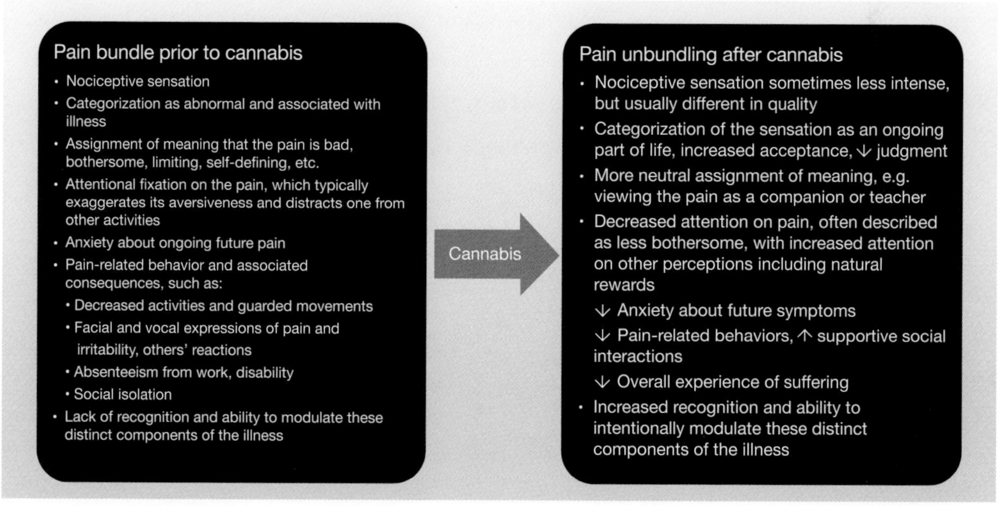

Pain bundle prior to cannabis
- Nociceptive sensation
- Categorization as abnormal and associated with illness
- Assignment of meaning that the pain is bad, bothersome, limiting, self-defining, etc.
- Attentional fixation on the pain, which typically exaggerates its aversiveness and distracts one from other activities
- Anxiety about ongoing future pain
- Pain-related behavior and associated consequences, such as:
  - Decreased activities and guarded movements
  - Facial and vocal expressions of pain and irritability, others' reactions
  - Absenteeism from work, disability
  - Social isolation
- Lack of recognition and ability to modulate these distinct components of the illness

Cannabis

Pain unbundling after cannabis
- Nociceptive sensation sometimes less intense, but usually different in quality
- Categorization of the sensation as an ongoing part of life, increased acceptance, ↓ judgment
- More neutral assignment of meaning, e.g. viewing the pain as a companion or teacher
- Decreased attention on pain, often described as less bothersome, with increased attention on other perceptions including natural rewards
- ↓ Anxiety about future symptoms
- ↓ Pain-related behaviors, ↑ supportive social interactions
- ↓ Overall experience of suffering
- Increased recognition and ability to intentionally modulate these distinct components of the illness

Source: Dustin Sulak

Most of my cannabis-naïve patients wish to experience symptom relief with minimal to no psychoactive effects, which we can typically accomplish using the dosing strategies suggested in this chapter. At some point during their follow-up, however, I explain that while symptom reduction is important, *healing* often involves a repatterning of perceptions, thoughts, and behavior and that the psychoactivity of cannabis, perhaps its most powerful medicinal property, can promote such changes, especially when intentionally used for that purpose.

Many patients assume that cannabis-induced psychoactivity is intense or hallucinogenic, which it can be at high doses, so I explain that the desired experience can be achieved with a mild effect, similar to 1–2 glasses of wine but typically more pleasurable. This context is reassuring and patients are usually willing to follow my instructions. Since my patients often use an oral or oromucosal dose of THC before bed to promote restorative sleep, I invite patients to, once weekly, take their before-bed dose of THC a couple of hours earlier than usual, turn off or set aside screens and communication devices, prevent other distractions, and prepare a safe environment conducive to gentle movement, meditation, reflecting, and journaling.* If they do not notice a shift in consciousness, I encourage them to increase the dose by 10%–25% each week until they do.

Treat the Patient, Not the Diagnosis

Clinicians are often surprised to learn that they might give similar cannabis dosing plans to patients with a wide range of diagnoses. Patients with Crohn's disease, multiple sclerosis, posttraumatic stress disorder, and chronic musculoskeletal pain may respond to similar regimens; conversely, two patients with the same condition may succeed with significantly different regimens. This challenges the way we think about condition-specific treatments and forces us to individually tailor treatment plans for our patients.

While this may seem complex and challenging, it actually simplifies the practice of cannabinoid medicine. The cannabis clinician typically becomes somewhat of a generalist, attracting refractory patients from all the other specialty fields, but we need not become experts in every field. While it is important to learn the basic pathophysiology of, and current conventional treatment options for, our patients' conditions, this information only sometimes impacts my cannabis recommendations. There are certainly clinical

---

* My patient education website Healer.com includes a section titled Wellness Activities with video instructions for gentle movements, meditations, and breathing practices I find useful for patients exploring the psychoactive benefits of cannabis.

pearls that can help with specific conditions and diagnoses that warrant caution or specific considerations, but the overall success of the cannabis clinician is largely based on one's general knowledge of dosing, delivery methods, and physiological effects of the various active constituents.

The most important information that will guide your individualized cannabis recommendations is an understanding of the patient and their context in life. Synchronize with their goals and personal preferences, understand their highest values, and identify high-impact opportunities for improving function and quality of life. Not only will this inform your therapeutic strategy, but the process of gathering this information will invoke trust and build the foundation for a therapeutic relationship, a partnership in healing.

When I begin an initial visit, I usually lead with these three questions to elucidate the goals and values of my patient:

- If you could get anything out of this visit, what would it be?
- Imagine you are much healthier 2 months from now: how is life different? Please paint the picture for me.
- Please describe your greatest successes and biggest challenges in dealing with this condition.

The responses help me craft two or three concrete goals that I always include in the patient's plan, which I print and provide to the patient at the end of their visit. If restorative sleep is lacking, that is always one of the goals at the end of an initial visit. I like the goals to include concrete details, demonstrating that I understand what makes my patients' lives more meaningful, whether it is "be able to tolerate and enjoy three hours of rabbit hunting," "be able to drive to work without stopping to use the bathroom," or "be able to enjoy your time with your grandchildren without being distracted by pain."

Dosing Strategies for Cannabis-Naïve Patients

For patients with no recent or historical experience with cannabis, my goal is to introduce and titrate cannabis with the greatest likelihood of benefits with the lowest risk of adverse effects, including mild adverse effects. Recall the basic principles of cannabis dosing that inform my strategy for the cannabis-naïve:

- broad safe and effective dosing range with interindividual variability and sometimes intraindividual variability (different symptoms responding to different doses)

- nonlinear dose–response effects, necessitating methodical titration and self-assessment
- narrow therapeutic window of THC, which can broaden over time and when combined with CBD

For patients with chronic, daily symptoms, I typically start with the oromucosal route of delivery, usually drops of infused oil, for easy titration, intermediate onset and duration, and overall efficacy and tolerability. I provide a starting dose intended to be sub-therapeutic, and I explain to the patient that by starting low and going slow we are most likely to achieve success. I provide a titration schedule and ask the patient to use the Inner Inventory, a scale I developed to help patients identify when they begin responding to dose adjustments (see Example Patient B box for details). At the minimal dose required to elicit a mild response, I instruct the patient to temporarily stop titration and continue at that dose for 3 days. Thereafter, if they are not satisfied with the therapeutic effects, they may resume titrating until they experience either satisfactory benefits, in which case they should stop titrating and continue on that dose, or adverse effects, in which case they should reduce their dose slightly.

I usually recommend three times daily dosing after meals, and unless there is a reason for a lower THC:CBD ratio, I start with 1:1, which is broadly effective, well-tolerated, and supported by a large body of (nabiximols) clinical trial data. The starting dose is usually 1–2 mg of THC with a corresponding dose of CBD if indicated. If the patient has disturbed sleep, this becomes our first therapeutic target. Because I have observed mixed results with CBD administration before bed, with some patients reporting enhanced sleep and others reporting disturbed sleep, I typically recommend THC-dominant, low-CBD formulas with sedating terpene profiles for this purpose.

I determine the frequency of titration based on my assessment of the urgency of the patient's need for relief, aversiveness to side effects, and self-efficacy. If the urgency is low, I may begin with before-bed dosing only and then proceed to daytime dosing after benefits are obtained, but for faster results, the day and night titration can occur simultaneously.

The accompanying boxes are examples of cannabis plan components that I print and provide to patients. I keep these as modifiable template items in my electronic health record so I can create custom recommendations for each patient. Please feel free to use them in your practice and modify as needed.

What Products Do I Need and How Do I Take Them?

Obtain a cannabis oil or tincture with a known potency and clear labeling so you can administer an accurate dosage using a dropper or oral syringe. For faster onset, hold the liquid in your mouth for 1–5 min before swallowing, and for better absorption, take after meals containing fat. If you purchase separate THC-dominant and CBD-dominant products, this will allow the ratio of these components to be adjusted if needed.

Driving, Adverse Effects, and Overdose

After starting cannabis and after each dosage increase, avoid driving or operating machinery until you know how a particular dose affects you. When a person is impaired from cannabis, they are usually aware of this impairment and able to make a good decision about whether they are safe to drive.

Unwanted side effects of cannabis are usually due to an excessive dose of THC. The most common mild adverse effects are dizziness, impaired coordination, dry mouth, and sleepiness. Overdose symptoms include confusion, nausea, vomiting, diarrhea, anxiety or panic, pain, and hallucination. Cannabis overdose is unpleasant but safe and resolves within 4–24 hr. The best treatment for accidental overdose is a calm, comfortable environment. Contact emergency medical services if you experience chest pain, palpitations, or trouble breathing or you suspect dehydration related to vomiting and/or diarrhea.

Example Patient A:
Cannabis-Naïve, Low Urgency, Slower Approach

Step 1: Address the need for restorative sleep.

- Take before bed (1–2 hr in advance for trouble falling asleep, right before bed for trouble staying asleep).
- Use a THC-dominant product, preferably made from sedating cannabis varieties.
- Take a starting dose of 2 mg.
- Increase the dose by 1 mg every 2–3 nights until you experience satisfactory restorative sleep and wake feeling rested. If you experience adverse effects like morning grogginess or disorientation in the middle of the night, reduce the dose by 1 mg.
- Until our next meeting, your maximum dose should be 15 mg.

Step 2: After restorative sleep is achieved, address daytime symptoms.

- Take in the morning and afternoon.
- Take a starting dose of 2 mg of THC and 2 mg of CBD.
- Increase the dose by 1 mg of THC and 1 mg of CBD every 3 days until you achieve satisfactory benefits or bothersome side effects. If you experience side effects, reduce the dose slightly.
- Until our next meeting, your maximum dose should be 10 mg of THC and 10 mg of CBD twice daily.

Example Patient B:
Cannabis-Naïve, Higher Urgency, Faster Approach

Step 1: Address the need for restorative sleep.

- Take before bed (1–2 hr in advance for trouble falling asleep, right before bed for trouble staying asleep).
- Use a THC-dominant product, preferably made from sedating cannabis varieties.
- Take a starting dose of 2 mg.
- Increase the dose by 1 mg every night until you experience satisfactory restorative sleep and wake feeling rested. If you experience adverse effects like morning grogginess or disorientation in the middle of the night, reduce the dose by 1 mg.
- Until our next meeting, your maximum dose should be 15 mg.

Step 2: Address daytime symptoms (can be concurrent with step 1).

- Take in the morning and afternoon.
- Take a starting dose of 2 mg of THC and 2 mg of CBD.
- Increase the dose by 1 mg of THC and 1 mg of CBD every day until you achieve a mild improvement in your Inner Inventory scores associated with the cannabis oil.
- Temporarily stop increasing and remain at this minimal noticeable dose for 3 days.
- Resume increasing the dose by 1 mg of THC and 1 mg of CBD every 3 days until you achieve satisfactory benefits or bothersome side effects. If you experience side effects, reduce the dose slightly.
- Until our next meeting, your maximum dose should be 10 mg of THC and 10 mg of CBD twice daily.

How to Check Your Inner Inventory:

Rate each item on a scale of 1 to 10 (1 = worst and 10 = best) before and 1–2 hr after taking each dose. Set an alarm reminder and record your scores for best results.

- **Breath:** How easy and smooth is your breath?
- **Body:** How comfortable and calm does your body feel? How easy is it to remain still and comfortable?
- **Mood:** How easy is it for you to feel a sense of contentment and appreciation? How easy is it for you to smile right now?
- **Symptoms:** How severe are your symptoms? (1 = minimal and 10 = severe)

I also appreciate the titration schedule of nabiximols oromucosal spray, which allows slow introduction starting with before-bed dosing and gives time for widening of the therapeutic window of THC using a slightly different method.[40] Prior to adopting this slower and lower dose titration schedule, previous nabiximols clinical trials yielded significantly higher rates of adverse effects.[41] In Table 17.1, each spray refers to THC (2.7 mg) + CBD (2.5 mg).

TABLE 17.1
Titration Schedule of Nabiximols Oromucosal Spray

	Number of sprays		
Day	In the morning	In the evening	Total per day
1	0	1	1
2	0	1	1
3	0	2	2
4	0	2	2
5	1	2	3
6	1	3	4
7	1	4	5
8	2	4	6
9	2	5	7

	Number of sprays		
Day	In the morning	In the evening	Total per day
10	3	5	8
11	3	6	9
12	4	6	10
13	4	7	11
14	5	7	12

Source. Sativex® Summary of Product Characteristics, https://www
.medicines.org.uk/emc/product/602. Accessed 9 October, 2020

For cannabis-naïve patients with episodic or infrequent symptoms that are more amenable to the inhaled route of delivery, such as migraine, nausea or vomiting, and acute spasms, I recommend starting with 1–2 inhalations, waiting 10–15 min, and then reassessing (using the Inner Inventory) whether another inhalation is needed. I advise my patients to be cautious when using flower vaporizers the first time; many will otherwise take several inhalations in a row while trying to determine if the device is turned on and set correctly. The respiratory sensations are much less noticeable and the exhalation is much less visible compared to smoking, so it is easy for novices to assume they did not receive a proper inhalation.

Dosing Strategies for Experienced Cannabis Users

I frequently encounter patients who have been using cannabis for psychoactive, social, creative, or spiritual purposes for years or decades prior to becoming ill. They consult me to learn how to modify their use pattern to achieve better symptom control with fewer side effects. I have found three strategies essential in helping such patients: reversing tolerance, noninhaled routes of delivery, and combining CBD with THC.

I first screen for signs of cannabis tolerance in daily users. It is common for the occasional cannabis smoker, who develops a symptom responsive to cannabis, to gradually increase the frequency and dosage until they are smoking all day every day. At first, they clearly note the increased intake is associated with symptomatic improvement, but over time the treatment loses efficacy. I explain the concept of biphasic dose–response, usually with a diagram (see Figure 17.4), and emphasize that by reversing cannabis tolerance they can achieve increased benefits and decreased side effects with significantly less expense.

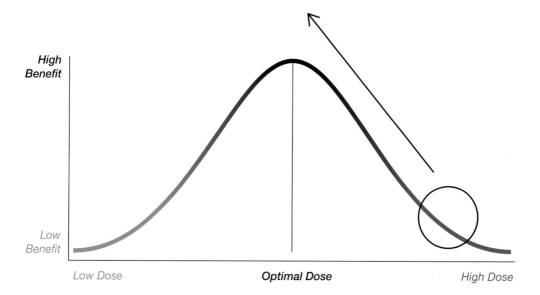

FIGURE 17.4

Biphasic Dose–Response

Source. Dustin Sulak

It is also common for experienced users to inappropriately rely on inhaled cannabis to treat persistent symptoms. I help them identify that they experience only temporary relief, and typically wait until the symptoms recur to an intensity that is significantly bothersome or limiting before deciding to readminister cannabis. The mental and physiological distress of breakthrough symptoms occurring numerous times daily is far from ideal. I explain that oromucosal and/or oral delivery can provide baseline relief so that the troughs between sessions of inhalation are less intense and the need to inhale is noticed less often (Figure 17.5). I also explain that many people who rely on inhalation to treat constant symptoms build tolerance and diminish the therapeutic power of their medicine.

Finally, I frequently meet experienced users who reserve cannabis for after work or on the weekends because they chose to avoid driving or working while impaired. As they age and their symptoms intensify, they find themselves suffering through the day and experiencing excellent relief at night. Some may have tried low or moderate doses of hemp-based CBD products with unsatisfactory results. I explain the concept of the therapeutic window of THC, that they can take a certain (usually oromucosal) dose of THC during the day with some relief and no impairment, and that adding CBD to the THC can improve their results and diminish potential impairment. Many experienced cannabis

FIGURE 17.5A AND FIGURE 17.5B

Dose Layering:
(A) Inhaled Only and
(B) Oromucosal and Inhaled

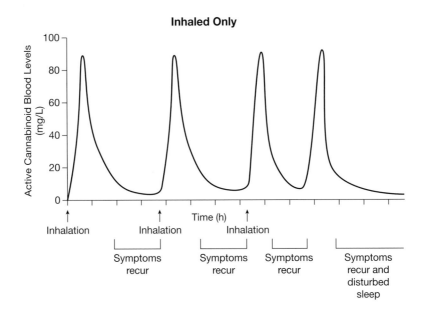

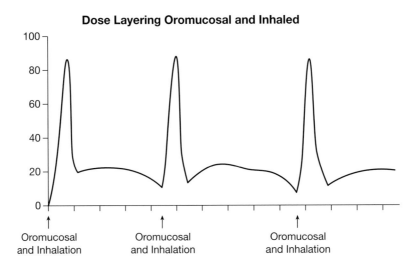

Source. Dustin Sulak

users fail to appreciate CBD until they try using it as an adjunct to THC and recognize the combination is fully compatible with their daily activities.

Cannabis Tolerance and How to Reverse It

I see many patients using cannabis with minimal benefit because they have built tolerance not only to the psychoactive or adverse effects but also to the therapeutic effects. For example, consider a 62-year-old woman with severe anxiety and chronic pain who smokes six joints daily: her symptoms are so severe she can barely leave the house to make an appointment, but she knows the cannabis must be helping because when she does not smoke she feels even worse. In this situation, layering in baseline treatment with oromucosal delivery or adding CBD will unlikely yield additional benefit. The priority, in this situation, is to first reverse her tolerance and then proceed with other dosing strategies.

Over the years I have interviewed hundreds of cannabis patients who have figured out how to reverse their own tolerance. Remarkably, most find a 2-day period of abstinence is all they need to experience stronger effects from a lower dose. This was confirmed by an imaging study that showed cannabis-dependent men had 15% lower CB1 receptor availability in the brain compared to healthy controls (significant in all brain regions except the thalamus and cerebellum), but after just 2 days of abstinence the cannabis-dependent subjects had no difference in CB1 availability compared to healthy controls. The CB1 availability increased only slightly between day 2 and day 28 of abstinence, and the magnitude of withdrawal symptoms was strongly inversely correlated with CB1 availability.[42] These findings suggest that avoiding and reversing cannabis tolerance is important not only for therapeutic efficacy but also for preventing dependence and withdrawal.

I developed a 6-day "sensitization protocol" that effectively helps patients reverse cannabis tolerance while developing self-awareness and self-efficacy, available free on Healer.com. In an email survey sent to my practice in 2012, 48 patients responded after completing the protocol. Five patients did not note benefit, but the other 43 reduced their dose by an average of 56% while universally reporting improvements in therapeutic effects. To help patients succeed, I include a variety of supports (and distractions) such as worksheets, exercises, and diet strategies.* The essential components of the protocol, however, are straightforward:

- **Days 1 and 2:** Begin with 48 hr of cannabis abstinence.†
- **Day 3:** Break the "cannabis fast" with the lowest dose required to produce a mini-

---

* www.healer.com/programs/sensitization-protocol/

† Can be modified to 24–36 hr in patients who cannot tolerate 48 hr.

mal noticeable response, using the Inner Inventory scale to help determine when this occurs.

- **Days 3–5:** Continue to administer cannabis up to three times daily to achieve only a minimal noticeable response.
- **Day 6:** Gradually increase the dose to achieve equal or superior therapeutic effects compared to those experiences prior to starting the protocol.

Interestingly, some patients report ongoing sensitization to cannabis during days 3–5. Perhaps they are simply becoming more aware of the subtle effects of cannabis by exercising their faculties of self-perception, or perhaps these minimal doses of THC are gently upregulating the sensitivity of the endocannabinoid system. Some preclinical data support the latter hypothesis: THC increased the production of endocannabinoids in brain cells;[43] coadministration of THC and morphine caused an upregulation of CB1 receptor levels in mouse spinal cords;[44] and an acute dose of THC increased cannabinoid receptor affinity in rats.[45]

When recommending the sensitization protocol, I am sure to emphasize several potential benefits, beyond improved efficacy, to help patients overcome their hesitancy about taking a break from their favorite medicine. Suggesting that they might reduce the monthly cost of their medicine by 50% or more is usually the most compelling, along with the likelihood of reducing adverse effects, especially fatigue.

For patients demonstrating some signs of problematic cannabis use, the sensitization protocol is an excellent exercise for regaining control over their relationship with cannabis. It provides a challenge they can usually overcome, contributing to self-efficacy; it often gives them a short experience of cannabis withdrawal, which can motivate them to avoid building tolerance in the future; and it helps reframe the relationship with cannabis, prioritizing the therapeutic effects.

Over the years, numerous patients have also reported that avoiding prolonged use of a particular chemovar helps prevent tolerance; rotating between several chemovars every 1–12 weeks seems to be helpful for many patients who use cannabis flower. It is possible that oromucosal and oral cannabis products that have some standardization for content of major constituents, but also have inherent variability in minor constituents related to batch differences in starting materials, may produce better results with greater retention of efficacy over time.

Summary: How to Craft Individualized Plans for Your Patients

Dosing principles:

- Wide safe and effective dosing range (0.01–50 mg·kg^{-1}·day^{-1}) with most patients responding in the 0.1–2 mg·kg^{-1}·day^{-1} range. Start low and go slow, but do not be afraid to go all the way.
- Biphasic and bidirectional dose–response effects are common. Methodical titration, self-awareness, and concrete goals are essential.
- The therapeutic window of THC is narrow in the cannabis-naïve. Use slow titration strategies and coadministration with CBD to improve tolerability and efficacy. Consider treating with a bedtime dose of THC for several days before starting daytime THC dosing.
- For those wishing to avoid psychoactive effects, use precision oromucosal dosing with a THC:CBD ratio ≤1:5, acidic cannabinoids, or topical products. Consider suggesting gentle psychoactive experiences at a follow-up visit.
- Expect most patients to eventually get best results with dose layering of various delivery methods to address baseline, breakthrough, and episodic symptoms.
- For patients who inhale cannabis frequently, suggest a flower vaporizer to minimize or eliminate potential harm. Avoid vape pens with oil cartridges until they are proven safe.
- Set concrete goals congruent with your patients' highest values and recognize that symptom amelioration may be less important than "restored self" and improvement in function.
- Prioritize correcting disturbed sleep, an essential element of healing that often potentiates other treatments. Because I often see mixed results in patients using CBD before bed, I suggest starting with low-dose oromucosal THC, which is much more often effective in my experience.
- Identify and reverse tolerance and problematic use by employing the sensitization protocol or intermittent 2-day periods of abstinence.

Elements of a cannabis plan:

- goal(s)
- route of delivery

- starting dose
- titration amount and frequency
- expectations and what to look for while titrating: signs of efficacy and adverse effects
- maximum dose (until the next follow-up visit)
- what to look for when selecting products compatible with the plan

Chapter 18

Adverse Effects and Cautions

THE ADVERSE EFFECTS PROFILE of appropriately dosed cannabis is well within the range of, and often superior to that of, many commonly used pharmacological agents. The ability to adjust dosage, chemovar, delivery method, and other factors provides opportunities for mitigating adverse effects while maintaining benefits; this typical clinical experience is absent from controlled clinical trials. I suspect that clinical data on pragmatic use of artisanal cannabis will demonstrate even greater tolerability.

One of the seldom-mentioned but perhaps most dangerous adverse effects of cannabis is directly linked to its efficacy: delay of diagnosis. Patients can effectively use cannabis as a home remedy to suppress symptoms that would otherwise have brought them to their clinician, and similarly, clinicians who treat patients without sufficient workup may mask a dangerous underlying diagnosis. I encourage caution, especially in cases of gastrointestinal symptoms and abdominal pain, and I encourage cannabis clinicians to review prior diagnostic efforts at the initial encounter.

Another frequently overlooked and often serious adverse effect of medical cannabis use may be forgotten by those reading this book, who likely work in a jurisdiction where cannabis is legal. Millions of cannabis users continue to do so illegally, risking fines, imprisonment, ineligibility for employment and higher education, and other grim consequences. In many cases, these legal consequences are far more dangerous than any risks associated with the substance itself. As medical professionals, our voices can influence the evolution of public health policy, and I believe our work is not done until individuals everywhere have the ability to legally grow, possess, and use this medicine. While strategies for safe and effective legalization and regulation of medical or adult-use cannabis can be complex, the simple decriminalization of small-scale cultivation and possession can, in my opinion, significantly improve public health; advocacy for this basic right is an inherent role for a cannabis clinician.

Toxicology

I searched for the longest and highest-dose animal toxicology data available on Δ^9-tetrahydrocannabinol (THC). The U.S. National Toxicology Program conducted 2-year toxicology studies in mice and rats of both genders to evaluate the long-term effects of high-dose THC administered orally in corn oil.[1] Mice received 0, 125, 250, or 500 mg of THC/kg of body weight, while rats received 0, 12.5, 25, or 50 mg of THC/kg of body weight. All the dosed rodents had similar survival rates as controls with the exception of the 500 mg/kg mouse group, which was somewhat lower. Mean body weights of all dosed groups were lower than those of the controls. As you can see in Table 18.1, no neoplastic effects were observed, and several tumors were found to have a reduced incidence in the dosed animals.

TABLE 18.1

Toxicology Data on Long-Term Oral THC in Rodents

Male rats	Female rats	Male mice	Female mice
NONNEOPLASTIC EFFECTS			
Convulsions and seizures, usually following dosing or handling	Convulsions and seizures, usually following dosing or handling	Hyperactivity, convulsions, and seizures following dosing or handling	Hyperactivity, convulsions, and seizures following dosing or handling
		Increased thyroid follicular cell hyperplasia, mostly in 125 and 250 mg/kg groups, somewhat in 500 mg/kg group	Increased thyroid follicular cell hyperplasia in 125 and 250 mg/kg groups
		Increased forestomach hyperplasia in all dosed groups; increased forestomach ulcer in 125 and 250 mg/kg groups but not 500 mg/kg group	

Male rats	Female rats	Male mice	Female mice
NEOPLASTIC EFFECTS			
None	None	None	None
DECREASED INCIDENCES			
Pancreatic adenoma, pituitary adenoma, testicular interstitial cell adenoma	Mammary fibroadenoma, uterine stromal polyp	Hepatocellular adenoma and carcinoma, eosinophilic foci, fatty liver	Hepatocellular adenoma and carcinoma, eosinophilic foci, fatty liver

Several primate toxicology studies have also been performed with oral doses of THC, but for shorter time periods. Single doses of THC up to 9,000 mg/kg in rhesus monkeys were nonlethal and produced no histopathological changes.[2] Daily doses of 50 mg/kg caused a moribund condition in one of six monkeys (day 16), and doses of 500 mg/kg caused a moribund condition in two of eight monkeys (days 10 and 14); the remaining animals survived the 28-day treatment. Interestingly, all six monkeys treated with 250 mg/kg THC survived the 28-day experiment.[3]

In regard to THC-dominant cannabis flowers, the median lethal dose (LD50) for dogs has not been established but is >3–9 g/kg of body weight.[4] Allometrically scaled, this suggests a lethal dose for a 10-kg child is no less than 16 g of cannabis flower consumed at once, or 116 g consumed by a 70-kg adult, both highly unlikely.

Large clinical trial data sets have shown that medically dosed cannabinoids are rarely linked with toxic or serious adverse effects. In nonmedical users, at least 35 cardiovascular emergencies, including 13 deaths, have been reported in people who had recently smoked cannabis.[5] While this is likely an underestimate of the true incidence of cannabis as a potential contributing factor to sudden death, considering the overall prevalence of nonmedical use, these numbers are extremely low.

Children, especially young children under 2 years of age, may be more susceptible to toxic and life-threatening effects of cannabis ingestion, including encephalopathy, respiratory insufficiency, arrhythmia, seizure, and coma.[6]

Cannabis intoxication in adults (summarized in Table 18.2) is typically self-limited and requires only supportive care: a calm, quiet environment with supportive reassurance and hydration. Substantial overdoses of THC can lead to more complicated clinical presentations that benefit from active pharmacological management and symptom-targeted therapy: sedative hypnotics (e.g., clonazepam or lorazepam), non-benzodiazepine anxiolytics (e.g., hydroxyzine) and antipsychotics, typically second-generation medications (e.g., risperidone or quetiapine), may be used in the emergency setting.

TABLE 18.2
Signs and Symptoms of Complications from Cannabis Intoxication in Adults[7]

Intensity	Signs and symptoms
	PHYSIOLOGICAL COMPLICATIONS
Mild	Conjunctival injection, pupil constriction, nystagmus, tachypnea, increased heart rate, sedation, increased appetite, headache
Severe	Orthostatic hypotension, palpitations, arrhythmia, urinary retention, nausea, vomiting, diarrhea, tremor, ataxia, lethargy
	PSYCHIATRIC COMPLICATIONS
Mild	"Abnormal" behavior or appearance, inappropriate affect, altered mood (depressed, expansive, euphoric), impaired memory
Severe	Disorganized thinking, delusions, hallucinations, impaired judgment, bizarre or dangerous behavior

Regarding cannabidiol (CBD) specifically, adverse effects in animal studies include developmental toxicity, embryo-fetal mortality, central nervous system inhibition and neurotoxicity, hepatocellular injuries, spermatogenesis reduction, organ weight alterations, male reproductive system alterations, and hypotension, but all of these occurred at doses higher than those recommended for human use. In rhesus monkeys, intravenous CBD at 150, 200, 225, 250, or 300 mg/kg for 9 days produced tremors and central nervous system (CNS) inhibition (depression, sedation, and prostration) at all doses. The LD50 was 212 mg/kg of CBD iv. Chronic treatment of rhesus monkeys with oral CBD at 30, 100, or 300 mg·kg^{-1}·day^{-1} for 90 days produced no behavioral changes, no definitive signs of CNS inhibition or stimulation, and no autonomic aberrations. Clinical measurements, eye examinations, and electrocardiogram recordings were all within normal limits. While growth rate and body weight were unaffected, researchers found increased size of the liver, heart, kidney, and thyroid, without any evidence of organ dysfunction, and decreased testicular size with inhibited spermatogenesis.[8]

High-dose human trials have shown lack of toxicity with pharmaceutical-grade CBD. Adult patients with psychosis received 1,000 mg daily for ~43 days and experienced a similar side effect profile to placebo.[9] In patients with treatment-resistant epilepsy with significant polypharmacy, doses of CBD up to 50 mg·kg^{-1}·day^{-1} were associated with somnolence, fatigue, lethargy, sedation, decreased or changed appetite, diarrhea, increased transaminases, status epilepticus, convulsions, diarrhea, weight loss, thrombocytopenia, hyperammonemia, and hepatotoxicity.[10]

Cardiovascular Adverse Effects

THC and other CB1 agonists exert significant cardiovascular effects via action in the central nervous system, where lower doses can stimulate the sympathetic and inhibit the parasympathetic systems. Higher doses can do the opposite, as well as having direct effects on cardiovascular tissues. The most common cardiovascular response is increased heart rate and decreased blood pressure, most pronounced in novice or occasional users who inhale cannabis and with inhalation of cannabis concentrates, but certainly observable with oral delivery. While these effects are tolerated by most patients using appropriate doses, those with sensitive cardiovascular status or those taking cardiovascular drugs could experience orthostatic hypotension, sinus tachycardia, and even potentially life-threatening effects such as arrhythmias, profound hypotension, myocardial infarction, and ischemic stroke.[11,12]

Clinicians should exercise caution in patients with angina or who are otherwise intolerant of increased cardiovascular demand. For example, in a study of 10 cannabis nonusers with stable exercise-induced angina, smoking one cannabis joint caused significantly decreased exercise performance associated with 48% earlier onset angina.[13] In studies of nabiximols, cardiovascular adverse events were seen occasionally in early studies with rapid titration and high doses, up to 130 mg of THC/day. These have become quite rare with the improved dosing protocol, up to 32.4 mg of THC/day with slower titration: tachycardia and hypertension, both well under 2% incidence, and orthostatic hypotension, 0.1–0.2% incidence.[14] At doses up to 97.2 mg of THC/day, nabimixols spray produced no corrected QT interval or other cardiac conduction abnormalities.[15]

Several animal studies have shown that CBD has a cardioprotective effect via scavenging of free radicals and reduction of oxidative stress, apoptosis, and inflammation.[16]

Pulmonary Adverse Effects[17,18]

Cannabis smoke contains numerous toxins and carcinogens, but even heavy smokers do not have increased rates of upper or lower respiratory cancers compared to those who do not smoke cannabis, after controlling for other factors like tobacco exposure.[19] This may be related to the anti-inflammatory or anticarcinogenic effects of the cannabinoids and other compounds in the cannabis smoke counteracting the effects of the toxins. Current cannabis smokers do have increased respiratory symptoms such as cough, sputum production, and wheezing but not shortness of breath. After quitting cannabis smoking, users experience a reduction in morning cough, sputum production, and wheezing compared to continuing smokers, and they had no increased risk of developing chronic bronchitis compared to nonsmokers at 10 years follow-up.

Inhaled cannabis causes an acute bronchodilator effect, seen in normal and asthmatic subjects and in asthmatics recovering from exacerbations. Chronic obstructive pulmonary disease (COPD) is typically diagnosed when a patient has an irreversible reduced forced expiratory volume in 1 s (FEV1) compared with forced vital capacity (FVC) on spirometry. Several large data sets have reported an increase in FVC with little or no change in FEV1 in long-term cannabis-only users, even after 20 joint-years of smoking.* It is unclear why heavy cannabis smoking does not cause COPD, but theories include a persistent bronchodilator effect (offsetting airway narrowing) or anti-inflammatory or immunomodulatory effects.

Several cases of spontaneous pneumothorax or pneumomediastinum have been reported in association with cannabis smoking, and several cases of large lung bullae have been reported in mostly heavy cannabis + tobacco smokers. Because the prevalence of bullous lung disease among marijuana smokers compared with that in the general population is unknown, no firm conclusions can be drawn as to whether or not bullous lung disease is causally linked to cannabis smoking.

Cases of pulmonary aspergillosis in immunocompromised patients have been associated with smoking contaminated cannabis. Smoking or vaporizing the cannabis flower is likely insufficient for sterilization and therefore not safe for immunocompromised patients.[20] One study evaluated hydrogen peroxide gas plasma sterilization (49 min, 51 °C, 30 Torr/40 mbar) and autoclave sterilization (50-min steam cycle and 30-min drying cycle, 135 °C, 316 kPa/3160 mbar) of cannabis flowers; both were effective but decreased the THC content of the flower by 12.6% and 22.6%, respectively.[21] Earlier data suggest that individuals can effectively sterilize aspergillus-contaminated cannabis by baking at 150 °C (300 °F) for 15 min before smoking or vaporizing.[22]

E-cigarette or vaping product use–associated lung injury (EVALI) is an evolving and poorly understood phenomenon, at the time of writing, and is cause for significant concern. With numerous hospitalizations, admissions to intensive care units, and confirmed deaths, around 80% of the cases involved THC-containing products, though some cases have been associated with only nicotine e-cigarette use.[23] Diluents, especially vitamin E acetate, are likely implicated in the toxicity. Until this condition is better understood, patients should avoid using cannabis e-cigarettes or vape cartridges.

---

* One joint-year is equivalent to 365 joints per year.

In general, patients using cannabis for therapeutic purposes who do well with pulmonary delivery should use a flower vaporizer, which delivers a comparable pulmonal uptake of THC[24] with drastic reductions in products of combustion.[25] Survey data show that cannabis users who vaporize report fewer respiratory symptoms than those who smoke, especially those who use larger amounts.[26]

Common Adverse Effects

Most common adverse effects can be prevented with individualized dosing and titration plans. The guidance of a cannabis clinician and access to diverse chemovars, formulations, and delivery methods allow for a distinct adverse effect profile compared to those seen in most controlled clinical trials. In the clinical setting, adverse effects are typically seen as a communication from the patient's physiology that can guide fine-tuning of their treatment plan.

The adverse effects listed in Table 18.3 were described in a systematic review of 79 randomized clinical trials (62 of which reported data on adverse effects) that compared cannabinoids (including inhaled cannabis, nabiximols, dronabinol, nabilone, CBD, and others) with usual care, placebo, or no treatment, arranged in order of highest odds.[27] None of the studies evaluated the long-term profile of adverse effects.

TABLE 18.3
Review of Adverse Effects in Clinical Trials

Adverse effect	Summary odds ratio	95% CI	No. of studies	No. of patients
Disorientation	5.41	[2.61–11.19]	12	1736
Dizziness	5.09	[4.10–6.32]	41	4243
Euphoria	4.08	[2.18–7.64]	27	2420
Confusion	4.03	[2.05–7.97]	12	1160
Drowsiness	3.68	[2.24–6.01]	18	1272
Dry mouth	3.50	[2.58–4.75]	36	4181
Somnolence	2.83	[2.05–391]	26	3168
Balance	2.62	[1.12–6.13]	6	920
Hallucination	2.19	[1.02–4.68]	10	898
Nausea	2.08	[1.63–2.65]	30	3579

Adverse effect	Summary odds ratio	95% CI	No. of studies	No. of patients
Paranoia[a]	2.05	[0.42–10.10]	4	492
Asthenia	2.03	[1.35–3.06]	15	1717
Fatigue	2.00	[1.54–2.62]	20	2717
Anxiety[a]	1.98	[0.73–5.35]	12	1242
Vomiting	1.67	[1.13–2.47]	17	2191
Diarrhea	1.65	[1.04–2.62]	12	2077
Depression[a]	1.32	[0.87–2.01]	15	2353
Psychosis[a]	1.09	[0.07–16.35]	2	37
Seizures[a]	0.91	[0.05–15.66]	2	42
Dyspnea[a]	0.83	[0.26–2.63]	4	375

[a] Not statistically significant (odds ratio confidence interval crosses 1).

Data on adverse effects of long-term oromucosal THC/CBD have been reported by an observational registry to collect safety data from patients receiving nabiximols in the United Kingdom, Germany, and Switzerland, where the drug is approved for the treatment of multiple sclerosis spasticity. The registry contained data from 941 patients with 2,214 patient-years of exposure, among which 123 cases of adverse effects were recorded as being treatment-related in the opinion of the prescribing physician.[28] The total treatment-related adverse effects by system, and the most common individual treatment-related adverse effects are summarized in Table 18.4. There were no signals to indicate abuse, diversion, dependence, or long-term cognitive impairment. Driving ability was reported to have worsened in 2% of patients but improved in 7%.

TABLE 18.4

Adverse Effects of Long-Term Nabiximols in Patients with MS

Treatment-related adverse effect	Percentage of patients in registry
NERVOUS SYSTEM DISORDERS	Total 5.8
Dizziness	2.3
Dysgeusia	1.0
Somnolence	0.9

Treatment-related adverse effect	Percentage of patients in registry	
GASTROINTESTINAL DISORDERS	Total	3.4
Nausea		1.1
PSYCHIATRIC DISORDERS	Total	2.9
Depressed mood		0.8
Anxiety		0.5
Depression		0.3
GENERAL DISORDERS AND ADMINISTRATION SITE CONDITIONS	Total	2.8
Fatigue		1.7
Falls requiring medical attention		0.6

Oral Health

Often overlooked as a potential adverse effect, detrimental effects on oral health have been associated with long-term cannabis use. For example, frequent cannabis use is associated with deeper periodontal pockets, greater attachment loss, and a higher risk of having severe periodontitis. Periodontitis may occur at earlier ages in cannabis users when compared to the general population. Cannabis users who also use tobacco may have higher incidence of caries on smooth tooth surfaces compared to tobacco-only users.[29,30]

Xerostomia is an independent strong risk factor for dental caries and is likely a major mechanism by which cannabis use can negatively impact oral health. CB1 signaling on salivary glands has been shown to reduce parasympathetic activity and saliva flow.[31] One study found 70% of participants reported dry mouth after smoking cannabis,[32] and another reported that dry mouth symptoms can last 1–6 hr after use.[33]

Most of the data on cannabis and oral health are derived from individuals smoking cannabis for nontherapeutic purposes, and implications may be different for those using oromucosal or oral delivery methods. I frequently ask my patients if they experience dry mouth in the period after using cannabis, and many report this initial side effect resolves after a couple of weeks of use. For those experiencing persistent dry mouth, I recommend a particular lozenge product containing hyaluronic acid and slippery elm bark, which keeps the oral cavity moist and lubricated.

Drug Interactions

Numerous in vitro and in vivo studies indicate that cannabinoids can act upon cyto-chrome P450 isozymes to affect the metabolism of various drugs. A systematic review showed that THC and cannabinol (CBN) are metabolized primarily by CYP2C9 and CYP3A4, and CBD is metabolized primarily by CYP2C19 and CYP3A4.[34] Cannabis smoking may induce CYP1A2, similar to tobacco smoking, which can increase clearance of theophylline.[35]

Beyond cytochrome P450 enzymes, in vitro interactions have been identified with membrane transporters: breast cancer–resistant protein, glycoprotein P, and multidrug resistance proteins. These transporters are upregulated with short exposure and down-regulated with chronic exposure to cannabinoids, but the concentrations of cannabinoids used in these studies are higher than those commonly measured in cannabis users, so the clinical relevance of these data is unknown.[36] Supraphysiological concentrations of CBD and CBN have been shown to inhibit UDP-glucuronosyltransferases (UGTs); on the basis of these data, cannabinoid–ethanol interactions are unlikely to occur in vivo. The effects of cannabinoids on other UGT substrates, such as some opioids and benzodiaze-pines, remain to be determined, both in vitro and in vivo.[37]

These predominantly preclinical data are limited in their relevance to clinical prac-tice. Results from the few available clinical studies indicate a risk for cannabis–drug interaction via inhibition of hepatic CYP2C19[38] (N-desmethylclobazam and hexobarbi-tal) and CYP3A4 (ketoconazole, a 3A4 inhibitor, and rifampicin, a 3A4 inducer) by CBD.[39] Case reports involving warfarin suggest a risk for interaction with cannabis via inhibition of hepatic CYP2C9.[40]

Additional clinical data on the interaction of CBD with antiepileptic drugs show increases in serum levels of topiramate, rufinamide, N-desmethylclobazam, zonisamide, and eslicarbazepine, and decreases in clobazam levels, with increasing CBD dose. Except for clobazam and N-desmethylclobazam, all mean level changes were within the accepted therapeutic range. Sedation was more frequent with higher N-desmethylcloba-zam levels in adults, and aspartate aminotransferase/alanine aminotransferase levels were significantly higher in participants taking valproate.[41]

Statins, though not mentioned in Table 18.5, are perhaps the most common and relevant drugs to consider for cannabis-related interactions. Most statins, including simvastatin, lovastatin, and atorvastatin, are metabolized by CYP3A4, and the risks of adverse effects, such as myopathy, increase when they are taken with drugs that inhibit CYP3A4.[42] Fluvastatin is primarily metabolized by CYP2C9 and may similarly interact with cannabis. Because I treat a large number of patients with chronic pain, including myalgia, who present already taking the maximum allowed daily dose of these agents, I frequently discuss alternatives with their prescriber, including switching to pravastatin (metabolized by other routes), reducing the dose of the current statin, or adding coenzyme Q10[43] to mitigate potential interactions or contributions of the statin to ongoing pain and fatigue.

Indomethacin has been shown to significantly attenuate the subjective "high" and the heart-rate-accelerating effects of THC and abolish the profound effect of THC on time estimation and production, but it does not affect the decremental effects of THC on word recall in humans.[44] In rabbits, indomethacin attenuated THC-induced decreases in intraocular pressure.[45] It is unclear whether other nonsteroidal anti-inflammatory drugs have similar interactions with THC, though many of my patients report additive benefits when they combine the two drugs.

Due to the anti-inflammatory and immunomodulating effects of cannabis, caution should be used in combination with immunotherapies, especially those designed to increase immune activity. For example, nivolumab, approved for the treatment of numerous types of cancer, is a monoclonal antibody to programmed cell death protein 1 that ultimately promotes immune system–mediated killing of tumor cells. Concomitant glucocorticoids and other immunosuppressants may alter the effectiveness of such treatments by undermining their mechanism of action, and these immunosuppressants are thus used sparingly and only when needed to address severe adverse effects (e.g., colitis, hepatitis, pneumonitis, nephritis, and encephalitis).[46] The impact of glucocorticoids on response rate (RR) has surprisingly been poorly monitored in cancer immunotherapy trials[47] but likely has a stronger impact than that of cannabinoids.

In a retrospective analysis of 140 patients (89 taking nivolumab alone, 51 taking nivolumab plus cannabis) with advanced melanoma, non-small-cell lung cancer, and renal clear cell carcinoma, cannabis was the only significant factor that reduced response rate to immunotherapy: 37.5% RR in nivolumab alone versus 15.9% RR in the nivolumab–cannabis group (p = .016, OR = 3.13, 95% confidence interval [CI] 1.24–8.1).[48] This potential interaction requires a delicate risk–benefit assessment, since in my clinical experience, I have found that low-dose cannabis may mitigate or prevent inflammatory adverse reactions to the immunotherapy, potentially allowing a patient to complete a course of treatment or avoid the use of glucocorticoids. I recommend that my patients avoid high-dose cannabis when taking nivolumab and other cancer immunotherapies and that they consider halting any cannabis use several days prior to and following the immunotherapy infusion.

Table 18.5 is adapted from the prescribing information of FDA-approved CBD (Epidiolex) and THC (dronabinol). Most online drug interaction checkers include these two drugs, and many include "cannabis" as well. Keep in mind that while these tools and the following information can be helpful, we still face many unknowns, likely complicated by the broad dosing range of cannabinoids, pharmacogenetic interactions, and diverse phytochemical composition of herbal preparations.

TABLE 18.5
Drug Interactions with Cannabis

Cannabinoid	Enzymes	Specific drug or class	Interactions
THC	CYP2C9, CYP3A4	Alcohol	THC may enhance the CNS depressant effect of alcohol.
		Amphotericin B	THC may displace amphotericin B from its protein-binding sites, leading to an increased concentration of active, unbound drug.
		Anticholinergic agents	These agents may enhance the tachycardic effect of THC-containing products.
		CNS depressants	THC may enhance the effects of CNS depressants.
		Cyclosporine (systemic)	THC may displace cyclosporine from its protein-binding sites, leading to an increased concentration of active, unbound drug.
		Ritonavir	Ritonavir may increase the serum concentration of THC.
		Sympathomimetics	THC may enhance the tachycardic effects of these drugs.
		Warfarin	THC may displace warfarin from its protein-binding sites, leading to an increased concentration of active, unbound drug.
CBD	CYP3A4, CYP2C19, CYP1A2, CYP2B6, CYP2C8, CYP2C9, UGT1A9, UGT2B7	Clobazam	Coadministration of CBD produces a 3-fold increase in plasma concentrations of *N*-desmethylclobazam, the active metabolite of clobazam (a substrate of CYP2C19). This may increase the risk of clobazam-related adverse reactions.

Cannabinoid	Enzymes	Specific drug or class	Interactions
CBD		Valproate	Concomitant use of CBD and valproate increases the incidence of liver enzyme elevations. Discontinuation or reduction of CBD or concomitant valproate should be considered.
		CNS depressants and alcohol	Concomitant use of CBD with other CNS depressants may increase the risk of sedation and somnolence.

On the basis of the preceding data and my clinical experience, clinicians should be most vigilant for drug interactions in patients who frequently use inhaled cannabis, since this produces higher serum concentrations of cannabinoids, or moderate to high-dose oral or oromucosal cannabinoids (≥ 1 mg·kg^{-1}·day^{-1}).

Problematic Use

Cannabis clinicians can play a role in identifying individuals with problematic cannabis use patterns and in remediating use patterns to reduce harm and improve benefit. While the risk of developing cannabis use disorder (CUD) among those using cannabis for therapeutic purposes under medical supervision appears to be low, any therapeutic agent with the potential for rewarding effects and withdrawal syndrome must be wielded with care.

The 2016 National Survey on Drug Use and Health[49] estimated that nearly 24 million Americans ages 12 and older were current cannabis users, defined as any use in the past month. This represents close to 9% of the household population in that age range, an increasing trend since 2002 attributed to an increase in adult use (age ≥ 18 years). Among youth ages 12–17, the trend decreased over the same time frame, from 8.2% reporting current use in 2002 to 6.5% in 2016. Of the 24 million current users, about 4 million (16.6%) met the criteria for CUD, corresponding to 1.5% of the U.S. population ages 12 and older.

Over the course of a lifetime, about 9% of people who ever use cannabis will develop CUD (i.e., either abuse or dependence), much lower than the rates of other substances with abuse potential (see Figure 18.1).[50] This rate of CUD is likely inflated by court-mandated drug treatment during cannabis prohibition: admitting to cannabis misuse and undergoing drug addiction education or treatment is a common alternative to more severe penalties for nonabusers caught with their medicine or substance of choice.

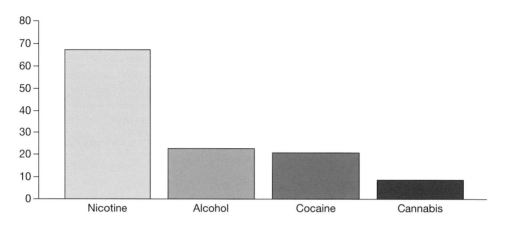

FIGURE 18.1
Lifetime Cumulative Probability Estimate:
Transition to Dependence

Note. Chart created by Dustin Sulak, with data from "Probability and predictors of transition from first use to dependence on nicotine, alcohol, cannabis, and cocaine: Results of the National Epidemiologic Survey on Alcohol and Related Conditions (NESARC)," by C. Lopez-Quintero, J. P. de los Cobos, D. S. Hasin, M. Okuda, S. Wang, B. F. Grant, and C. Blanco, 2011, *Drug and Alcohol Dependence*, 115(1–2), pp. 120–130 (https://doi .org/10.1016/j.drugalcdep.2010.11.004). Copyright © 2011 by Elsevier.

A comprehensive report in 2017 by The National Academies of Sciences, Engineering and Medicine reviewed the literature to identify risk factors involved in the development or exacerbation of problematic cannabis use;[51] these are summarized in Table 18.6.

TABLE 18.6
Risk Factors for Problematic Cannabis Use

Risk factor	Not a risk factor
SUBSTANTIAL EVIDENCE	
Male gender	Stimulant treatment of attention deficit hyperactivity disorder (ADHD) during adolescence
Cigarette smoking	
Initiation of cannabis use at an earlier age	
Increase in cannabis use frequency	
MODERATE EVIDENCE	
Major depressive disorder	Anxiety, personality disorders, and bipolar disorders

Risk factor	Not a risk factor
Exposure to the combined use of abused drugs	Adolescent ADHD
History of psychiatric treatment	Alcohol or nicotine dependence
In adolescents: 　Frequent cannabis use 　Oppositional behaviors 　Younger age of first alcohol use 　Nicotine use 　Parental substance use 　Poor school performance 　Antisocial behaviors	
Childhood sexual abuse	

How common is it for medically supervised cannabis users to transition to cannabis use disorder? While the answer is not clear, existing data suggest this is very uncommon. Beyond the risk factors listed above, I believe failure to regularly follow up, declining self-management strategies, and other expressions of low self-efficacy are the most important warning signs for problematic use.

Inhaled THC-dominant cannabis is the fastest onset and most rewarding delivery method, so patients with a history of substance abuse, other addictive tendencies, or the risk factors described above who require inhaled cannabis need closer monitoring. In my experience, joint smoking, dabs, and vape pens are most likely to build tolerance, while flower vaporizers and single inhalations from a pipe are often used more responsibly at the lowest effective dose. This is not to say that patients with addiction history must abstain from inhaled cannabis; the rapid onset of effects may be the best harm reduction strategy for mitigating cravings and preventing relapse with more dangerous substances.

Noninhaled delivery is likely the safest route for patients at risk for problematic use. In a long-term registry of 941 patients using nabiximols for MS-related spasticity with 2,214 patient-years of exposure, there were no signs of abuse, dependence, or diversion.[52] A postmarketing review of dronabinol did not find the drug associated with abuse or diversion and described very low abuse potential.[53]

Though it may not show up in long-term nabiximols and dronabinol data, another study does suggest abuse potential for oral and oromucosal routes of delivery, at least in high doses. In a single-dose, randomized, double-blind, crossover study, 23 heavy cannabis users were given nabiximols THC + CBD (THC content 10.8, 21.6, or 43.2 mg) or dronabinol (THC content 20 or 40 mg), compared with placebo, with subjective and cognitive or psychomotor abuse potential measures administered over 24 hr postdose. The low dose of nabiximols was not significantly different from placebo on any primary abuse potential end points. The middle dose had significantly greater scores only on Drug Liking and Subjective Drug Value compared with placebo, and the high dose was significantly different from the placebo on all primary end points other than Drug Liking. When roughly equivalent THC doses of nabiximols and dronabinol were compared, abuse potential measures were higher in the dronabinol groups.[54] While THC (10 mg) + CBD (10 mg) was the lowest dose of nabiximols in the study, I would consider this a moderate single dose in my practice, and it is comforting that this dose showed no abuse potential. The data also suggest that combining CBD with THC reduces the abuse potential.

In my experience, patients at risk for problematic use are easily identified in their initial or first follow-up visit. While I do infrequently see patients in my practice who abuse cannabis, I do not think I have ever observed this in a patient who gave no warning signs at the beginning of our relationship. Unlike many of the agents cannabis frequently replaces (e.g., opioids and benzodiazepines), I have not observed cannabis leading patients with no clear risk factors or abuse history down the slippery slope of dependence and addiction.

Cannabis Use Disorder

The *Diagnostic and Statistical Manual of Mental Disorders, Fifth Edition* (*DSM-5*), of the American Psychiatric Association defines cannabis use disorder as a problematic pattern of cannabis use leading to clinically significant impairment or distress, as manifested by at least two of the following, occurring within a 12-month period:

- Cannabis is often taken in larger amounts or over a longer period than was intended.
- There is a persistent desire or unsuccessful efforts to cut down or control cannabis use.
- A great deal of time is spent in activities necessary to obtain cannabis, use cannabis, or recover from its effects.
- Craving, or a strong desire or urge to use cannabis, is experienced.
- Recurrent cannabis use results in a failure to fulfill major role obligations at work, school, or home.
- Cannabis use continues despite having persistent or recurrent social or interpersonal problems caused or exacerbated by the effects of cannabis.
- Important social, occupational, or recreational activities are given up or reduced because of cannabis use.

- Cannabis is used recurrently in situations in which it is physically hazardous.
- Cannabis use is continued despite knowledge of having a persistent or recurrent physical or psychological problem that is likely to have been caused or exacerbated by cannabis.
- Tolerance is experienced, defined by either (1) a need for markedly increased amounts of cannabis to achieve intoxication or desired effect or (2) markedly diminished effect with continued use of the same amount of cannabis.
- Withdrawal is experienced, manifested by either (1) the characteristic withdrawal syndrome for cannabis or (2) use of cannabis to relieve or avoid withdrawal symptoms.

Withdrawal

Cannabis withdrawal occurs reliably in rodents, nonhuman primates, and a subset of cannabis users following abrupt cessation of frequent cannabis use. Symptoms of cannabis withdrawal are mostly behavioral and affective: they include irritability, anger, or aggression; nervousness or anxiety; sleep difficulty (e.g., insomnia, strange or vivid dreams); decreased appetite or weight loss; restlessness; and depressed mood. Physical symptoms include abdominal or stomach pain, shakiness or tremors, sweating, fever, chills, and headache, but these are experienced less frequently.[55]

Symptoms emerge within 24–48 hr after cessation, reach peak intensity on days 2–5, and resolve within 2–3 weeks, though sleep difficulties may persist. Compared with other drug withdrawal syndromes, cannabis withdrawal is most similar to tobacco withdrawal, but with a more gradual emergence and peak intensity. Some data have demonstrated sex differences in cannabis withdrawal: women may experience increased symptom intensity and number of symptoms, especially nausea, compared to men.[56]

The prevalence of withdrawal is difficult to determine, but clearly not all regular cannabis users experience withdrawal symptoms upon cessation. In a survey of 469 adult non-treatment-seeking cannabis smokers who had made attempts to quit, only 42.6% reported ever having experienced withdrawal.[57] The authors reviewed previous studies that reported prevalence in the range 15.6%–95.5%, and they suggested these differences are related to differences in the rates of true cannabis dependence and in substance abuse and psychiatric comorbidity among the various study populations. Diagnostic criteria for cannabis withdrawal are summarized in Table 18.7.

TABLE 18.7
DSM-5 Cannabis Withdrawal Diagnostic Criteria[58]

Criterion	Description
A	Cessation of cannabis use that has been heavy and prolonged (i.e., usually daily or almost daily use over a period of at least a few months)
B	Three (or more) of the following signs and symptoms develop within approximately 1 week after Criterion A: 1. Irritability, anger, or aggression 2. Nervousness or anxiety 3. Sleep difficulty (e.g., insomnia, disturbing dreams) 4. Decreased appetite or weight loss 5. Restlessness 6. Depressed mood 7. At least one of the following physical symptoms causing significant discomfort: abdominal pain, shakiness/tremors, sweating, fever, chills, or headache
C	The signs and symptoms in Criterion B cause clinically significant distress or impairment in social, occupational, or other important areas of functioning
D	The signs or symptoms are not attributable to another condition and are not better explained by another mental disorder, including intoxication or withdrawal from another substance.

Source. Reprinted with permission from the Diagnostic and Statistical Manual of Mental Disorders, Fifth Edition, (Copyright © 2013). American Psychiatric Association. All Rights Reserved.

Among medical users, withdrawal prevalence is even more difficult to discern due to the baseline symptoms, which may cause functional impairment and are likely exacerbated with cannabis abstinence. A recent study surveyed 665 patients using medical cannabis to treat chronic pain at least once weekly over 3 months, 87% of whom endorsed daily or near-daily use. Sixty-seven percent of respondents reported experiencing at least one moderate or severe withdrawal symptom. The most commonly observed symptom was sleep difficulties (50.3%), followed by anxiety (27.8%), irritability (26.7%), and appetite disturbance (25.2%). Only 1.8% of the sample met the Alcohol, Smoking and Substance Involvement Screening Test threshold of having a probable cannabis use disorder.[59]

In my experience, patients who build tolerance to cannabis are the most likely to experience withdrawal, probably due to CB1 receptor downregulation. Supporting this observation, an imaging study in cannabis-dependent men found that lower CB1 receptor density (presumably due to greater CB1 receptor downregulation) was associated with more severe cannabis withdrawal symptoms on the second day of abstinence, the time when peak withdrawal effects are typically observed.[60] While most publications compare cannabis withdrawal to nicotine withdrawal, several of my patients familiar with both dispute the similarity, preferring to compare cannabis withdrawal to caffeine withdrawal.

Not surprisingly, pharmaceutical cannabinoids (nabilone, dronabinol, nabiximols) have been shown to be relatively safe and effective for treating cannabis withdrawal.[61] I suspect with further study these agents will also prove effective for treating cannabis use disorder, primarily because they are inherently medically supervised, less rewarding, and less likely to build tolerance than inhaled cannabis.

Impairment and Driving

Similar to the use of any psychoactive medication, patients using cannabis are instructed to avoid driving or engagement in any hazardous activity until they know how a particular dose of a particular cannabis formulation affects them. While cannabis can certainly produce psychomotor disturbances that impair driving, regular users of specific doses often experience tachyphylaxis to these adverse effects while maintaining therapeutic efficacy.

Two recent meta-analyses have reviewed the extensive data on the association between cannabis use and driving accidents. One found no significant association between driving under the influence of cannabis and the risk of various unfavorable traffic events.[62] Another found cannabis-impaired driving was associated with a statistically significant increased risk of motor-vehicle crash of low-to-moderate magnitude: OR = 1.36 (95% CI 1.15–1.61).[63]

To put this in perspective, texting while driving was associated with more than double the risk of crash (OR 2.22, 95% CI 1.07–4.63)[64]; in older adults ≥70 years, cell phone use was associated with almost a 4-fold increase in the likelihood of having a major crash (OR = 3.79, 95% CI 1.00–14.37).[65] Though it is clear that cell phones are a greater driving hazard than cannabis, I do not mean to suggest that cannabis is harmless.

Like the other adverse effects of cannabis and as demonstrated by studies on cannabis and impairment, the risk of a cannabis-related accident is greatest in the cannabis-naïve, after a dosage increase, or during the acute effects of inhaled THC. Based on driving simulation data, cannabis-related impairment typically involves tracking tasks, for which drivers can compensate by reducing the difficulty of the task, that is, by slowing down. Higher cognitive functions and integration processes, such as divided attention tasks, are less likely to be impacted by cannabis. Importantly, simulation studies show that drivers under the influence of cannabis are aware of their impairment, allowing them to compensate by slowing down or avoiding driving.[66] This is distinct from those under the influence of alcohol, who are often unaware of their impairment, which does impact higher cognitive functions and integration tasks.

The most commonly reported changes in driving associated with cannabis use are decreased speed and variability in lane position and headway. A recent study in young nondaily cannabis users did not find any residual effects 24 and 48 hr after smoking and found only decreased speed 30 min after smoking.[67]

Unlike alcohol, but like most other psychoactive substances, there is no blood level of THC that can determine impairment. Several jurisdictions have adopted per se policies limiting blood THC to <5 µg/L. This limit is unscientific due to the pronounced variability in results depending on blood collection time after inhalation; THC is rapidly metabolized to 11-OH-THC and COOH-THC. Among 302 toxicologically confirmed cannabis-only cases that underwent Drug Recognition Expert (DRE) examination, compared to controls, the 5 µg/L per se limit was irrelevant. The finger-to-nose and Modified Romberg Balance eyelid tremor results were the best tests to predict cannabis impairment.[68]

The goals of people using cannabis for nontherapeutic purposes (e.g., euphoria) are often different than those of medical cannabis patients, who typically use cannabis in an effort to improve function. Depending on the symptoms being addressed by cannabis, this may include improvement in driving function. A review of nabiximols driving studies and real-world registries found no evidence of an increase in motor vehicle accidents associated with THC/CBD oromucosal spray.[69] The majority of patients reported an improvement in driving ability after starting THC/CBD oromucosal spray, perhaps due to reduced spasticity or better cognitive function.

Other experts have also observed that medical cannabis patients, using daily, appropriate low doses of THC, develop tolerance and experience minimal if any impairment.[70]

More concerningly, in a cohort of 790 patients using cannabis for chronic pain, 56.4% reported driving within 2 hr of using cannabis; driving while "a little high" was reported by 50.5%, and driving while "very high" was reported by 21.1%.[71] While the term "very high" lacks a concrete definition, I suspect that most of these respondents were at increased risk for crash while driving in that state.

Some patients and clinicians may expect that using CBD in conjunction with THC will mitigate the potential driving risks. This was not the case in a randomized, double-blind crossover trial of 14 healthy volunteers with a history of light (≤2 times/week in the previous 3 months) cannabis use. Vaporization of 125 mg of THC-dominant (11% THC, <1% CBD), THC/CBD equivalent (11% THC, 11% CBD), or placebo (<1% THC/CBD) cannabis were compared. Both active cannabis groups had increases in lane-weaving but no detriment on other driving performance measures. Subjects performed worse on two of the cognitive assessments with THC/CBD, and peak plasma THC concentrations were higher following THC/CBD, likely a pharmacokinetic interaction.[72]

In summary, it is important to remind patients not to engage in driving or hazardous activity after an adjustment to their cannabis dosage. Regular users should also be cautious after taking >24-hr break and may choose to restart at a slightly lower dose. Patients with diminished judgement or self-awareness are more likely to put themselves and others at risk, while most patients impaired by cannabis are able to recognize their impairment and compensate accordingly. Per se THC blood level limits are not supported by science, and the presence of CBD may not mitigate THC-related driving impairment. Patients appropriately using cannabis may experience improvements in driving ability, and if legal to do so in their jurisdiction, appropriately dosed THC and CBD can safely be used before driving.

Impact on Mental Health

Are medical cannabis users more likely to develop mental or cognitive health disorders? While the literature on medical use of cannabis and mental health outcomes is substantially less developed than that of nonmedical use, one 2017 systematic review comprehensively evaluated studies of cannabis for therapeutic purposes (CTP) for outcomes related to anxiety, depression, and neurocognition:[73]

- **Anxiety:** Of the eight cross-sectional studies that evaluated anxiety as a primary or secondary end point, all reported anxiolysis, and one reported recurrence of anxiety upon cessation of cannabis.
- **Depression:** Of the nine cross-sectional studies that evaluated depressed mood, seven noted mood improvement among the beneficial effects of CTP, with benefits consistent across pain, multiple sclerosis, and other diverse conditions. One study reported a positive association between depression severity and problematic CTP use.
- **Neurocognition:** One high-quality prospective cohort study of CTP for management of noncancer chronic pain, with 200 participants using a median of 2.5 g daily, reported no significant differences in neurocognitive functioning between cannabis users and controls at 1 year poststudy. Among studies that compared users of nonmedical cannabis to nonusers after 25 days or more of supervised abstinence, there were no lasting residual effects on neurocognitive performance, perhaps in parallel to the reversal of downregulation of cannabinoid receptors from chronic cannabis use.

Several studies have evaluated correlations between cannabis use and neurocognition in people with human immunodeficiency virus (HIV). This population, which experiences higher rates of neurocognitive decline than the general population, may illustrate the complex interaction between cannabis-related impairment and neuroprotection. In one study of 952 individuals, 71% with HIV and 16% who used cannabis, cannabis was associated with less neurocognitive impairment in the people living with HIV, who had similar rates of neurocognitive impairment to both cannabis users and nonusers without HIV.[74] Other studies have found null or adverse effects of cannabis on cognition in people living with HIV, but the adverse findings occurred selectively among frequent cannabis users (3+ times per day), on specific cognitive domains (delayed recall, learning), and in those with advanced or symptomatic HIV.[75,76] Two of the studies correlated cannabis use with higher performance in verbal fluency.

In the first neuroimaging study of medical cannabis users, 22 patients, average age 50 years, who elected to use cannabis to treat pain, anxiety, posttraumatic stress disorder (PTSD), sleep, and other conditions, were evaluated with functional magnetic resonance imaging and neurocognitive tests prior to and 3 months after initiation of cannabis use. Remarkably, brain activation patterns normalized after treatment, appearing more similar to those exhibited by healthy controls than the pretreatment patterns. The changes were accompanied by improved task performance as well as positive changes in ratings of clinical state, impulsivity, sleep, and quality of life, as well as notable decreases in their use of conventional medications, including opioids.[77]

Does cannabis use, medical or nonmedical, cause psychosis? High doses of THC can absolutely induce transient, acute psychotic symptoms in psychiatrically well individuals. Intravenous THC (2.5 mg) given to healthy men, which resulted in average blood THC levels (Cmax) of 177 ng/ml, caused an increase in positive psychotic symptoms, unrelated to anxiety,[78] and negative psychotic symptoms, unrelated to sedation.[79] Both resolved within 2 hr. While these blood levels are similar to those seen with cannabis inhalation, I suspect the rapid peak levels of iv administration, even faster than inhalation, contributed to the intensity of effects. I have observed high doses of inhaled cannabis cause psychotic symptoms in a psychiatrically well cannabis-naïve individual, but after interviewing thousands of cannabis patients over a decade, this appears to be infrequent. Subjects with experience using cannabis in the past (but not within 24 hr of the study) demonstrated fewer psychotic symptoms in the aforementioned study. While this may be related to cannabis tolerance, I suspect it had more to do with developing a greater ability to maintain cognitive function under cannabis-induced nonordinary states of awareness.

Does cannabis use, medical or nonmedical, cause psychotic disorders? This question has been the subject of much debate, epidemiological studies, and numerous review articles. Several studies have identified an association between cannabis use and schizophrenia. Some data indicate cannabis use during adolescence may cause an earlier age of onset of psychosis than would have occurred in the absence of cannabis use.[80] One study found a direct association between age of onset of cannabis use and age of onset of psychosis;[81] another found an association between self-reported cannabis use and future hospital admission for schizophrenia, with a dose-dependent relationship between frequency of cannabis use and risk for schizophrenia.[82]

None of these associations provide strong evidence of causality, and several studies dispute the theory that cannabis causes psychosis, but it is important to note that it would be difficult to prove causality without experimental control of cannabis use and the numerous behaviors associated with cannabis use in large populations. Instead of assuming causality, which was done but barely mentioned in a highly publicized 2019 multicenter case–control study that concluded 12% of psychosis could be prevented by prohibiting high-potency cannabis,[83] and instead of refuting causality, a deeper look into a complex topic is warranted.

Epidemiological data from a different perspective dispute causality. Numerous studies have found that increases in population cannabis use have not been associated with increases in psychotic incidence, which has generally been stable over time.[84] While other factors may account for this discrepancy, one would imagine that a consistent increase in population cannabis use would produce a signal in schizophrenia prevalence if there were a causal relationship.

One creative study compared four cohorts: 87 nonpsychotic controls with no drug use, 84 nonpsychotic controls with adolescent cannabis use, 32 patients with a schizophrenia spectrum psychosis with no drug use, and 76 patients with a schizophrenia spectrum psychosis with adolescent cannabis use. None of the subjects used any other substance except alcohol (one distinguishing aspect of these data). On the basis of their findings and previous data, the authors concluded that in genetically vulnerable individuals, while cannabis can hasten the onset and modify the severity and outcome of psychotic disorders, there was no evidence that cannabis can cause the psychosis. Rather, there was an increased risk for psychotic disorders in relatives of both cannabis-using and non-cannabis-using patients with this condition.[85]

A 2016 review of recent data evaluated the two main hypotheses explaining the relationship between cannabis and schizophrenia: cannabis as a contributing cause and shared vulnerability. The authors concluded that the evidence reviewed did not support the contributing cause hypothesis, but it much more strongly supported the theory that early and heavy patterns of cannabis use are more likely in individuals with a vulnerability to a variety of other problem behaviors, like early or heavy use of other drugs and poor school performance, and that in some individuals the same vulnerability also results in increased risk for psychosis or other mental disorders. They suggested that early or heavy cannabis use and associated problem behaviors may be prodromal signs of psychotic and other mental disorders.[86]

Two gene polymorphisms appear to modulate the association between cannabis use and psychotic disorders. The C/C genotype of a specific polymorphism (rs2494732) in the gene that codes for AKT1, a pathway stimulated by CB1 and CB2 agonism that is involved in a number of cellular processes, is associated with higher overall rates of psychotic disorders, higher rates of cannabis use in schizophrenic patients, higher rates of psychosis in cannabis users, and increased cognitive side effects from cannabis use. The Val158/108Met genotype of COMT, an enzyme that degrades catecholamines, results in more rapid degradation of dopamine. In a large prospective study, individuals with the Val/Val allele had 10 times the risk of developing psychosis in association with cannabis use, and two experimental studies have found that this allele increases the likelihood of acute psychosis with exposure to THC. Numerous and better-powered subsequent studies, however, have failed to confirm these findings.[87] I suspect that complex interactions between genetics and environment may increase one's susceptibility to either or both the contributing cause or shared vulnerability hypotheses.

Other authors have suggested that patients with subclinical psychotic disorders attempt to self-medicate with cannabis, contributing to the temporal association with age of first use of cannabis, typically occurring 5 or more years before the first psychotic episode. This is supported by data that associate cannabis use in schizophrenic patients with less negative symptomatology.[88,89,90]

If cannabis does cause schizophrenia, how many individuals prevented from using cannabis would be required to prevent one case? According to data from a meta-analysis that found an adjusted risk ratio of 2.1 between "heavy cannabis users" and psychosis outcome compared to nonusers, combined with epidemiological data from England and Wales, the number needed to prevent psychosis ranges from 2,800 in the highest risk group (men age 20–24) to 10,870 in the lowest risk group (women age 35–39).[91] I hope these numbers give confidence to clinicians that a cannabis-related iatrogenic cause of a psychotic disorder is very unlikely.

I strongly suspect that one's cannabis use pattern significantly modulates this and other mental health–related risks. If a person predisposed to mental illness overuses cannabis, downregulating the endocannabinoid system (ECS) and undermining the nervous system's capacity for homeostasis, I would not be surprised if this could worsen or hasten the onset of their condition. Conversely, if appropriately dosed cannabis is used to reduce symptoms, improve function, improve sleep, and modulate neurological inflammation, I suspect this would be protective.

In summary, the impact of medically supervised cannabis use on mental health outcomes is likely different from that of nonmedical or problematic use. Appropriately treated medical users are more likely to experience improvements than deteriorations in anxiety, depression, and neurocognition. A causal link between nonmedical cannabis use and psychotic disorders has not been proven, though there are likely some genetic and environmental factors that increase the potential for cannabis to hasten the onset of psychotic disorders. Individuals with a family history of psychotic disorders may be more vulnerable to this very low risk. Patients with personal or family history of mental illness warrant closer monitoring, collaboration with their mental health providers, and guidance to avoid building tolerance to the therapeutic effects of cannabis.

Fertility

Evidence that cannabis use has clinically significant adverse effects on human male or female[92] fertility is lacking. The hypothesis that cannabis use impacts fertility is based on preclinical data showing that cannabinoids can alter endocrine function, that ECS signaling is critical in all stages of pregnancy, and that chronic cannabinoid administration can impair reproductive function. The strongest human findings related to fertility are alterations in sperm function and semen parameters.[93] Studies have found reduced sperm count and concentration, morphological changes, reduced motility and viability, and decreased fertilizing capacity in animals and humans exposed to cannabis or cannabinoids. Some data suggest that while cannabis may increase the libido of men in some cases, chronic use may be associated with decreased erectile function.[94]

It is possible that the effects of cannabis use on sperm and semen function may cross the threshold of clinically relevant among those whose fertility is already impaired, but the results of human research in this context are limited and inconsistent. When treating either male or female moderate to heavy cannabis users with impaired fertility, I consider a period of cannabis abstinence a worthwhile trial to improve fertility. For the general population using cannabis for medical purposes, I do not believe the current data support discussing impaired fertility as a potential adverse effect.

Pregnancy

Our understanding of the impact of cannabis use during pregnancy and lactation is limited to observational data and therefore full of confounders, since experimental research would be unethical. As such, causality of any associated outcomes cannot be proven. In most cases, the observational data lack information on dosage, delivery method, trimester, and duration of cannabis use, providing little guidance in our understanding of the risks associated with medically supervised, maternal use of nonsmoked cannabis.

Furthermore, most of the observational data rely on self-reported cannabis use. There are many reasons why a mother would choose not to disclose her cannabis use, and I suspect behavioral characteristics that may make a mother more or less likely to do so could impact other outcomes. In a 2019 retrospective cohort study that included urine toxicology data in 90.5% of 1206 pregnant young women, perhaps the highest rate published, cannabis use was self-reported in only 78 of the 211 cannabis users.[95] Unfortunately, the unreliability of maternal self-reporting makes the following findings much less informative.

The 2017 National Academies of Sciences, Engineering and Medicine (NASEM) report[96] performed an analysis of the available data, with an emphasis on data since 1999, and reached the following conclusions:

- There is limited evidence of a statistical association between maternal cannabis smoking and pregnancy complications for the mother.
- There is substantial evidence of a statistical association between maternal cannabis smoking and lower birth weight of offspring.
- There is insufficient evidence to support or refute a statistical association between maternal cannabis smoking and later outcomes in offspring (e.g., sudden infant death syndrome, cognition, academic achievement, and later substance use).

Regarding maternal complications, increased risk of anemia was the only complication that had a significant association with exposure to cannabis (pooled odds ratio 1.36; 95% CI = 1.10–1.69), but this association lacks any clear mechanism of action and is not likely causal. The following outcomes were not associated with cannabis use: maternal diabetes, rupture of membranes, premature onset of labor, use of prenatal care, duration of labor, placental abruption, secondary arrest of labor, elevated blood pressure, hyperemesis gravidarum, maternal bleeding after 20 weeks, antepartum or postpartum hemorrhage, maternal weight gain, maternal postnatal issues, duration of maternal hospital stay, or hormone concentrations.[97]

Pertaining to the association with low birth weight, the NASEM authors noted these changes in birth weight are consistent with the effects of noncannabinoid substances in smoked cannabis and with cigarette smoking. After adjustment for any smoking exposure, there was no association between cannabis and offspring being small for gestational age (defined as a birth weight less than the 10th percentile). Two subsequent studies[98,99] and a meta-analysis[100] have also found that the associations between cannabis use and lower birth weight, head circumference, or gestational age disappear after controlling for tobacco use; conversely, other studies[101,102] have found this association to be significant. Overall, the evidence points to smoking as a contributing factor to low birth weight, not the cannabis itself.

Concerning other neonatal outcomes, the NASEM review did not find any to be associated with maternal cannabis use. There is evidence suggesting a higher rate of neonatal intensive care unit (NICU) admissions for children of cannabis-using mothers, but this likely reflects hospital policies that commonly require NICU admissions for infants whose mothers fail a drug toxicology screening test, a theory supported by the absence of an increased length of hospital stay for cannabis-exposed neonates. This practice, which interrupts bonding and breastfeeding, has no scientific basis and should be abolished.

We do know that THC readily crosses the placenta, though fetal exposure may be limited compared to maternal exposure, likely due to active transport in the placenta. Human data do not yet exist to establish a quantitative relationship between maternal and fetal cannabis levels, but we do know that endocannabinoid signaling is critical in development, and disrupting that signaling could have adverse consequences. Cannabis does not act as a classical teratogen and is not associated with morphological abnormalities at birth, but animal models have associated fetal exposure to cannabinoids with behaviors consistent with anxiety.[103]

In 1994, Melanie Dreher and colleagues[104] published data on 24 cannabis-exposed and 20 nonexposed neonates. They found no significant differences between the two groups at day 3, but at 1 month the exposed infants showed better physiological stability. The offspring of the 10 heavy-cannabis-using mothers, in fact, had the best scores on autonomic stability, quality of alertness, irritability, and self-regulation and were judged to be more rewarding for caregivers. The authors attributed this difference to cultural positioning and socioeconomic characteristics of mothers that select for cannabis use and also promote neonatal development, not the cannabis itself, though it is plausible that phytocannabinoids directly contributed to the benefits in neurological function and behavior.

Compared to THC, very few data exist about prenatal exposure to CBD. One mouse study found that a single 50 mg/kg dose on day 18 of gestation resulted in slightly lower brain and hypothalamic concentrations of norepinephrine, dopamine, and sero-tonin in male offspring; prenatal THC exposure did not influence these levels.[105] In a study of zebrafish embryos, CBD did not induce teratogenicity or neurotoxicity.[106] In a rodent model of gastroschisis, CBD has been shown to cross the placenta and impart anti-inflammatory and altered protein expression effects in the fetus, and ex vivo models have demonstrated CBD-related changes in protein expression in placental and umbilical vein endothelial tissue.[107]

Do we need to be concerned about late effects in the offspring of pregnant cannabis users? This is an important question in a risk–benefit assessment of medically super-vised cannabis use during pregnancy.

The NASEM review did not find enough evidence to support or refute an association between prenatal exposure and later outcomes in life, mostly because studies on conse-quences of maternal cannabis use on child development beyond the neonatal period are sparse. Some of the data suggested associated adolescent outcomes such as increased delinquency, more tobacco and cannabis use, and perhaps increased mental health symptoms, but numerous confounders preclude an understanding of whether or not this has anything to do with the prenatal cannabis exposure.

More recent data from 5,903 children in the Netherlands, evaluated at age 7–10, highlight this point: externalizing problems (such as aggression and rule breaking) but not internalizing problems (such as anxiety, depression, withdrawal, and somatic com-plaints) were associated with maternal cannabis use but were also similarly associated with paternal cannabis use, including paternal use in the absence of maternal use.[108] This suggests an effect due to shared familial or genetic factors, not in utero exposure. Other findings have also been reported, such as a slight increase in psychosis proneness test scores during middle childhood (in this case without any evidence of an association with internalizing or externalizing symptoms).[109] Not all associated outcomes are adverse; for example, prenatal cannabis exposure was associated with significantly improved global motion perception at age 4.[110]

A systematic review of 1,001 publications from 3 decades that compared subjects with and without prenatal cannabis exposure found that of the 1,004 cognitive outcomes assessed, children with prenatal cannabis exposure performed more poorly on 34 (3.4%) and better on 9 (0.9%) vs. control group. The clinical significance is limited because cog-nitive performance scores of cannabis-exposed groups overwhelmingly fell within the normal range when compared against normative data; only 1 article found the exposed group scored lower than the normal range.[111]

Overall, there is no clear signal that prenatal exposure increases risk of any adverse health outcome later in life, though I suspect that heavy maternal use could, to some extent, disrupt ECS signaling and predispose offspring to problems. This as-yet-theoretical concern must be considered in the real-world context of evaluating whether or not to treat a pregnant woman with cannabis.

The most common indications I have treated in pregnancy are hyperemesis gravidarum (HG), chronic pain, and PTSD. These conditions are often refractory to conventional treatment but may respond very well to low-dose cannabis. For example, in 40 women with HG (not strictly defined) who used cannabis to treat their nausea, 37 considered the cannabis to have been "extremely effective" or "effective" in controlling their symptoms.[112] Four other published cases of HG showed highly significant improvement in emesis and quality of life with cannabis use.[113] I have observed similar results in my practice.

It is important to note the well-established association between maternal stress and adverse outcomes, including preterm birth[114] and neurocognitive, behavioral, endocrine, and motor development aberrations in the offspring.[115,116] It is also clear that standard treatments for maternal stress have more clear adverse effects than cannabis. For example, opioid analgesics,[117] benzodiazepines,[118] and selective serotonin reuptake inhibitors[119] cause neonatal abstinence syndrome; cannabis does not.[120]

Historically, cannabis has been used commonly to aid in childbirth. Morris Fishbein, a past editor of the *Journal of the American Medical Association*, espoused cannabis in childbirth to aid in a painless labor with no adverse events for the baby.[121] I have also witnessed cannabis tincture used in this setting with excellent results.

Ina May Gaskin, known as the "mother of authentic midwifery," led the lay midwives at The Farm, an intentional community where cannabis was frequently used during pregnancy, labor, and lactation. Of over 1900 births from 1970 to 1994, the total incidence of small for gestational age and placental insufficiency was 0.002% (four births). Prematurity incidence was 0.01% (22 births).[122] In a recent survey of 71 mothers (average age 66) reporting on 178 children born at The Farm, 25% reported smoking cannabis daily, 55% reported several times weekly, and 20% reported rare use during pregnancy and lactation. Fifty percent smoked during labor, with most comments describing beneficial effects, though one woman reported that smoking cannabis stalled her labor, with progress resuming only after the effects wore off. This is certainly plausible considering the autonomic and muscle relaxant effects of THC. Among the offspring, 5% were reported to have significant mental illness, similar to the general population, and 3% had addiction disorders, lower than the national average.[123]

For patients not already using it before becoming pregnant, I would not initiate cannabis until after exhausting safer options. For example, for nausea I start with ginger,[124] acupressure (Neiguan point P6),[125] osteopathic treatment, acupuncture,[126] vitamin

B6,[127] or homeopathy (typically *Nux vomica* or *Sepia succus*). Depending on the urgency of the case, I might try all of the above options, often in combination, before a cannabis trial. I would, however, turn to cannabis before ondansetron, which has been associated with an increased risk for cardiac septal defects.[128] It is also important to consider the patient's personal preference for conventional versus complementary and alternative treatments when defining a treatment course that precedes a cannabis trial.

When might the potential benefits of medically supervised cannabis during pregnancy outweigh the potential risks?

- substitution for opioids, benzodiazepines, selective serotonin reuptake inhibitors, or other drugs that cause neonatal abstinence syndrome or other risks to mother and child
- for HG, consider before invasive procedures such as parenteral nutrition or potentially teratogenic drugs like ondansetron
- mitigation of high levels of maternal stress due to pain or psychological distress.
- in patients with prepregnancy medical use for a clear indication with excellent response at low or moderate doses, consider continuing the treatment with cannabis instead of discontinuing or trying other options.

How can the clinician minimize risk and maximize benefit while treating pregnant patients?

- Explain that cannabis can be abused, describe problematic use, and advise against it.
- Advise the patient to avoid smoking, dabs, and electronic cigarettes (vape pens).
- Recommend the use of flower vapor for rapid-onset antiemetic effects; otherwise recommend oromucosal or enteral delivery.
- Consider prescribing cannabis tea, which delivers very low doses of acidic cannabinoids and even lower doses of their neutral counterparts. The acidic cannabinoids are often extraordinarily effective for nausea in low doses.
- Recommend the lowest effective dose to avoid building tolerance to THC.
- Supervise closely and ensure use patterns are appropriate and optimal.
- Assess and mitigate any legal risks related to child protection agencies, uninformed medical providers, nosy neighbors, estranged husbands, and the like.

Lactation

Human breast milk is an extraordinarily complex biofluid evolutionarily designed to meet the infant's nutritional requirements for growth and development. Endocannabinoids and, when present in the mother's circulation, phytocannabinoids are transferred into breast milk. Data suggest that 2-arachidonoylglycerol (2-AG) content in breast milk has a role in establishing the suckling response of the newborn by activating oral-motor musculature needed for milk suckling (via CB1) and that other endocannabinoid constituents in breast milk may also play a role in infant health and development.[129]

The presence of THC and other phytocannabinoids in breast milk may therefore have either desirable or undesirable impacts on the infant. Excessive levels that potentially downregulate or disrupt appropriate endocannabinoid signaling in the infant would certainly be undesirable, but appropriate maternal consumption directed at correcting a physiological disturbance in the mother could theoretically convey more ideal cannabinoid activity to breast milk.

How much of the mother's phytocannabinoid intake makes its way into breast milk? Several studies have investigated this. Early data suggested that infants are exposed to 0.8% of the mother's exposure to THC per kilogram of body weight when exclusively breastfeeding.[130] In a more recent study measuring breast milk THC concentrations after inhalation of 100 mg of cannabis (23% THC), the authors calculated that exclusively breast-fed infants receive 2.5% of the maternal dose of THC per kilogram of body weight; breast milk THC concentration peaked at 1 hr and receded over 4 hr.[131]

Low levels of THC, 11-OH-THC, and CBD can be found in breast milk several days after the mother's last use, but these may not be enough to impact infant physiology, unless perhaps when maternal use is very high. One study found THC levels in breast milk ranging from 1 to 323 ng/ml (median 9.47 ng/ml) after 6 days of maternal abstinence;[132] in comparison, the average level of 2-AG in mature breast milk is 312 ± 119 ng/ml.[133]

Do infants exposed to phytocannabinoids via breast milk have adverse outcomes? Human data to answer this question are sparse. One study reported mild psychomotor deficits at 12 months in 68 infants breastfed by cannabis-using mothers during their first month of life, compared to 68 matched unexposed infants. This effect was observed only with daily or near-daily consumption, and occasional maternal cannabis use during breastfeeding was not associated with any significant effects on infant development; the association remained significant after controlling for maternal smoking, drinking, and cocaine use during pregnancy and lactation, but the study was unable to control for prenatal cannabis use.[134] Another study found no differences in motor or cognitive development at 12 months in 27 cannabis-exposed infants compared to 35 unexposed infants.[135]

Though I was unable to find human data supporting this hypothesis, I believe that lactating mothers who use the oromucosal route of delivery, which leads to much lower phytocannabinoid blood levels than smoking, will expose the infant to significantly lower doses.

Should lactating cannabis users, whether medically supervised or not, discard their milk produced in the 4–6 hr after inhaling cannabis? As cannabis becomes legal in more jurisdictions, and because many perceive cannabis as safer than alcohol and other psychoactive substances during pregnancy and lactation, this becomes an important question. In the United States, cannabis is now the most commonly reported recreational drug used by lactating women, with a high prevalence in some populations: among clients of the Special Supplemental Nutrition Program for Women, Infants, and Children in one of the largest health departments in Colorado, a state with legal adult-use cannabis, of the women who reported any history of marijuana use (past, ever, or current), 35.8% reported having used marijuana at some point in their pregnancy, and 18% report having used it while breastfeeding.[136]

The American Academy of Pediatrics advises against cannabis use during lactation but does not recommend stopping breastfeeding or discarding contaminated milk.[137] With the benefits of breast-feeding to mother and child so clearly established and the risks of phytocannabinoid exposure in breast milk so uncertain, I agree. When cannabis is clinically indicated for a specific therapeutic purpose, the best strategy is to mitigate potential risk by encouraging lactating mothers to use the lowest effective dose for a specific health-related goal, avoid smoking and use a noninhaled route of delivery if possible, and avoid THC-related impairment that may jeopardize infant safety.

Unfortunately, even in states where cannabis is legal, pregnant and breastfeeding users can be subject to child welfare investigations if they have a positive cannabis result on urine drug toxicology screens. A 2013 review article in the journal *Obstetrical & Gynecological Survey* concluded that "Based on these findings, mandatory reporting of marijuana use during pregnancy and punitive measures related to the use of this drug during pregnancy or breast-feeding do not seem medically warranted. A consistent message of 'breast is best' seems appropriate for mothers who continue to use marijuana while breast-feeding."[138]

Recommendations on Cannabis and Breast-Feeding

The American Academy of Pediatrics 2018 recommendations on cannabis and breast-feeding are as follows:[139]

- Present data are insufficient to assess the effects of exposure of infants to maternal marijuana use during breast-feeding. As a result, maternal marijuana use while breast-feeding is discouraged. Because the potential risks of infant exposure to marijuana metabolites are unknown, women should be informed of the potential risk of exposure during lactation and encouraged to abstain from using any marijuana products while breast-feeding.
- Pregnant or breast-feeding women should be cautioned about infant exposure to smoke from marijuana in the environment, given emerging data on the effects of passive marijuana smoke.

Pediatrics

Expertise in medical cannabis can turn one's practice into a magnet for patients with rare and refractory conditions, including children of all ages. In our practice, my colleagues and I have seen pediatric patients with rare congenital conditions, cancer, seizures and other neurological disorders, behavior disorders and more. Our pediatric cases are usually severe, highly refractory, and emotionally challenging since parents and referring providers tend to consider cannabis as a last resort.

This is unfortunate, because I believe that in many situations a careful risk–benefit assessment would show that cannabis is safer than many first- and second-line therapies, and in some conditions (for example, seizures; see Chapter 25 for more information) the chance of success with cannabis is much higher than with another pharmaceutical after first-line agents have failed. Despite the demanding nature of these cases, I estimate that 90% receive some benefit from cannabis, results commonly affirmed by colleagues in the field and research publications. In a series of 272 patients with epilepsy refractory to multiple medications, for example, 86% of patients experienced some improvement with cannabis and 10% became seizure-free, while only 4% experienced an exacerbation.[140] Compare this to a study of 470 adolescents and adults with newly diagnosed epilepsy: 47% became seizure-free on the first antiepileptic agent, 13% on a second monotherapy, but only 1% on the third agent;[141] these data are the basis for polytherapy as a standard of care in refractory epilepsy. Perhaps a cannabis trial, which typically involves less risk of adverse effects and higher likelihood of beneficial side effects, is indicated after the first or second drug failure.

The thought of a child taking cannabis may, for some, conjure images of teenage illicit cannabis smoking, which clearly has many potential risks. More recently, with the approval of a CBD-based medication in the United States for two rare seizure disorders, the medical community is beginning to accept the idea that CBD can be helpful for some children, yet THC is still considered forbidden territory. It is essential that we set aside these notions and consider the therapeutic and palliative potential of cannabis without bias.

How do we safely recommend cannabis for pediatric patients, and for which indications? Clinical evidence supports the use of THC for chemotherapy-induced nausea and vomiting and CBD for seizures.[142] Smaller studies have shown efficacy of THC for seizures, autism, encephalopathies, spasticity, and other neurological conditions.[143,144] In my pediatric patients with cancer, I typically observe pain relief, improvement in sleep, and excellent palliative effects at the end of life. Rare and highly refractory conditions may similarly benefit. Before recommending, clinicians need to be able to describe potential risks and benefits as they obtain informed consent.

What are the potential risks? First, it is important to distinguish the adverse effects of a medically supervised, judiciously dosed pediatric trial from the known detrimental effects of adolescent illicit cannabis smoking. The latter has been associated with adverse neuropsychiatric outcomes in adulthood, though the association has not proven to be causal.[145]

In controlled pediatric trials, THC most commonly led to side effects of drowsiness and dizziness, with severity associated with higher doses; no major side effects were reported with dose reduction. The most common side effects with high-dose CBD are somnolence, diarrhea, and decreased appetite.[146] This is similar to a systematic review of adult data, which found dizziness and somnolence as the most commonly reported adverse events.[147] Among published 29 cases of accidental overdose of cannabis containing THC in children, the most frequent symptoms were sinus tachycardia (58.6%), mydriasis (48.3%), drowsiness (24%), hypoventilation (20.6%), and agitation (10.3%). Four children (13.8%) experienced seizures before admission. Thirty-four percent had a decreased level of consciousness (<12 on the Glasgow coma scale) and were admitted to a pediatric intensive care unit for 12–24 hr. All patients had ingested hashish.[148]

Unfortunately, there are few data that shed light on the potential long-term adverse effects of medically supervised pediatric cannabis use, highlighting the importance of frequently reevaluating the effects of cannabis on overall function, capacity to participate in school and other activities, sleep, nutrition, and other factors that influence growth and development. While there may be some theoretical risk of impairing neurological development and causing a long-term deficit in cognitive performance, the benefits of, for example, resolving daily seizures, reversing failure to thrive, relieving chronic pain, or promoting restorative sleep, in my opinion, outweigh the potential risks, in terms of both quality of life and support of healthy development.

In my clinical experience, and that of several colleagues, we have found that children are less likely than adults to experience adverse psychoactive effects from THC. The late Ester Fride, PhD, who pioneered exploration of the ECS in early development, reported that the gradual postnatal increase of CB1 receptors and anandamide is accompanied by a gradual maturing response to the psychoactive potential of THC (or anandamide) in postnatal mice between birth and weaning.[149] This is supported by frequent mentions in the 19th-century literature that children often tolerated heroic doses of cannabis medicines that would produce incapacitation in an adult.[150] Examples are also found in the modern literature: in a clinical trial with sublingual Δ^8-THC, up to 0.64 mg·kg^{-1}·dose^{-1}, for chemotherapy-induced nausea or vomiting, the treatment was virtually totally effective and free of side effects.[151]

In my experience with pediatric palliative and end-of-life care, I have found THC to be extraordinarily useful for relieving pain and anxiety, drying secretions, and fostering a sense of peace and acceptance. It is well-tolerated, even at high doses. I encourage readers to consider this compassionate option in your pediatric patients when needed.

Summary:

- Clinical studies support pediatric use of THC for chemotherapy-induced nausea and vomiting and CBD for seizures.
- Smaller studies have shown efficacy with THC for seizures, autism, encephalopathies, spasticity, and other neurological conditions.
- The risks of medically supervised pediatric cannabis use are distinct from those of adolescent illicit cannabis smoking, though little is known about long-term effects on development.
- Similar to adults, the most common adverse effects of THC in pediatrics are dizziness and somnolence.
- The most common adverse effects of CBD in pediatrics are somnolence, diarrhea, and decreased appetite, typically occurring only at high doses. I also observe restlessness and hyperactivity in some patients at low doses.
- Children are less likely to experience adverse psychoactive effects of THC, likely due to gradual maturation of the ECS.

Cannabis Allergy

Several reports of cutaneous and respiratory allergies to cannabis have been published, though the prevalence of cannabis allergy is unknown. Airway symptoms include nasal and pharyngeal pruritis, lacrimation, nasal congestion, rhinitis, cough, dyspnea, and wheezing. Hypotension, palpitations, vertigo, nausea, vomiting, abdominal cramping, and cutaneous reactions including pruritis, urticaria, eczema, and angioedema have been reported. Anaphylaxis has been reported from ingestion of hemp seed, drinking cannabis tea, and smoking.[152]

It is important to distinguish smoke-related symptoms from true cannabis allergy; several patients who describe upper and/or lower respiratory symptoms from inhaled cannabis do well with oral delivery. In my 11 years in practice, I believe I have seen no more than five cases in which an allergic-type reaction to cannabis precluded its use as a medicine, though I did not confirm these cases as true cannabis allergy with skin or immunoglobulin E testing.

Direct handling of cannabis plants has been reported to cause contact urticaria, generalized pruritus, contact dermatitis, and periorbital edema. This has been commonly reported by my patients, most of whom are able to inhale or ingest cannabis without a reaction.

Cannabis pollen inhalation has been noted to cause symptoms of allergic rhinitis, conjunctivitis, and asthma. This can be significant in regions where hemp is grown; one study in Nebraska found cannabis pollen comprised 36% of the total pollen count during mid- to late-August.[153]

While the allergic components of cannabis are not well-elucidated, Can s 3, its nonspecific lipid transfer protein, is likely a major culprit, especially in flower or leaf (nonpollen) sensitivity cases.[154] One Spanish study found 124 out of 130 patients with a primary cannabis allergy were sensitized to Can s 3.[155] Nonspecific lipid transfer proteins are ubiquitous in the plant kingdom; thus, sensitization to Can s 3 could be associated with cross-reactivity to a number of foods and other plants, such as cherry, tangerine, orange, peach, apple, tomato, hazelnut, walnut, banana, wheat, latex, and tobacco. One study found a high degree of cross-reactivity between tomato and cannabis leaf extract,[156] and another found cross-reactivity with banana, tomato, citrus, and grapefruit.[157] Fungal contamination of cannabis is common and may contribute to an allergic response in some individuals.

Cannabinoid Hyperemesis Syndrome

Cannabinoid hyperemesis syndrome (CHS), first reported in 2004,[158] is characterized by cyclic nausea and vomiting in the setting of chronic, high-dose cannabis use. It is often associated with frequent high-temperature bathing, which temporarily ameliorates symptoms in most cases, and it resolves with cannabis abstinence. CHS can be difficult to identify because it may present in patients who have been successfully using cannabis for years without a significant change in their use patterns.

CHS presents in three stages: prodromal, hyperemetic, and recovery.[159] The prodrome is often characterized by anxiety, nausea (sometimes only present in the morning), and autonomic symptoms like sweating, flushing, and increased thirst. This stage can last for months before any vomiting begins. The hyperemetic phase includes severe abdominal pain, nausea, and vomiting that typically does not respond to conventional antiemetics. Patients often discover that hot bathing or showering provides effective relief, and bathing behavior can become compulsive and frequent. Higher temperatures provide better relief, and some cases have even reported superficial skin burns from bathing. In most cases, the hyperemetic phase ends and the recovery phase begins within 2 days of conservative management and cannabis abstinence, but in some cases patients' symptoms have taken up to a month to resolve.

CHS shares several clinical features with cyclic vomiting syndrome (CVS), and the two can be difficult to distinguish at the time of presentation. Controversially, the Rome IV criteria even list CHS as a subset of CVS (see Table 18.8). Although the Rome IV does not include hot bathing in the CVS criteria, non-cannabis-using patients with CVS have also reported relief with this behavior: in one study of CVS patients, 34% of cannabis nonusers endorsed hot bathing, compared to 71% endorsement among cannabis users with CVS.[160]

TABLE 18.8

Rome IV Diagnostic Criteria for Cyclical Vomiting Syndrome and Cannabinoid Hyperemesis Syndrome[161]

Cyclical vomiting syndrome (CVS)	Cannabinoid hyperemesis syndrome (CHS)
Acute onset of stereotypical vomiting episode that lasts less than 1 week	Stereotypical vomiting episodes similar to CVS
At least three episodes in the previous year, two episodes in the last 6 months at least 1 week apart	Presentation following sustained excessive cannabis use

Cyclical vomiting syndrome (CVS)	Cannabinoid hyperemesis syndrome (CHS)
No vomiting between episodes	Relief from vomiting after abstinence from cannabis
Symptoms must be present for 3 months with onset 6 months earlier	Symptoms must be present for 3 months with onset 6 months earlier
Supportive criteria: history of migraine headaches	Supportive criteria: pathological bathing behavior (prolonged hot baths or showers)

Further clarifying the diagnostic criteria for CHS, a recent systematic review of the literature identified the following frequency of characteristics in published cases:[162]

- history of regular cannabis for any duration of time (100%)
- cyclic nausea and vomiting (100%)
- age less than 50 at onset of illness (100%)
- at least weekly cannabis use (97.4%)
- resolution of symptoms after stopping cannabis (96.8%)
- compulsive hot baths with symptom relief (92.3%)
- abdominal pain (85.1%)
- history of regular cannabis use for >1 year (74.8%)
- male predominance (72.9%)

I have observed the development of CHS in a handful of patients. It can occur in patients who are using cannabis appropriately without ongoing adverse effects and in those without previous gastrointestinal (GI) disorders. The prodromal morning nausea or vague and mild abdominal pain is a useful warning sign.

I have also seen non-cannabis-using patients with true CVS, refractory to all standard antiemetics, respond extremely well to cannabis taken at the earliest onset of a vomiting episode or migraine. Thus, it is important to distinguish the two entities, which may have opposite treatments: cannabis abstinence for CHS and episodic cannabis use for CVS.

Atypical variants of CHS also exist. I published one of two cases that involved lower GI symptoms including diarrhea, no vomiting, no response to hot bathing, but resolution with cannabis abstinence.[163] Interestingly, both patients were also triggered by CBD-dominant, low-THC cannabis. This suggests there may be a spectrum of episodic cannabis-related GI adverse effects that share some clinical and physiological features with CHS.

In both cases, the patients were able to resume using cannabis at a low dose, after a period of abstinence, without triggering a hyperemetic episode. I have seen other patients with CHS similarly able to resume using cannabis at a lower dose and frequency, sometimes taking periodic breaks of several days if they suspect the development of prodromal symptoms.

The pathophysiology of CHS is unknown and likely multifactorial since this condition only develops in a small subset of regular cannabis users. A variety of theories have been proposed, including genetic vulnerability, ECS dysregulation, delayed gastric emptying, dysfunctional stress response, altered thermoregulatory and TRPV1 systems, and abnormal allostatic regulation of the hypothalamic–pituitary–adrenal axis and sympathetic nervous system.[164,165]

Others have suggested noncannabis culprits, such as pesticide contamination, though this is unlikely because pesticide poisoning presents differently and because CHS can develop in users of synthetic cannabinoids,[166] which are produced in laboratories and would be unlikely to contain pesticides.

Acute treatment of CHS involves supportive care and hydration. Traditional antiemetics are often ineffective; benzodiazepines and antipsychotic medications (e.g., haloperidol) seem to be the most effective for emetic phases of CVS and CHS.[167] Some data suggest that application of topical capsaicin to the abdomen can help improve acute symptoms.[168] This may be due to a common mechanism of action with hot bathing: TRPV1, which can be activated by both heat and capsaicin, can produce antiemetic effects.

Problematically, I have found some local emergency medicine providers may overdiagnose CHS in cannabis-using patients who present to the emergency department (ED) with GI complaints. In all fairness, early identification of CHS in the ED is useful to save health-care resources: a 2012 observational study of CHS patients followed over 2 years found the median charge for ED visits and hospital admissions was $95,023.[169] Unfortunately, I have had several patients who perceive discrimination in the ED setting based on their reported medical use of cannabis, sometimes discharged without sufficient workup or treatment.

CHS is yet another example of bidirectional effects in cannabis. It can be disabling on its own and even worse when it precludes the ongoing use of a previously effective treatment for other chronic symptoms, though CHS is uncommon in medical-only users and especially in those who do not use inhaled cannabis. Perhaps CHS is the expression of a patient's physiology demanding a shift in one's relationship with cannabis, toward lower and less frequent dosing, and a lesson to cannabis clinicians emphasizing the use of the lowest effective dose.

I encourage readers to remain vigilant for new-onset prodromal symptoms in patients who regularly use cannabis for over a year. When it is unclear if a patient has CHS or CVS, a 1-month period of cannabis abstinence, followed by the challenge of resuming cannabis use, is usually sufficient to differentiate these syndromes. For patients with a previous therapeutic response to cannabis, it can be worthwhile to carefully explore reintroducing low-dose cannabis after a 1–3-month period of abstinence.

Chapter 19

Strategies for Improving Efficacy and Access

IN MY CLINICAL EXPERIENCE, I've found cannabis to frequently potentiate or be potentiated by non-pharmacological treatments and other herbs. For patients who are unable to access cannabis, off-label use of synthetic cannabinoids and treatment with exogenous *N*-Palmitoylethanolamine are additional options for modulating the endocannabinoid system.

Cannabis as an Adjunct to Nonpharmacological Treatments

Beyond symptom management, I have observed that cannabis can potentiate nonpharmacological treatments, including psychological and physical therapies. Examples of this potential synergy have been reported in the literature. For example, in an observational study of 290 patients with multiple sclerosis treated with nabiximols (oromucosal Δ^9-tetrahydrocannabinol [THC]/ cannabidiol [CBD] spray), the 210 who participated in physiotherapy were 2.6 times more likely to reach a clinically relevant response to nabiximols (≥ 30% improvement), and were less likely to discontinue nabiximols, than those without physiotherapy.[1]

Several experimental human studies have indicated that cannabinoids could be helpful in fear (i.e., threat) extinction and consolidation, processes inherent in the success of many cognitive-behavioral approaches to anxiety and posttraumatic stress disorder (PTSD). For example, a single 7.5-mg dose of THC administered 2 hr before threat extinction learning, compared to placebo, resulted in significantly decreased threat responses 1 day and 1 week later, accompanied with functional imaging data showing a significant effect on the connectivity of threat-detection networks.[2] Another study found that 32 mg of inhaled CBD enhanced consolidation of fear extinction learning in humans.[3] Both suggest that cannabinoids may have potential as an adjunct to extinction-based therapies for anxiety disorders. In a cohort of 136 individuals receiving cognitive behavioral therapies for co-occurring PTSD and substance use disorders, higher cannabis use was associated with greater PTSD symptom severity early in treatment but lower PTSD symptom severity later in treatment; the authors suggested that cannabis may interact synergistically with psychological treatment to reduce PTSD symptoms.[4]

Many of the most common physical diseases in modern society co-occur with mental health conditions, and both can be caused or exacerbated by chronic stress. Similar to the versatile effects of cannabis on diverse diagnoses, a large body of evidence shows that mindfulness—both as a dispositional trait and as a skill-based training—can reduce patient-reported symptoms and improve coping and quality of life across many physical health conditions, including cardiovascular disease, diabetes, and musculoskeletal conditions.[5] Several of my patients have reported synergistic therapeutic effects when combining cannabis with mindfulness and other forms of meditation, a long-held tradition in Indian tantra and yoga.[6]

Mindfulness is commonly defined as an awareness and acceptance of one's present experience. In theory, the ability to mindfully observe one's present-moment experience with clarity and equanimity enables more effective appraisals of stressors, which, in turn, facilitates conscious, healthy decisions and prevents automatic, unhealthy, habitual reactions.

Savoring, a form of mindfulness focused on recognizing and appreciating positive experiences, may be an especially powerful adjunct to cannabis, both to enhance therapeutic effects and to prevent problematic use. Hedonic dysregulation, a blunted response to natural rewards, is known to drive addictive behavior and is especially implicated as a contributing factor to opioid misuse in patients with chronic pain. Mindfulness-oriented recovery enhancement (MORE) is an intervention that integrates mindfulness, cognitive restructuring, and positive emotion regulation. Studies on MORE have shown that mindful savoring, by increasing responsiveness to natural rewards, may decrease prescription opioid misuse and craving.[7,8] Savoring behavior, assessed by the Savoring Beliefs Inventory, was also shown to negatively correlate with problematic cannabis use in a survey of 195 cannabis users.[9]

I believe that patients with anhedonia can potentially employ the psychoactive effects of cannabis in combination with an intentional practice of mindful savoring to reverse hedonic dysregulation, restore the pleasure response to natural rewards, reduce chronic stress and associated pathophysiology, and improve quality of life. This intervention could also prevent problematic cannabis use. This theory is supported by a functional magnetic resonance imaging study on 11 healthy individuals, which found that vaporized THC alters brain function in relevant networks and reduces negative bias in emotional processing.[10] This suggests THC could help shift a patient's psychological orientation from stimuli that have a negative effect toward stimuli that have a positive effect.

While some patients may do best with training sessions to build mindfulness and savoring skills, I find that a straightforward suggestion to spend 5–15 min intentionally savoring some natural reward, such as the sunrise or sunset, a piece of classical music, or a bouquet of flowers, can be adequate. The simple practice of checking the Inner Inventory (see Chapter 17) before and after cannabis administration also promotes mindfulness.

Herbal Adjuncts to Cannabis

In traditional Ayurveda, Arabic medicine, and other ethnobotanical systems, cannabis is frequently used in combination with, and considered synergistic with, other herbs.[11] Without requiring expertise in herbal medicine, there are a few useful adjuncts to cannabis that can be readily employed to enhance its therapeutic effects and mitigate certain side effects (see Table 19.1).

TABLE 19.1

Potential Uses and Mechanisms of Herbal Adjuncts to Cannabis

Herb	Potential candidates	Mechanism of action	Dosage	Cautions
Tulsi (holy basil)	Patients with a weak, depleted constitution, cannabis-related fatigue	Numerous: general adaptogenic, anti-inflammatory, antioxidant, and antimicrobial agent	One cup of tea 1–2 times daily; tincture or capsules twice daily (follow package instructions)	None
Calamus (sweet flag)	Patients sensitive to anxiogenesis, excessive mental activity, memory impairment, and other adverse psychoactive effects of cannabis; chronic dry mouth; GI hypomotility and other GI symptoms	Inhibition of acetylcholinesterase, N-methyl-D-aspartate, and others	Small piece of rhizome or root (0.5 cm diameter) chewed and held in mouth 1–3 times daily; tincture or capsules 1–3 times daily (follow package instructions)	North American and European varieties are safer; Asian varieties may have significant quantities of carcinogenic β-asarone

Herb	Potential candidates	Mechanism of action	Dosage	Cautions
Kratom	Patients with chronic pain not fully responding to cannabis; may be a safer alternative to pharmaceutical opioids; adjunct to cannabis in the setting of opioid withdrawal	Partial agonist at μ-opioid and α_2-adrenergic receptors	½ tsp to 3 Tbsp of leaf powder in a slurry up to 4 times daily (titrate slowly)	Dependence, tolerance, and withdrawal upon cessation; unlikely to cause cardiorespiratory depression, even in high doses; concern about quality and consistency of commercially available products
5-hydroxytryptophan (Griffonia simplicifolia)	Patients with anxiety, depression, or sleep disturbance not fully responding to cannabis	Direct precursor to serotonin	50–100 mg 2–3 times daily for daytime symptoms, 100–300 mg at bedtime for promoting sleep; bedtime dosing may also be effective for depression without daytime dosing	Avoid or introduce cautiously in patients with nausea, diarrhea, or other GI symptoms; use caution in combination with other serotonergic agents

Tulsi (*Ocimum sanctum* L.), also known as holy basil, is a highly revered culinary and medicinal aromatic herb that has been used in Ayurvedic medicine for more than 3,000 years. Numerous preclinical studies demonstrate potent pharmacological actions that include adaptogenic (improving resilience or adaptation to stress), metabolic, immunomodulatory, anticancer, anti-inflammatory, antioxidant, hepatoprotective, radioprotective, antimicrobial, and antidiabetic effects. The leaf contains several bioactive compounds including eugenol, ursolic acid, β-caryophyllene, linalool, and 1,8-cineole, plus vitamins and minerals. Typically taken as a tea, tincture, or capsule, holy basil is composed of three cultivars (Rama tulsi, Krishna tulsi, and Vana tulsi), each with distinct morphology and phytochemical composition and frequently combined in commercially available products. In a review of 24 human studies on metabolic disorders, cardiovascular disease, immunity, and neurocognition, all studies remarkably reported favorable clinical outcomes with no significant adverse events, supporting the traditional use of tulsi for lifestyle-related chronic diseases including psychological stress, metabolic syndrome, and diabetes.[12]

I frequently recommend tulsi to patients who have a weak, depleted constitution or experience fatigue as a side effect from cannabis. One of my Ayurveda teach-ers explained that cannabis is associated with Shiva, the archetype of destruction and change: it has great power to transform imbalances and suffering, though it can utilize and deplete one's core vitality while doing so. Cannabis may be combined with tulsi or other herbs associated with Vishnu, the archetype of preservation and protection, to pre-vent depletion. I often recommend 1–2 cups of tulsi tea daily, which has a pleasant taste and is readily available in most grocery stores in the United States, or tincture or capsule preparations 1–2 times daily.

Calamus (*Acorus calamus*), also known as sweet flag, has been traditionally used in Ayurvedic, Chinese, and Native American medicine to treat a variety of conditions, espe-cially psychoneurological conditions such as insomnia, hysteria, epilepsy, and memory loss. It is considered a rejuvenator for the brain and nervous systems. In low doses, it is commonly used for the treatment of gastrointestinal symptoms such as heartburn, dyspepsia, constipation, and anorexia, while in high doses it can be used as an emetic. Calamus is also used in treating spasticity, upper and lower respiratory symptoms, den-tal conditions, topically for wounds,[13] and to support tobacco cessation. Many of these traditional uses correlate with its known pharmacology as an inhibitor of the acetylcho-linesterase enzyme and the *N*-methyl-d-aspartate receptor.[14] While acute and chronic animal toxicology studies of whole-herb calamus ethanolic extracts have demonstrated no safety concerns, one of the active constituents, b-asarone, is potentially toxic and carcinogenic. The content of β-asarone correlates with the polyploidy of the plant; the North American and European diploid varieties completely lack this constituent and are thus considered safer than the Asian varieties.[15]

Combining calamus with cannabis dates to ancient India; according to Ayurvedic medical texts, calamus "balances" and "neutralizes the toxic side effects" of cannabis.[16] I sometimes recommend calamus for my cannabis-using patients who experience dry mucous membranes, anxiety, or racing mental activity as adverse effects, which are likely ameliorated by the procholinergic effects of calamus. A small piece of the root can be chewed and held in the mouth, or it can be taken as a tea, tincture, or capsule. Some can-nabis users have been known to smoke a mixture of ground calamus root with cannabis flower, reportedly decreasing memory deficits and psychotropic effects while increasing feelings of calm and centeredness.[17] Alternatively, patients desiring this effect can seek out chemovars with high levels of α-pinene, another acetylcholinesterase inhibitor.

Kratom is a controversial herb derived from the leaves of *Mitragyna speciosa*, a tree in the coffee family native to Southeast Asia, where it is commonly used for a variety of symptoms including pain, fatigue, depression, and anxiety and as a substitute for alcohol, opioids, and other drugs. Like cannabis, kratom exhibits biphasic dose–response trends, with smaller doses producing mild stimulant like effects and larger doses producing opioid like effects. Importantly, there is little to no evidence of respiratory depression associated with kratom use, which is consistent with the characterization of its main active alkaloid, mitragynine, as a partial agonist of the μ-opioid receptor and competitive antagonist at κ- and δ-opioid receptors.[18]

While few clinical studies on the use of kratom exist, many users consider kratom a safer and less addictive alternative to synthetic opioids for managing pain and opioid dependence. An online survey of kratom users (2867 current users and 157 former users) indicated that the herb was used primarily to relieve pain (48% of respondents); for anxiety, PTSD, or depression (22%); to increase energy or focus (10%); and to help cut down on opioid use or relieve withdrawal (10%). Adverse reactions (12.6%) were predominantly gastrointestinal and were mostly mild and self-managed.[19] Kratom has been associated with a number of serious adverse effects and even death, though most of those cases have been in the context of polysubstance abuse. Some kratom products have also been found to be contaminated with salmonella.

A number of my patients have successfully combined cannabis and kratom to treat chronic pain with excellent results. Simultaneously targeting cannabinoid and opioid signaling pathways has been shown to produce synergistic analgesic effects in numerous preclinical and some clinical studies, and the use of a partial μ-opioid agonist like kratom may be safer than synthetic, stronger opioids. Kratom users in my practice typically consume a slurry of kratom leaf powder, with doses as low as ½ tsp and as high as 3 Tbsp taken 2–4 times daily.

Griffonia simplicifolia is a shrub native to West Africa whose seeds contain high levels of 5-hydroxytryptophan (5-HTP), an endogenous metabolite of tryptophan and direct precursor of serotonin that is readily absorbed when taken by mouth and crosses the blood–brain barrier. Supplemental use of 5-HTP thus holds promise for conditions in which serotonergic dysfunction or reduced central serotonin levels may play a role, including depression, anxiety, and sleep disturbance. A number of my patients have noted benefit when combining cannabis with 5-HTP for these symptoms. In one controlled trial, 300 mg of 5-HTP daily was shown to effectively reduce symptoms of fibromyalgia, including pain, morning stiffness, sleep disturbances, and anxiety.[20] For insomnia, a single 100-mg nighttime dose of 5-HTP was sufficient to improve the duration and depth of sleep in one placebo-controlled trial.[21]

I consider suggesting a trial of 5-HTP in patients with ongoing anxiety, depression, or sleep disturbance despite optimal use of cannabis, but I avoid suggesting it for patients with gastrointestinal symptoms since nausea and diarrhea are the most common adverse effects of 5-HTP. I usually start with 50–100 mg and increase as needed to a maximum of 300 mg/day.

N-Palmitoylethanolamine

Clinicians who don't have access to cannabis, may wish to explore *N*-Palmitoylethanolamine (PEA). PEA is the first endogenous endocannabinoid-like compound commercially available as a nutritional supplement. Interestingly, PEA is naturally produced in many plants (making it arguably also a phyto-cannabinoid), and the biosynthesis and degradation pathways of PEA in plants and humans are nearly identical. Lecithin is likely the best dietary source of PEA.

The therapeutic effects of PEA are conveyed via synergistic interactions among several mechanisms of action. Though it lacks direct activity at CB1 and CB2, data suggest that PEA acts upon these receptors indirectly via "entourage" effects such as inhibition of fatty acid amide hydrolase and stimulation of diacylglycerol lipase. It has a direct activity at the peroxisome proliferator-activated receptor α (PPAR-α) nuclear receptor and GPR55; both are targets for anti-inflammatory effects. PEA acts indirectly on transient receptor potential vanilloid 1 (TRPV1) channels, enhancing TRPV1 activation induced by anandamide and TRPV1 desensitization induced by 2-arachidonoylglycerol, possibly through allosteric effects. PEA also has been shown to indirectly activate TRPV1 via a PPAR-α mechanism.[22]

PEA tends to have poor oral bioavailability, but preliminary studies on micronized and ultramicronized formulations show promise for increased absorption. Several preclinical and some clinical studies have evaluated therapeutic use of PEA in neurological, inflammatory, and painful conditions; the following is a nonexhaustive review that illustrates the potential clinical utility of this agent, which has demonstrated excellent safety and tolerability. The most commonly reported adverse effects of PEA are mild gastrointestinal symptoms.

In a single case report of a patient with amyotrophic lateral sclerosis (ALS), 600 mg of ultramicronized PEA administered orally twice daily improved respiration, both subjectively and as measured by electromyography.[23] A clinical study on 64 patients with ALS randomly assigned to receive either 600 mg of ultramicronized PEA plus 50 mg of riluzole (a drug used to treat ALS and delay the onset of ventilator dependence or tracheostomy) twice daily or riluzole alone showed slower worsening of respiratory function, less death, and less tracheostomy in the PEA group.[24] The addition of ultramicronized PEA to patients with Parkinson's disease receiving levodopa therapy significantly reduced most motor and nonmotor symptoms over the course of a year.[25] An observational study in which a co-ultramicronized composite containing PEA (700 mg) and the antioxidant flavonoid luteolin (70 mg) was administered twice daily to 250 stroke patients demonstrated improvement in neurological status, spasticity, cognitive abilities, pain, and independence in daily living activities after 30 days of treatment.[26] A randomized trial of 70 children with moderate to severe autism were treated with risperidone, with or without PEA; those receiving PEA experienced improved irritability and hyperactivity compared to risperidone alone.[27]

As of 2019, 19 studies and five randomized controlled trials (RCTs) evaluated PEA as an adjunctive analgesic therapy for neuropathic pain. PEA was shown to reduce pain from diabetic neuropathy, chemotherapy-induced neuropathy, idiopathic axonal neuropathy, nonspecific neuropathy, and sciatic and lumbosacral spine disease, improving the effects of pregabalin, oxycodone, and codeine analgesia. Multiple studies of PEA in carpal tunnel syndrome demonstrate improvement in symptoms and objective improvement in nerve function. PEA was effective in reducing pain from fibromyalgia, burning mouth syndrome, temporomandibular joint disease, and molar extractions.[28]

PEA may also be helpful for arthritic pain. In an RCT of 110 patients with knee osteoarthritis who received PEA (300 or 600 mg) or a placebo twice daily, there was a significant reduction in pain, stiffness, and anxiety compared to placebo and improvement in function in the PEA groups; results were improved at the higher dose.[29]

PEA also shows promise in treating depression. In an RCT that added 1200 mg/day PEA or placebo to citalopram in 58 patients, depression scores in the PEA group improved at 2, 4, and 6 weeks compared to placebo. The response rate, defined as a 50% reduction in the Hamilton Rating Scale for Depression, was 100% for PEA and 74% for placebo at 6 weeks.[30]

PEA has also been shown to reduce mast cell recruitment and activation, with potential application in the growing awareness of mast cell activation syndrome and related conditions characterized by excessive mast cell activity, including irritable bowel syndrome. In one study of 54 patients with irritable bowel syndrome and 12 healthy controls, compared to placebo, treatment with PEA and polydatin, a resveratrol precursor, markedly improved abdominal pain severity.[31]

In summary, PEA is well tolerated, currently available over the counter, and has promising therapeutic potential as an adjunct to conventional therapies, and potentially to cannabis, in the treatment of neurodegeneration, pain, inflammation, and other conditions.

Off-Label Use of Prescription Cannabinoids

Treatment with herbal cannabis is typically not allowed in hospital settings, rehabilitation facilities, nursing homes, and other residential facilities (excepting some progressive facilities),[32] nor is it currently allowed in interstate and international travel. Other patients are unable to use herbal cannabis due to prohibition by employers, professional licensing (e.g., commercial drivers, medical providers in some jurisdictions), and correctional probation and parole. In these situations, I have found that off-label use of prescription cannabinoids can be a useful tool.

Dronabinol is synthetic THC obtainable by prescription in the United States (schedule III controlled substance) and several other countries. It is available in 2.5-, 5-, and 10-mg capsules as well as a 5 mg/ml oral solution and is indicated for anorexia associated with weight loss in patients with AIDS and chemotherapy-induced nausea or vomiting refractory to conventional antiemetics. In my experience, patients who have used herbal cannabis report similar but somewhat less effective therapeutic results with dronabinol and sometimes stronger psychoactive side effects, and they often comment on the erratic onset and duration of the capsules. Instructing patients to chew the capsules (which contain sesame oil and THC) and hold in the mouth for a few minutes prior to swallowing, or changing to the oral solution, can mitigate this problem.

Nabilone is a synthetic analogue of THC, with similar activity at CB1 and CB2. Approved in the United States and Canada for the treatment of chemotherapy-induced nausea and vomiting, and sometimes used in Canada off-label and in clinical trials for treating pain and PTSD, nabilone is available in 1-mg capsules because it has higher oral bioavailability and clearer dose linearity than THC.[33]

Epidiolex is a cannabis-derived 100 mg/ml CBD oral solution. It may contain trace amounts of other phytoconstituents; though official reports claim it is devoid of THC, they also report it can cause a patient to test positive on a urine drug test (which does not test for CBD or its metabolites).[34] According to one third-party lab analysis paid for and provided by a patient's parent, the solution contained 0.5 mg/ml THC; I have not seen other independent analyses of this agent. Indicated for Dravet syndrome and Lennox-Gastaut syndrome, two rare seizure disorders, Epidiolex has also demonstrated efficacy in clinical trials with other seizure etiologies.

While caring for patients with chronic pain, orthopedic surgeries requiring hospital admission and/or inpatient rehabilitation are common. In my clinical experience, continuing treatment with cannabinoids in the postoperative course can potentially spare opioid analgesics, improve sleep, and prevent potential cannabis withdrawal symptoms such as anorexia, irritability, and sleep disturbance. When my cannabis-using patients are expecting an inpatient stay, I usually coordinate with their attending physicians to provide an as-needed order for dronabinol, typically administered three times daily, with THC dosage similar to their outpatient herbal use. If a patient is exclusively using inhaled cannabis in the outpatient setting, an approximate conversion scale of 2.5 mg of dronabinol po for 1–2 inhalations/session, 5 mg for 3–5 inhalations, 7.5 mg for 6–8 inhalations, and 10 mg for >8 inhalations can provide a starting point for subsequent titration.

I also care for several physically and/or mentally disabled patients who live in skilled nursing and assisted living facilities that prohibit cannabis on their premises, based on a theoretical risk of being denied federal funding. In these situations, starting with a dronabinol prescription is often the easiest path forward. I care for several pediatric patients with autistic spectrum disorder whose aggressive or self-injurious behaviors respond very well to THC; while school nurses will not administer herbal cannabis, dronabinol can provide an effective midday dose to prevent breakthrough symptoms in the afternoon.

Despite being approved for only two narrow indications, dronabinol and nabilone have been described in case reports, case series, and clinical trials as effective treatments for a wide variety of conditions and symptoms, as one would expect with agents that target the ubiquitous endocannabinoid system. These are old, relatively safe drugs available in generic formulations that offer potential treatment alternatives in patients who may benefit from but lack access to cannabis, after informed consent is obtained for the off-label use of a controlled substance.

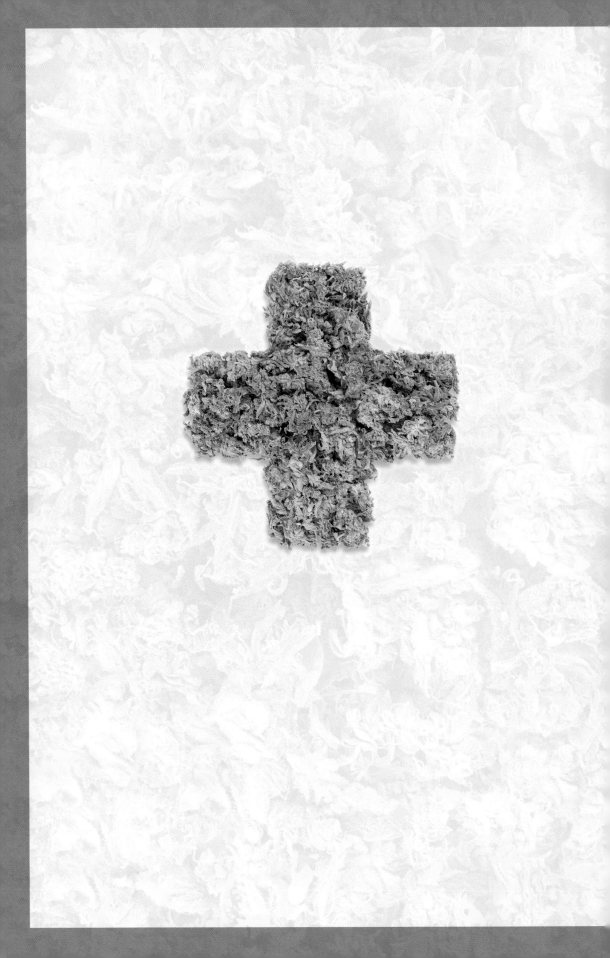

Part 5

Common Clinical Applications

Chapter 20

Chronic Pain and Spasticity

CHRONIC PAIN, frequently accompanied by varying degrees of muscle tension or spasticity, is the most common condition I have treated with cannabis. Pain is the most common reason people use cannabis for therapeutic purposes in the United States.[1] In the 2017 National Academies of Sciences, Engineering, and Medicine (NASEM) report, chronic pain was one of three conditions for which authors found substantial or conclusive evidence that cannabis could be an effective treatment.[2]

Chronic pain is a common medical condition for which conventional treatments are often inadequate or unsafe. According to the 2016 National Health Interview Survey, an estimated 20.4% (50.0 million) of U.S. adults had chronic pain, defined as pain on most days or every day in the past 6 months, and 8.0% of U.S. adults (19.6 million) had "high-impact chronic pain," defined as chronic pain that limited life or work activities on most days or every day during the past 6 months.[3] Prevalence of chronic pain was similar in India, at 19%,[4] and higher in the United Kingdom: a meta-analysis found 35%–51% of the population had chronic pain and 10%–14% had moderately to severely disabling chronic pain.[5] In all three countries, chronic pain is more common in women.

The economic burden of the health-care and indirect costs of chronic pain (e.g., lost wages and productivity) is difficult to calculate but amounts to many trillions of dollars globally each year ($560 billion each year in the United States).[6] Thus, reducing the prevalence of chronic pain by even 1% would have an enormous impact on financial and health-care resources around the world and would improve quality of life for hundreds of millions of people. In our work as clinicians, mitigating chronic pain and related disability is clearly a priority.

Unfortunately, recognition of this need without sufficiently safe and effective treatments in the conventional repertoire, mingled with opportunistic economic forces, gave rise to the overuse of opioid analgesics and the subsequent opioid crisis, with its own high costs of death, disability, and resources. A 2017 report by the Council of Economic Advisers estimated that the opioid crisis cost American taxpayers $504 billion in total economic burden in 2015, 2.8% of the gross domestic profit.[7] The human cost of the opioid crisis for its victims and their loved ones is immeasurable.

Because of the stigma of cannabis among patients and a lack of education among clinicians, it is often a last-resort treatment for chronic pain, considered only after failure to benefit from surgery or opioids. This needs to change. In my experience, the medically supervised use of cannabis is safer and more effective than any individual opioid or non-opioid pharmacotherapy, and not because it is a superior analgesic.

The ability of cannabis to decrease pain intensity is often modest at best. The utility of cannabis is more related to its holistic effects on both nociceptive and affective components of pain, spasticity, inflammation, sleep, mood, anxiety, self-perception, and symptom unbundling (see Chapter 17) and to its versatility in composition and delivery methods, allowing for highly individualized treatments. Patients who use cannabis to treat pain usually experience more self-empowerment and active involvement in their treatment, with greater freedom to titrate and adjust their treatment compared to traditional pharmacotherapies. In patients with coexisting opiate use disorder and chronic pain who are taking methadone or buprenorphine, I've often found that cannabis is the best choice for analgesia and other symptoms.

Clinical Evidence

Several meta-analyses have been performed on data using cannabis or cannabinoids for chronic pain, with most, but not all, reporting significant benefit.

The 2017 NASEM report mentioned earlier based its conclusions primarily on a 2015 review, which evaluated 28 randomized trials on 2,454 participants with varied etiology, including neuropathy (17 trials), cancer pain, fibromyalgia, and others. Of the eight parallel group trials (seven with nabiximols and one with inhaled cannabis), cannabinoid treatment increased the odds of >30% pain reduction by approximately 40% over placebo (*OR* 1.41, 95% confidence interval [CI] 0.99–2.00). Inclusion of the 20 crossover trials in the analysis yielded similar results.[8]

The same meta-analysis reviewed 14 placebo-controlled studies on 2,280 participants with spasticity due to multiple sclerosis (MS) or paraplegia caused by spinal cord injury. Cannabinoids produced an improvement on the Ashworth scale,* an objective measure of resistance to passive movement, but this did not reach statistical significance, with a weighted mean difference of −0.12 (95% CI −0.24 to 0.01). The subjective numeric rating scale of spasticity yielded stronger, significant improvements (mean difference −0.76, 95% CI −1.38 to −0.14), as did the subject global impression of change (OR 1.44, 95% CI 1.07–1.94).

A 2014 review of 34 studies, published by the American Academy of Neurology, found similar results: oral cannabis extract was effective for reducing subjective measures of spasticity in MS, probably ineffective for reducing objective (Ashworth) measures of spasticity at 12–14 weeks, and possibly effective for reducing objective measures of spasticity at 1 year. The authors acknowledged that ≥30% subjective improvement best correlates with a clinically important change, and they suggested the difference between subjective and objective measures may be explained by improvements in feelings of well-being or pain relief that allowed increased mobility. The same review found oral cannabis effective for central pain and spasticity-related pain and probably effective for reducing bladder complaints in MS.[9]

In my clinical experience, I have found inhaled cannabis to be much more effective than oral cannabis for producing objective improvements in spasticity and tremor. A crossover trial on 30 patients with MS using low-quality cannabis cigarettes (4% Δ[9]-tetrahydrocannabinol [THC]) versus placebo cigarettes smoked once daily for 3 days confirmed my observations: reduction on the modified Ashworth scale by an average of 2.74 points more than placebo ($p < .0001$) and reduced visual analogue scale (VAS) pain scores by an average of 5.28 points more than placebo ($p = .008$).[10]

A 2015 review of five randomized trials using inhaled cannabis in 178 participants with chronic neuropathic pain found the number needed to treat to achieve ≥30% short-term subjective improvement in chronic pain was 5.6 patients.[11] These studies were confounded by the use of low-quality cannabis supplied by NIDA and by short-term treatment; I suspect that longer trials using higher-quality medicine would produce even better results.

----

* The Ashworth scale has been criticized as unreliable and insensitive to other forms of spasticity and therapeutic benefit (Pandyan et al., 1999; Wade et al., 2010).

Cannabis for Research Purposes

At the time of writing, the University of Mississippi, funded through the National Institutes of Health and the National Institute on Drug Abuse (NIDA), is the sole facility licensed by the Drug Enforcement Agency to cultivate cannabis for research purposes in the United States. Thus, most federally funded research in which participants consume cannabis relies on NIDA-supplied product. The cannabinoid levels in NIDA research-grade cannabis (~5% THC) have been shown to be significantly divergent from commercially available cannabis from Colorado, Washington, and California (averaging ~18% THC); NIDA samples also contained 11–23 times more CBN than state samples.[12] Furthermore, a majority of commercially available "drug-type" cannabis was genetically very distinct from NIDA samples; NIDA research-grade cannabis was found to genetically group with hemp samples along with a small subset of commercial drug-type cannabis.[13] The substantial differences between NIDA and commercially available cannabis raises significant questions about whether research conducted with federal cannabis is indicative of the experience of our patients.

Cannabis offers many benefits to patients with chronic pain or spasticity, often best achieved by dose layering of different products and delivery methods to maximize an individual's response. As mentioned in Chapter 16, a survey of 1,321 cannabis-using patients with chronic pain found 93.4% used two or more administration routes and 72.5% used three or more.[14] To evaluate the true efficacy and tolerability of real-world medical cannabis treatments, we need pragmatic study designs using commercial-grade cannabis products.

Interestingly, the clinical trials do not suggest any etiology of pain more likely to respond to cannabis, perhaps due to its activity at multiple sites controlling nociception and pain perception. Chronic neuropathic, musculoskeletal, and inflammatory pain can all be ameliorated with cannabis.

Acute pain, however, is less likely to respond and more likely to be exacerbated by cannabis. Eleven randomized controlled trials of cannabinoids for experimentally induced or acute postoperative pain on 238 participants showed no or weak analgesic effects from a variety of cannabinoid doses and routes of administration. The best results were achieved in the medium dose range, and several studies found cannabinoids increased the intensity of acute pain.[15] There is some evidence that analgesic effects are more likely in experienced cannabis users and hyperalgesia effects in cannabis-naïve patients; I have observed this in my clinical practice. Furthermore, many of my experi-

enced patients report bidirectional effects on acute pain, especially with inhaled cannabis: a brief increase in pain intensity may be followed by relief.

Not all meta-analyses have concluded that cannabis is effective for chronic pain. A
2018 review, often cited by cannabis adversaries, that ambitiously compiled data from
47 controlled and 57 observational trials, with a total of 9,958 participants, concluded
that (1) it is unlikely that cannabinoids are highly effective medicines for chronic noncancer pain, with a high number needed to treat to benefit and a low number needed to treat
to harm, and (2) there is minimal evidence that cannabinoids are effective in improving
emotional or physical functioning in patients with chronic noncancer pain. Interestingly,
their conclusions were not exactly congruent with their results. Among nine randomized
controlled trials, the *OR* of ≥30% pain reduction was 1.46 (95% CI 1.16–1.84) and the
Patient Global Impression of Change standard mean difference was 2.0 (95% CI 1.37–
2.94) on a 7-point scale. Several of the authors reported financial conflicts of interest
involving research funding from the opioid industry.[16] This is a perfect example of the
importance of reading the entire paper, including the authors' disclosures, and not just
the abstract, as described in Chapter 4.

Preclinical Evidence and Mechanisms of Action

The antinociceptive effects of cannabis have been demonstrated in animal models since
the 19th century, and a substantial body of evidence has accumulated since then that
demonstrates cannabinoid agonists of CB1 and/or CB2 cannabinoid receptors decrease
pain signaling in models of acute pain and chronic pain of varying etiologies.[17] Analgesia
is considered a primary indicator of CB1 agonism, one of four effects that comprise the
"tetrad model" of CB1 agonist drug discovery (along with hypolocomotion, hypothermia,
and catalepsy).[18]

The endocannabinoid system actively modulates pain signaling throughout the central and peripheral nervous systems at spinal, supraspinal, and peripheral sites of action,
and much of the activity of exogenous cannabinoids mimics the endocannabinoid effects.

Descending Pain Inhibitory Pathway

The "top-down" regulation of pain signaling begins in the periaqueductal gray, a brain
region with high densities of cannabinoid and opioid receptors, and projects into the ros-
tral ventromedial medulla and then to the dorsal horn of the spinal cord. This pathway
enables the brain to dampen nociceptive input and, under certain conditions, entirely suppress pain signaling. While this is essential to our ability to function and survive in the set-

ting of acute injury and is involved in preventing central sensitization and the conversion of acute to chronic pain, the descending inhibitory pathway must not be overly active— otherwise we would fail to experience sufficient pain to protect ourselves from injury. Thus, the descending pain inhibitory pathway includes inhibitory interneurons to dampen its activity. Cannabinoids have been shown to suppress the activity of these GABA-releasing interneurons via CB1 activation, thereby increasing activity of the descending inhibitory pathway and decreasing pain perception, a mechanism similar to opioids.[19]

Ascending Pain Pathway

At the site of an injury, nociceptors begin the ascending signaling that is eventually inter-preted in the brain as pain. The nociceptors are activated and sensitized by a variety of signaling molecules released by damaged tissue (K^+ and H^+ ions, bradykinins, and adenosine triphosphates), leukocytes (histamines, prostaglandins, leukotrienes, and pro-inflammatory cytokines), leukocyte-activated platelets (5-hydroxytryptamine), neighboring autonomic nerves (norepinephrine), and the nociceptor itself (substance P and calcitonin gene-related peptide). If uncontrolled, this process can cause peripheral sensitization, hyperalgesia, and allodynia.

CB1 receptors are present in the distal terminal of nociceptors,* where they open potassium channels and make the nerve less likely to fire, and in the peripheral tissues, where they decrease the release of the aforementioned activators and sensitizers. CB2 receptors in local mast cells and macrophages also decrease the release of activators and sensitizers. The activity of the endocannabinoid system produces a first line of defense against pain at the site of an injury; exogenous cannabinoids reproduce this activity.[20]

CB1 receptors are also present in presynaptic nociceptor terminals in the dorsal horn, where they decrease glutamate signaling and dampen afferent nociceptive signaling.

Affective Component of Pain

In addition to the somatosensory elements of pain processing, pain perception involves a number of psychological processes involving cortico-limbic striatal circuits. These include cognitive appraisal of the meaning of the sensation, attentional orientation to the painful sensation and its source, and the subsequent emotional, behavioral, and psy-

---

* As described in Chapter 11, interrupting axonal transport of CB1 receptors from the dorsal root ganglia, where they are produced, to the nociceptor terminal can interfere with the analgesic effects of cannabinoids in the periphery.

chophysiological (autonomic and inflammatory) reactions: all are sources of feedback to influence pain perception (Figure 20.1).[21]

FIGURE 20.1

Influence of Cannabis on Nociception, Pain Perception, and the Biobehavioral Response to Pain in the Nervous System

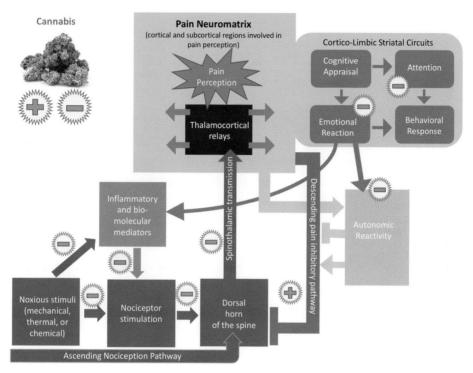

Note. Adapted from "Pain processing in the human nervous system: A selective review of nociceptive and biobehavioral pathways," by Eric L. Garland, 2012, *Primary Care: Clinics in Office Practice, 39*(3), pp. 561–571. Copyright © 2012 by Elsevier. Reprinted with permission.

Ascending nociceptive signaling is often considered as two parallel pathways. The anterior cingulate cortex is part of the "medial" stream, involved in processing affective aspects of pain. The somatosensory cortex is considered part of the "lateral" stream, involved in the sensory aspects of pain processing, though it is clear that these two pathways are heavily interconnected. A recent small human randomized controlled trial on patients with chronic radicular neuropathic pain treated with THC and evaluated with functional magnetic resonance imaging found that THC-induced analgesia was correlated with reduced functional connectivity between the anterior cingulate cortex and the sensorimotor cortex.[22]

These results suggest that THC can induce analgesia, in part by helping disconnect cognitive-emotional functions from sensory signaling, and that the potential benefit of THC may be greater in patients with higher baseline connectivity between the sensory and affective pathways. As described in Chapter 17 (in the section titled Adverse and Beneficial Psychoactive Effects), cannabis can help patients disengage from an experience of pain consuming their life (attentional fixation) and subsequently reengage in more supportive patterns of emotion and behavior (restored self).

CB2-Related Analgesia[23]

Selective CB2 agonists produce antinociceptive effects in animal models of acute and persistent pain. The impact of CB2 on pain signaling is most pronounced in models involving inflammation, likely related to the ability of CB2 to suppress inflammatory cytokine production. CB2 receptors are also found on primary afferents where they suppress nociception in the absence of inflammation, perhaps by stimulating release of β-endorphin. When the sensory nerves are injured, CB2 receptor expression increases significantly, especially in painful neuromas.

Noncannabinoid Receptor Mechanisms

Cannabidiol (CBD) conveys analgesic effects, though they are typically less pronounced than those of THC. The antinociceptive and antiallodynic effects likely occur via TRPV1 agonism, and affective/anxiolytic effects likely occur via 5-HT1A agonism.[24] CBD has been shown to suppress neuropathic pain in rats with spinal nerve injury via the α3 glycine receptor[25] and to reduce chronic inflammatory pain via the α1 glycine receptor.[26] The antihyperalgesic effects of cannabidiolic acid are also likely mediated by TRPV1.[27]

Several of the terpenoids found in cannabis, such as β-myrcene and linalool, convey their own analgesic properties.[28] Furthermore, the numerous anti-inflammatory effects of cannabinoids and terpenoids, including inhibition of tumor necrosis factor α, are likely indirectly involved in the analgesic effects.[29]

Antispasmodic Mechanisms of Action

Animal models of MS have demonstrated that the antispasmodic effects of cannabis are dependent on CB1 signaling,[30] though the exact neural pathways involved have not been well elucidated. CB1 receptors are densely represented in cortical and basal ganglia areas subserving motor control, in their corresponding cerebellar counterparts, and in interneurons of the spinal cord and neocortex that may relate to pathophysiolog-ical mechanisms of spasticity.[31] The antispasmodic effects of CBD are likely related to its indirect activity on CB1 signaling through inhibition of anandamide breakdown and transport, but CBD may also work via indirect activity at glycine receptors.[32]

Cannabinoid–Opioid Interactions

Cannabinoid and opioid receptors are colocalized in pain signaling regions of the brain and spinal cord. The two signaling pathways clearly interact with each other, producing synergistic (greater than additive) antinociceptive effects.[33] In a recent meta-analysis of 19 preclinical studies, 17 reported cannabinoid–opioid synergy. Remarkably, the median effective dose (ED50) of morphine administered in combination with THC was 3.6 times lower than the ED50 of morphine alone, and the ED50 for codeine administered in com-bination with THC was 9.5 times lower than the ED50 of codeine alone.[34]

Even subanalgesic doses of THC have been shown to potentiate opioid analgesia, prevent opioid withdrawal, and, importantly, prevent opioid tolerance.[35] Animals treated with THC and morphine retained analgesic efficacy and had an increase in μ-opioid receptor proteins in the spinal cord; long-term treatment with opioids alone typically results in tolerance, loss of efficacy, and m-opioid receptor downregulation.[36] THC has even been shown to restore opioid analgesia after loss of efficacy.[37]

Several studies have shown that CB1 receptors modulate the release of endog-enous opioids, and THC has been shown to increase levels of β-endorphin and other endogenous opioids. Other potential mechanisms of synergy between these two sys-tems include receptor heterodimerization and signaling transduction overlap.[38] Clearly, our endogenous cannabinoid and opioid systems interact significantly in our response to pain; treatment strategies with exogenous agents can learn from this example.

Human experimental evidence confirms the ability of cannabis to potentiate opioid analgesia. In 18 healthy cannabis users, the cold pressor test, an experimental model of pain threshold and tolerance, was used to evaluate the analgesic effects of combining various doses of oxycodone (0, 2.5, and 5 mg) and cannabis cigarettes (0.0% and 5.6% THC). Administered alone, only the 5-mg dose of oxycodone increased pain threshold and tolerance compared to placebo; when combined with active cannabis, the 2.5-mg dose of oxycodone effectively increased pain threshold and tolerance compared to pla-cebo and to active cannabis alone. The authors also evaluated the abuse liability of com-bined cannabis and oxycodone by asking about likeability and desire to take the drug again; interestingly, participants preferred the 2.5 mg of oxycodone + cannabis condition more than 5 mg of oxycodone ± cannabis.[39]

A similar study using oral THC (0, 2.5, and 5 mg) administered 1 hr before oxyco-done (0, 5, and 10 mg) in 10 non-cannabis-using healthy participants failed to show any enhancement of the analgesic effects of oxycodone in four experimental models of acute pain (cold pressor, pressure algometer, hot thermode, and cold hyperalgesia). THC did increase the subjective effects of oxycodone, including ratings of feeling high and drug liking. These results are unsurprising; as mentioned previously, cannabis-naïve patients are much less likely to experience the analgesic effects of THC in acute pain.

It is important to note that models of acute pain in healthy patients likely do not adequately reflect the clinical use of combined cannabinoid–opioid therapy in patients with chronic pain. In an inpatient study on 21 patients with chronic pain on sustained-release opioids, cannabis (3.56% THC) vaporized 3 times daily decreased pain by an average of 27%.[40] In a study on 30 patients with chronic pain refractory to >6 months of treatment with opioids, single oral doses of THC (10 or 20 mg) improved pain intensity compared to placebo; both doses were equally effective (Figure 20.2a). A subsequent open-label titration trial in the same patients relieved pain, reduced pain bothersome-ness, and increased satisfaction compared with baseline (Figure 20.2b).[41]

FIGURE 20.2A

Average Hourly Pain Intensity Ratings with Dronabinol

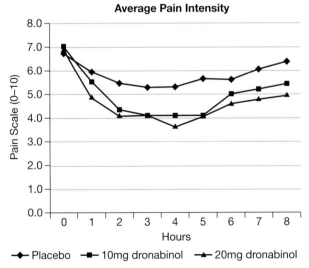

Note. From "Efficacy of dronabinol as an adjuvant treatment for chronic pain patients on opioid therapy," by S. Narang, D. P. Gibson, A. D. Wasan, E. L. Ross, E. Michna, S. S. Nedeljkovic, and R. N. Jamison, 2008, *The Journal of Pain, 9*(3), pp. 254–264 (https://doi.org/10.1016/j.jpain.2007.10.018). Copyright © 2008 by American Pain Society. Reprinted with permission.

FIGURE 20.2B

Average Pain Intensity Ratings with Dronabinol over 4 Weeks

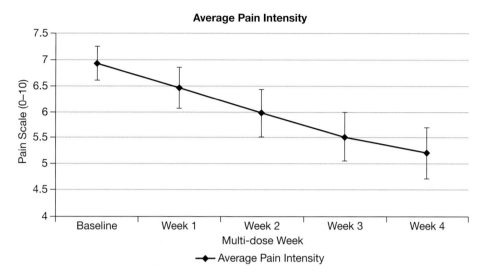

Average Pain Intensity

Note. From "Efficacy of dronabinol as an adjuvant treatment for chronic pain patients on opioid therapy," by S. Narang, D. P. Gibson, A. D. Wasan, E. L. Ross, E. Michna, S. S. Nedeljkovic, and R. N. Jamison, 2008, *The Journal of Pain, 9*(3), pp. 254–264 (https://doi.org/10.1016/j.jpain.2007.10.018). Copyright © 2008 by American Pain Society. Reprinted with permission.

There is also some preclinical evidence that CBD can potentiate opioid analgesia. In a mouse model of neuropathic pain, CBD had analgesic effects at 1 mg/kg but not at 2 mg/kg, a notable biphasic dose response. A subanalgesic dose of morphine (0.1 mg/kg) produced analgesic effects when combined with 1 mg/kg CBD and even stronger effects, comparable to those of 2.5 mg/kg morphine alone, when combined with 2 mg/kg CBD.[42]

Human evidence of CBD–opioid synergy is sparse; in an 8-week observational study of 97 patients with moderate to severe chronic pain that was refractory to >1 year of opioid treatment, adding gel caps of approximately 15 mg of CBD-dominant hemp oil twice daily was associated with improved quality of life in 94% of subjects, complete cessation of opioids in two subjects, and numerous reports of ability to skip opioid doses among other subjects.[43] Though not necessarily related to analgesia, high-dose CBD (400 or 800 mg) has been shown to reduce cue-induced craving and anxiety in abstinent heroin users.[44]

A large and ever-growing body of observational human evidence consistently documents the opioid-sparing effects of cannabis in real-world setting (see Chapter 28 for more details). Though most cannabis specialists experience significant selection bias in our patient populations, attracting those who are highly motivated to decrease or discontinue their opioid drugs, I have been sincerely impressed with the ability of cannabis to spare opioids or provide superior results when used in combination.

I collected survey responses from 525 patients with chronic pain who had used prescription opioid medications continuously for at least 3 months from my practices in Maine and our sister site in Massachusetts. Upon addition of medical cannabis, 40.4% (n = 204) reported that they stopped all opioids, 45.2% (n = 228) reported some decrease in their opioid usage, 13.3% (n = 67) reported no change in opioid usage, and 1.1% (n = 6) reported an increase in opioid usage. Almost half (48.2%, n = 241) reported a 40%–100% decrease in pain, 8.6% (n = 43) had no change in pain, and 2.6% (n = 13) had worsening pain. The majority reported improved ability to function (80.0%, n = 420) and improved quality of life (87.0%, n = 457) with medical cannabis.

Treatment Strategies for Clinicians

- Establish concrete functional goals tailored to a patient's individual values; create realistic expectations and explain that reductions in pain interference and bothersomeness are usually more pronounced than reductions in pain intensity.
- Prioritize correcting sleep disturbance, which contributes to hyperalgesia,[45] with THC-dominant preparations. In cannabis-naïve patients, I sometimes start with 3–14 days of evening-only dosing. This can widen the therapeutic window and improve analgesic response when daytime dosing is started.
- For chronic pain, begin baseline daytime treatment with oral or oromucosal dosing in the morning and repeat in the afternoon if needed.
- Combination THC/CBD is usually best for daytime treatment; adjust the ratio based on sensitivity to the psychoactive effects of THC.
- CBD-dominant treatment may be helpful in some patients but likely requires higher doses than combined THC/CBD and may be cost-prohibitive.
- Use inhaled cannabis for breakthrough symptoms, opioid craving, and sleep latency.
- For episodic pain like migraine and other nondaily headaches, use inhaled cannabis at the earliest signs of an episode.
- For localized pain, consider topical cannabis products.
- Use cannabis to potentiate nonpharmacological treatments (see Chapter 19) like physical therapy and mindfulness. Savoring practices may be especially effective for patients with opioid dependence or anhedonia.
- In patients with spasticity or muscular hypertonicity, inhaled cannabis may be more effective than oral or oromucosal routes.
- In addition to opioids, I have observed many patients who are able to use cannabis to spare gabapentinoids (which require slow taper), benzodiazepines, nonsteroidal anti-inflammatory drugs, and skeletal muscle relaxants.

- For patients who wish to use cannabis to spare opioid analgesics, I have found the following strategies effective:
    - Take an oral or oromucosal dose of cannabis with every opioid dose. This can be below the threshold of impairment or undesirable psychoactive effects.
    - Use inhaled cannabis for opioid cravings and withdrawal symptoms.
    - Identify and reverse cannabis tolerance before tapering opioids (see Chapter 17).
    - Titrate the oromucosal cannabis until the patient begins to feel potentiation of analgesia or sedation, then taper the opioid.
    - Many patients are able to drastically reduce their opioid dose in the first 2 weeks of combination treatment (often by 50%–80%), followed by more gradual taper or dose stabilization.
    - Others do well with a slow, gradual taper, with temporary small increases in cannabis dosage in the days following an opioid dose reduction.
    - Some patients find the cannabinoid–opioid combination treatment superior to opioid monotherapy but are unable to reduce their opioid dose; I consider this an acceptable outcome. The addition of cannabis usually stabilizes their response to a consistent dose of opioids and halts previous trends of dose escalation.
    - Some patients do not experience analgesia potentiation with low to moderate doses of cannabis but do well by titrating up to high doses of cannabinoids (e.g. 100–500 mg po, three times daily). These benefits may be more related to decreasing reward signaling and anti-inflammatory effects.

Cautions

- The absence of cannabinoid receptors in brain-stem cardiorespiratory centers makes it improbable that adding cannabis to opioids will increase the risk of cardiorespiratory suppression, an adverse effect that has never been reported in the literature or observed in my clinical experience. It is more likely that adding cannabis to opioids improves the therapeutic index of the opioids. The ability of THC to increase endogenous opioid secretion, however, could plausibly increase the risk of opioid-related adverse effects.
- The combined muscle-relaxant and analgesic effects of cannabis can predispose people to injury when cannabis is combined with physical therapy, yoga, etc. While patients often report that cannabis augments the benefits of these modalities, patients and their therapists should use caution to avoid excessive stretching into the range of motion barrier.

Chapter 21

Anxiety and Trauma-Related Disorders

ANXIETY DISORDERS are the most common type of psychiatric disorders, with a lifetime prevalence of up to 33.7% and double the prevalence in women compared to men.[1] A large number of patients report using cannabis and related products to treat anxiety symptoms or disorders: in a pooled sample from 13 survey studies of cannabis use (*N* = 6,665), 52% reported using cannabis for anxiety, making it the second most commonly treated symptom, following pain.[2]

According to the *Diagnostic and Statistical Manual of Mental Disorders*, 5th edition (DSM-5), anxiety disorders share features of excessive fear, anxiety, and related behavioral disturbances. These disorders include separation anxiety disorder, selective mutism, specific phobia, social anxiety disorder, panic disorder, agoraphobia, generalized anxiety disorder, substance- or medication-induced anxiety disorder, and anxiety disorder due to another medical condition.[3] While most anxiety disorders are functional psychiatric disorders, organic causes such as substance-induced anxiety, acute and chronic infections, and hyperthyroid-related anxiety should be considered.

Environmental factors such as trauma increase the risk of developing anxiety disorders, as do several genetic factors.[4] A polymorphism in *CNR1*, the gene that codes for the human CB1 receptor, has been associated with the development of posttraumatic stress disorder (PTSD), potentially related to its impact on the function of the hypothalamic–pituitary–adrenocortical (HPA) axis.[5]

Symptoms vary depending on the specific anxiety disorder. *Generalized anxiety disorder* is characterized by excessive and difficult-to-control anxiety and worry associated with at least three of the following six symptoms, occurring more days than not for at least 6 months: restlessness, fatigue, difficulty concentrating, irritability, muscle tension, and sleep disturbance. *Social anxiety disorder* features impaired function due to excessive fear of social or performance situations and includes avoidance behavior, anticipation, and distress.

Panic disorder features recurrent panic attacks, with one or more attacks followed by at least 1 month of fear of another panic attack or significant maladaptive behavior related to the attacks. A panic attack is an abrupt period of intense fear or discomfort accompanied by four or more systemic symptoms (e.g., palpitations, sweating, trembling, shortness of breath, or fear of losing control or going crazy).

Scientific understanding of the brain circuits and regions associated with anxiety disorders is growing. The amygdala is key in modulating fear and anxiety, and patients with anxiety disorders often show heightened amygdala response to anxiety cues.[6] Many of the symptoms of anxiety disorders described above are related to activation of the sympathetic nervous system.[7,8] These areas represent targets for pharmacotherapy: it is well-established that CB1 receptors occur with high density in certain amygdala nuclei associated with anxiety signaling[9] and that cannabinoid signaling can suppress excessive sympathetic activity[10] and HPA axis signaling.[11]

The use of cannabis and CB1 agonists has been associated with both anxiolytic effects at lower doses and anxiogenic effects at higher doses.[12] This may explain why, though cannabis users widely report its anxiolytic benefits, one meta-analysis found that cannabis use is associated with anxiety ($OR = 1.24$, 95% confidence interval [CI] 1.06–1.45, $p = .006$; $N = 15$ studies) after controlling for confounding factors (demographics, other substance use, or other psychiatric comorbidity); this association infers causality.[13] Conversely, several other papers have failed to show an association between cannabis use and anxiety disorders.[14,15,16]

While the bidirectional effect on anxiety may be most evident for cannabis dominant in Δ^9-tetrahydrocannabinol (THC), pharmaceutical-grade cannabidiol (CBD) has also demonstrated similar dose–response trends.[17] For example, in one study of healthy subjects, a 300-mg dose of CBD was associated with improvements in anxiety scores compared to placebo during public speaking, while a 900-mg dose was associated with increased anxiety scores compared to placebo.[18]

Though they are closely related to anxiety disorders, the DSM-5 created a new category for "trauma- and stressor-related disorders" that includes acute stress disorder and PTSD. These conditions develop as an aberrant adaptation to a traumatic event and are characterized by intrusive symptoms such as nightmares and flashbacks, avoidance of trauma-related stimuli, negative alterations in cognition and mood, and alterations in arousal and reactivity like hypervigilance and irritability. The pathophysiology of trauma-related disorders is similar to that of anxiety disorders, involving increased responsivity in the amygdala and decreased volume in the prefrontal cortex and hippocampus, resulting in hyperarousal and anxiety, dysfunction in the HPA axis coordination of the neuro-endocrine stress response, and dysregulation of neurotransmitters, such as increases in norepinephrine and glutamate and decrease in serotonin.

Some evidence suggests dysfunction of the endocannabinoid system in trauma-related disorders. Reduced peripheral levels of anandamide (AEA), abnormal CB1 receptor-mediated AEA signaling, and compensatory increase of CB1 receptor avail-ability are implicated in PTSD etiology and degree of intrusive symptoms.[19] Among 46 individuals in close proximity to the World Trade Center at the time of the 9/11 attacks, those who met diagnostic criteria for PTSD (n = 24) had significantly lower levels of cir-culating 2-arachidonoylglycerol (measured at 8 A.M.) than those who did not. AEA levels exhibited a negative relationship with the degree of intrusive symptoms within the PTSD sample, consistent with animal data indicating that reductions in AEA promote retention of aversive emotional memories.[20]

PTSD is often resistant to traditional antidepressant and anxiolytic medications, in part because these treatments failed to address memory alterations, such as the inability to extinguish learned fear responses, to suppress episodic traumatic retrieval, to acquire safety signals, and to dampen the overconsolidation process taking place right after reexperiencing symptoms. Cannabinoids are promising for treating PTSD due to their dual anxiolytic and memory-modulating effects. Preclinical and early clinical research has produced encouraging results targeting the enhancement of extinction learning, which could "reduce the conditioned fear and anxiety responses triggered by trauma reminders, increasing patients' general ability to actively cope with the trauma without affecting the original memory trace."[21]

I have observed this benefit in some of my patients. For example, a 34-year-old vet-eran who was injured by a roadside explosive returned to civilian life with recurrent epi-sodes of extreme distress most commonly triggered by visual stimuli while driving, such as a red flag tied to the end of lumber extending from the back of a pickup truck. He explained that every time this happened, he would pull over, take an inhalation or two of THC-rich cannabis from a pipe he kept in his car, and then meditate for 15–30 min before continuing on his way (assuring me he avoided driving until any potential impairment had subsided). One day he was proud to report that seeing a red flag on the way to our office visit, for the first time since his injury, elicited no adverse response. Perhaps his use of cannabis with every trigger enhanced extinction learning; human studies supporting this hypothesis are reviewed in Chapter 19.

Clinical Evidence

Little research has directly evaluated the effects of medical cannabis on symptoms in patients with anxiety and trauma-related disorders.

A few studies have evaluated the use of nabilone in patients with anxiety and PTSD. Nabilone was found to be effective for reducing anxiety in both an open-label dose range study of five men with psychoneurotic anxiety, which found the optimum dose to be 3 mg daily, and a 28-day double-blind study (N = 20). Improvement of anxiety occurred within 3 days, symptoms of depression also improved.[22] A double-blind trial of 20 patients with anxiety treated with nabilone (1 mg three times daily) demonstrated dramatic improvement in anxiety in the nabilone group when compared with placebo (p < .001).[23] An observational study of nabilone in six patients requiring multiple antidepressants for mixed anxiety and mood disorders, titrated from 0.25 mg to 1 mg at bedtime, showed an average improvement in Generalized Anxiety Disorder 7-item scores of 26.5% over 6 months.[24] This supports my observation that some patients with anxiety are able to use cannabis in the evening with residual improvements in symptoms the following day.

In a retrospective study of 104 male inmates with serious mental illness, treatment with nabilone (average of 4 mg daily) led to significant improvement in PTSD-associated insomnia, nightmares, PTSD symptoms, and Global Assessment of Functioning scores (as well as subjective improvements in chronic pain). Medications associated with greater risk for adverse effects or abuse than nabilone, most often antipsychotics, sedatives or hypnotics, and antidepressants, could often be discontinued, and there was no evidence of nabilone abuse or diversion. The authors found it particularly noteworthy that, in virtually all subjects, nabilone targeted several symptoms simultaneously (average 3.5 symptoms per participant), likely reducing polypharmacy risk.[25]

An open-label pilot study carried out in 10 patients with chronic PTSD, on stable medication, found that adding on 5 mg of THC twice a day led to statistically significant improvements in global symptom severity, sleep quality, frequency of nightmares, and PTSD hyperarousal symptoms.[26] A placebo-controlled crossover trial of nabilone (0.5–3 mg at bedtime) in 10 military personnel with PTSD demonstrated a significant reduction in nightmares, improvement general well-being, and improvement in Clinical Global Impression of Change scores.[27]

At the time of writing, no published controlled trials had evaluated the use of herbal cannabis for anxiety or trauma-related disorders, though at least two randomized controlled trials are underway in patients with PTSD.[28,29] Eight cross-sectional studies reported relief of anxiety as a primary or secondary benefit of cannabis for therapeutic purposes, with one reporting recurrence of symptoms upon cannabis cessation.[30]

In one placebo-controlled study of 24 treatment-naïve patients with generalized social anxiety disorder, pretreatment with 600 mg of CBD before a simulated public speaking test significantly reduced anxiety, cognitive impairment, and discomfort in speech performance.[31]

A large case series found that CBD at doses of 25–175 mg/day reduced anxiety scores in 57 of 72 patients.[32] Another case series on 11 adult patients with PTSD found an average of around 50 mg of CBD, added to their routine psychiatric care, reduced symptoms in 10 patients by an average of 28%, as measured by the PTSD Checklist for DSM-5, after 8 weeks of treatment.[33]

A survey of 271 medical cannabis users in Canada found that 16% reported using cannabis as a substitute for benzodiazepines and 12% for antidepressant drugs.[34] In a survey of 2,774 patients who used cannabis to treat various medical conditions, 58% substituted prescription medications with cannabis; 13.6% of patients substituted anxiolytic and benzodiazepine medications with medical cannabis, the second most substituted drug class following narcotics and opioids (35.8%).[35] Another survey of dispensary members (N = 1,513) revealed that 71.8% of respondents reduced their intake of anti-anxiety medications.[36]

Some data suggest better outcomes in patients with PTSD who use cannabis. A retrospective study analyzing PTSD symptoms collected during 80 psychiatric evaluations of patients applying to the New Mexico Medical Cannabis Program during 2009–2011 identified >75% reduction in Clinician-Administered PTSD Scale for DSM-IV symptom scores when patients with PTSD were using cannabis compared to when they were not.[37]

Data from the 2012 Canadian Community Health Survey-Mental Health of over 24,000 respondents, after control for demographic characteristics, mental health, and substance use comorbidities, demonstrated that, among cannabis nonusers, PTSD was significantly associated with recent major depressive episodes (adjusted *OR* 7.18, 95% CI 4.32–11.91) and suicidal ideation (adjusted *OR* 4.76, 95% CI 2.39–9.47). Importantly, PTSD was not associated with either outcome among cannabis-using respondents.[38]

Conversely, other observational data do not support improvement in PTSD symptoms among cannabis users. A cross-sectional study of 350 cannabis-using military veterans with PTSD and 350 matched non-cannabis-using controls found no significant differences in mean PTSD scores.[39]

While the bidirectional effects of cannabis on anxiety are clearly related to dosage, among cannabis-using patients, specific chemovars are commonly considered more likely to produce anxiolytic effects. One study surveyed 442 patients (60% who reported anxiety as a symptom for which they use medical cannabis and 15% who reported being diagnosed with a specific anxiety disorder) who received medical cannabis from a single source. The chemovars most effective for treating anxiety were Bubba Kush, Skywalker OG Kush, Blueberry Lambsbread, and Kosher Kush. Compared to the least effective chemovars, these contained higher levels of THC, lower levels of CBD, higher levels of *trans*-nerolidol, and lower levels of terpinolene and guaiol. Among the respondents, 14.2% reported an anxiogenic side effect of the cannabis. While this study had many limitations, it began to shed light on the complex entourage effects of cannabis phyto-constituents in relation to anxiolytic activity.[40]

Preclinical Evidence

Several studies have demonstrated that acute administration of low doses of CB1 ago-nists can reduce anxiety behaviors in a variety of animal models,[41,42] likely through acti-vation of CB1 receptors on glutamatergic nerve terminals.[43] Conversely, for example, 12 days of high-dose cannabinoid treatment (100 µg/kg HU-210 synthetic cannabinoid) increased anxiety behaviors and neuroendocrine responses to acute stress in rats.[44] Thus, preclinical studies support the hypothesis that low doses or infrequent exposure to THC-predominant cannabis can reduce feelings of anxiety and stress but that chronic overuse can increase anxiety.

Most rodent studies demonstrate anxiolytic effects of CBD in a biphasic dose–response pattern, with moderate doses producing the best results. Preclinical data have also demonstrated the ability of CBD to mitigate the anxiogenic effects of THC in certain doses.[45]

A large body of preclinical research has investigated and demonstrated the utility of cannabinoids in several different models of PTSD:

- Cannabinoid administration in the immediate aftermath of a trauma may reduce the impact of the subsequent traumatic memory by interfering with the memory consol-idation process (the process taking place in a limited time window immediately after an experience that allows an initially labile memory trace to become stabilized into long-term memory).
- Cannabinoids may reduce traumatic memory by interfering with the memory retrieval process. After a memory trace has been reactivated, it becomes labile again and requires a new wave of consolidation (or reconsolidation) to be updated in the long-term memory. A poorly retrieved memory is less prone to be reconsolidated.
- Cannabinoids may enhance extinction learning (the form of learning that allows a stimulus, previously paired with a negative emotional experience that triggers fear

and anxiety responses, to become nonthreatening again). The case I presented above (34-year-old veteran) is a likely example of this intervention.

Among these three potential applications, the third has the most supporting preclinical evidence and arguably the highest likelihood for successful translation to human studies.[46]

Rodent studies have also demonstrated pharmacodynamic synergy between THC and benzodiazepines,[47,48] suggesting that coadministration of cannabis with this drug class could offer benzodiazepine-sparing effects and support drug tapers.

Treatment Strategies for Clinicians

- Low to moderate oromucosal dosing 2–3 times daily is usually the best strategy for preventing anxiety and trauma-related symptoms. Many patients do well with CBD-dominant preparations in the daytime (10–50 mg) and THC-dominant preparations before bed (5–20 mg).

- Carefully titrated low-dose inhaled cannabis can be helpful for breakthrough anxiety symptoms and, in the experienced user, to abort panic attacks and intense reexperiencing symptoms. This can be especially effective when the inhaled cannabis is followed by an autogenic relaxation technique.

- I have observed nearly universal clinical success reducing or resolving trauma-related nightmares and sleep disturbance with THC-dominant oral preparations. This essential priority often yields global improvements in symptoms around the clock.

- For patients who inhale THC-dominant cannabis, appropriate chemovar selection can be crucial. Some THC-dominant chemovars are known for their anxiolytic effects, while others are commonly anxiogenic.

- Some patients report anxiolytic effects from inhaled CBD-dominant chemovars without risk of anxiogenesis or impairment.

- For THC-sensitive individuals who experience exacerbations of anxiety even with low-dose oromucosal delivery, consider a trial of CBD-dominant cannabis or CBD isolate in the 10–200 mg range, 2–3 times daily.

- Concurrent nonpharmacological treatments, such as cognitive and behavioral therapies, biofeedback, and physical exercise, are likely to improve self-efficacy and improve safety and efficacy.

- For patients who wish to use cannabis to help taper benzodiazepines, concurrent use is unlikely to increase cardiorespiratory suppression but is likely to increase anxiolysis and sedation. I typically titrate up to an effective dose of cannabis prior to tapering benzodiazepines.

- Consider adjunctive anxiolytic herbs (see Chapter 19), especially calamus for patients with gastrointestinal symptoms, 5-hydroxytryptophan for those with co-occurring depression and/or insomnia, kava for patients striving to avoid benzodiazepines, and tulsi for those with fatigue and depleted constitution ("wired but tired").

Cautions

- High doses and inhaled delivery of THC-dominant cannabis, including cannabis concentrates, are most likely to acutely increase anxiety, likely via autonomic dysregulation.
- Long-term, high-dose cannabis use that leads to tolerance may worsen baseline anxiety symptoms over time and increase the likelihood of anxiety symptoms during withdrawal.
- Pharmacodynamic interactions between THC and anticholinergic drugs may increase the likelihood of an anxiogenic response.
- Patients with higher levels of self-efficacy are most likely to be successful using cannabis to treat anxiety. Patients with low self-efficacy and histories of substance misuse require closer monitoring.
- In certain patients, cannabis use can increase avoidant behaviors. Be sure to monitor functional goals in addition to anxiety severity.
- An individual's anxiolytic or anxiogenic responses to cannabis can change drastically over time. Patients who once enjoyed anxiolytic effects may fail to recognize that their cannabis use is currently causing anxiety, or they may choose to tolerate short periods of increased anxiety followed by decreased anxiety (often concurrent with euphoria, analgesia, or other benefits). Conversely, those who experienced an anxiogenic response in their youth are often able to achieve anxiolysis with appropriate dosing later in life.

Chapter 22

Sleep Disorders

SLEEP IS AN ESSENTIAL COMPONENT of health, healing, and quality of life, and from a practical standpoint, I rarely see patients significantly improve their physical and mental health when they are not getting restorative sleep. Sleep disruption is a common problem, and while cannabis is not a hypnotic agent per se, I have seen excellent clinical responses due to its ability to mitigate symptoms disturbing sleep (like anxiety, pain, and restless limbs), promote physical relaxation and stillness, and allow the mind to wander away from ruminating and stress thoughts. I have also observed consistently impressive results in reducing trauma-related nightmares that disrupt sleep. I prioritize improving sleep in all of my patients who sleep poorly, and I have been overwhelmingly impressed by the efficacy and high response rate when cannabis is dosed appropriately.

Insufficient sleep is reported in 30%–35% of the general population[1] and is strongly associated with higher rates of chronic illness, including obesity, diabetes, hypertension, coronary heart disease, stroke, asthma, and arthritis, as well as frequent mental distress, and these associations remain strong even after controlling for age, sex, ethnicity, education, and obesity. For example, in a population of 375,653 U.S. adults, those with the worst reported sleep, compared to those with no sleep disturbance, had 1.48 adjusted *OR* for having diabetes, 2.18 adjusted *OR* for having coronary heart disease, 2.08 adjusted *OR* for having stroke, and 2.52 adjusted *OR* for having arthritis.[2] While these associations likely have reciprocal and bidirectional causality, the potential to reduce morbidity, mortality, and health-care costs by improving sleep is profound.

Higher-order cognition is negatively impacted by sleep deprivation; small reductions in sleep (≤7 hr of sleep per night for 1 week) result in decreased speed on cognitive tasks, and larger disruptions (≤5 hr of sleep per night for 1 week) result in decreased accuracy.[3]

In tasks requiring judgment, risky behaviors increase as the total sleep duration is limited to 5 hr per night.[4]

Depression and anxiety have high rates of comorbidity with sleep problems and the aforementioned chronic diseases, and poor sleep is more common in people with mental health disorders. Though often viewed as a symptom or epiphenomenon of psychiatric disorders, increasing evidence suggests that disturbed sleep has a contributory causal role in these conditions and that sleep promotion can be used as an intervention. In the OASIS trial, perhaps the largest randomized controlled trial (RCT) of a psychological intervention, 3,755 university students with insomnia received either 10 weeks of digital cognitive behavioral therapy (CBT) for insomnia or usual care; the odds ratios for depressive disorder, anxiety disorder, mania, and ultrahigh risk of psychosis were markedly reduced and highly statistically significant in the treatment group, and function and well-being scores increased.[5]

Sleep quality and duration are intimately related to pain signaling. Experimental data strongly demonstrate that disturbed sleep can cause hyperalgesia and the development or exacerbation of spontaneous pain symptoms, and it is a risk factor in the development of chronic pain. The reciprocal relationship between sleep deficiency and pain perpetuates both in a vicious cycle in patients with chronic pain: a bad night's sleep enhances pain, which in turn disturbs sleep, and the cycle continues and amplifies over time. Numerous endogenous mechanisms are involved in this relationship, including opioid, monoaminergic, orexigenic, hypothalamus–pituitary–adrenocortical axis, pineal melatonin, and endocannabinoid systems.[6]

While the causal relationship of sleep and pain is bidirectional, sleep status is a more reliable predictor of pain than pain is of sleep,[7] and stand-alone sleep interventions have been shown to improve pain. For example, a systematic review of RCTs of pharmacological and nonpharmacological sleep interventions in patients with low back pain found a pooled mean difference on the visual analogue pain scale of −12.77/100; there was, however, no significant difference in pain in a similar analysis of osteoarthritis.[8]

Nonpharmacological interventions like CBT, considered first-line therapy for insomnia, and sleep hygiene education cannot be replaced by pharmacotherapy, including cannabis. CBT for insomnia is, according to a recent review, the most effective at addressing sleep disturbance in patients with chronic pain and, interestingly, has been shown to reduce levels of inflammatory markers like C-reactive protein and interleukin 6. The pathophysiology of sleep disturbance involves brain inflammation, and anti-inflammatory and immunomodulatory treatments, such as anti–tumor necrosis factor therapies in rheumatological conditions, have been shown to improve sleep even in the absence of pain improvement.[9] Thus, a pharmacotherapy approach that can modulate inflammation, promote sleep, and enhance the effects of CBT is appealing; cannabis likely fits this description.

Cannabis is also frequently able to spare or replace medications known to disturb sleep, especially opioids. Acute and chronic opioid use generally disrupts sleep, as indicated by reduced slow-wave sleep, REM sleep suppression, and increased awakenings and arousal during sleep, and chronic opioid use increases both daytime sedation and the prevalence of breathing disorders, particularly central sleep apnea.[10] Even worse, preclinical studies suggest that sleep disturbance counteracts the analgesic effects of opioids,[11] a factor contributing to loss of efficacy, dose escalation, hyperalgesia, and augmentation of this vicious cycle.

In the last decade, our understanding of the blood–brain barrier has grown immensely, revealing a complex system that regulates both blood-to-brain and brain-to-blood transport and immune function, and sleep has been shown to be a factor influencing blood–brain barrier function and dysfunction. The recently described glymphatic system, paravascular pathways in which cerebrospinal fluid circulates through brain parenchyma, exchanges with interstitial fluid, and exits along paravenous pathways, facilitates both clearance of interstitial central nervous system (CNS) waste and distribution of glucose, lipids, amino acids, growth factors, and neuromodulators. Incredibly, cortical interstitial space has been shown to increase by 60% during natural sleep, the time when most glymphatic activity occurs.[12]

Sleep, glymphatic function, and neurodegenerative disorders are intimately related. Sleep problems are both early symptoms and contributing factors in several neurodegenerative disorders, most of which are associated with a toxic buildup of waste products in the nervous system, and glymphatic function has been shown to remove contributing proteins like amyloid-β, a component of innate response to CNS infection and also a pathogenic marker of Alzheimer's disease. Accumulating data suggest an infectious component of neurodegenerative disorders: herpes simplex virus type 1, *Chlamydia* pneumonia, and spirochetes like *Borrelia* can remain dormant in the CNS until immune activity weakens.[13] Activation of human endogenous retroviruses has also been strongly implicated in neurodegenerative diseases.[14] Thus, effective treatment and prevention of neurodegenerative conditions requires both adequate clearing of CNS toxins and adequate immune activity to suppress latent CNS infections.

The direct effects of sleep on immune function and inflammation have been clearly demonstrated. For example, immune response to vaccination is markedly impaired in people with chronic sleep deprivation.[15] Other indirect detrimental immune and inflammatory effects of poor sleep are mediated by mental distress, obesity, and lifestyle factors. It is likely that disturbed sleep in aging and neurodegenerative conditions limits both detoxification and innate defense against infection in the CNS. A pharmacotherapy approach for sleep that also provides neuroprotection and potential anti-infectious and immune-balancing effects in the CNS is appealing, especially in patients who have, or are predisposed to, neurodegeneration. Again, cannabis fits this description.

Sleep Cycle Stages[16]

Normal sleep is divided into non–rapid eye movement (NREM) and rapid eye movement (REM) sleep. NREM sleep is further divided into progressively deeper stages of sleep: stages N1 through N4. As NREM stages progress, metabolism and vital signs decrease, and stronger stimuli are required to result in an awakening. The restorative theory proposes that growth hormone is secreted during stages N3 and N4, promoting protein synthesis, tissue healing, and restoration.[17] NREM sleep is also believed to consolidate memory and remove redundant or excess synapses via oscillating depolarizations and hyperpolarizations.[18]

REM sleep also plays a role in memory retention and consolidation, as well as removing useless information from memory, but this effect likely occurs indirectly via promotion of slow-wave sleep.[19] REM sleep has parasympathetically driven tonic components (no eye movements, decreased electroencephalogram [EEG] amplitude, and atonia) and sympathetically driven phasic components (rapid eye movements, distal muscle twitches, cardiorespiratory variability, and middle ear muscle activity). REM sleep follows NREM sleep, occurring 4–5 times during a normal 8-hr sleep period and becoming progressively longer through the night. The NREM–REM cycles vary in length from 70–100 min initially to 90–120 min later in the night.

Stage N1: Dozing

- EEG recordings show a low-voltage fast activity mixed with slower waves within the theta frequency band (4–7 Hz).
- Muscle activity is present but considerably reduced.
- Slow rolling, but not rapid, eye movements may occur.

Stage N2: Light sleep

- EEG shows sleep spindles (bursts of alpha waves lasting 0.5–1 s) and K complexes (high-voltage biphasic waves usually present at the beginning or the end of a sleep spindle).
- Muscle activity is diminished but still present.
- Slow rolling ocular movements are rare.

Stages N3 and N4: Deep sleep (i.e., slow-wave sleep, sometimes grouped together as stage N3)

- EEG shows that high-voltage slow delta waves (0.3–3 Hz) occupy 20–50% of the tracing in stage 3 and surpass 50% in stage 4.
- Muscle activity is much reduced or absent.
- Eye movements are absent.

REM sleep

- EEG activity is practically indistinguishable from the "mixed activity" present in stage N1.
- REMs are present, either isolated or grouped in bursts.
- Complete absence of muscular activity (atonia) is typical of REM sleep, but sudden recovery of muscle tone may randomly occur in some muscular groups (muscular twitches), usually coinciding with REMs.

Clinical Evidence

The phytoconstituent profile, dose, route of administration, and timing all play an important role in the capacity of cannabis to promote or interfere with sleep. Thus, clinical polysomnographic studies are often inconsistent. Some studies have shown that Δ^9-tetrahydrocannabinol (THC) decreases sleep latency. There is some evidence that cannabis reduces stage 3 but increases stage 4 and total slow-wave sleep, but contradictory results have also been reported, and the significance of these alterations is questionable. THC has more consistently been associated with decreased total REM sleep and REM density. Some studies suggest that long-term cannabis use can result in some tolerance to its effects on sleep. Paradoxical arousing effects are likely with high doses of THC in naïve users, and sleep disruption is a common symptom of cannabis withdrawal.[20]

Historical accounts of the benefits of cannabis for sleep appear in premodern and modern medical literature. For example, German physician Bernhard Fronmüller reported his tests of "Indian hemp" in 1,000 patients with sleep disturbance in 1869: 53% experienced a curative effect, 21.5% experienced a partial cure, and 25.5% felt little or no effect.[21]

RCTs of cannabinoids for primary sleep disorders are limited but supportive. One double-blind crossover trial in nine patients with insomnia compared THC (10, 20, and

30 mg) with placebo. The 20-mg dose produced the greatest reduction in time to fall asleep (mean 62 min faster than placebo, $p < .01$).[22] A double-blind crossover study of pure CBD in 15 patients with insomnia found that 160 mg of CBD improved sleep duration, though no improvement was seen with 40- or 80-mg doses. All doses decreased dream recall.[23]

A double-blind four-way crossover polysomnography study of eight healthy young adults compared cannabis extracts containing 15 mg of THC, 5 mg of THC + 5 mg of CBD, and 15 mg of THC + 15 mg of CBD. The 15-mg dose of THC caused no changes in sleep architecture but did cause memory impairments the following day; the 5 mg combination treatment caused a decrease in stage 3 sleep but not total stage 3 + 4 sleep; and the 15 mg combination treatment similarly caused a decrease in stage 3 sleep but not total stage 3 + 4 sleep, but did result in increased nighttime wakefulness.[24] Another polysomnography study in 27 healthy volunteers found that 300 mg of CBD, compared to placebo, did not alter sleep architecture or subjective measures of sleep.[25]

While the results of these small studies in healthy volunteers may not apply to patients with sleep disorders, the findings suggest that doses of THC that are titrated to avoid impairment the following day are unlikely to disrupt sleep architecture, low doses of CBD may disturb sleep, and high doses of CBD may be less likely to disturb sleep.

Interestingly, obstructive sleep apnea (OSA) appears to respond to THC. In a parallel group trial of 73 patients with moderate or severe OSA comparing dronabinol (2.5 or 10 mg) and placebo 1 hr before bedtime for 6 weeks, dronabinol dose-dependently reduced the apnea–hypopnea index (approximate 50% reduction in the 10 mg group); the 10-mg dose also reduced Epworth Sleepiness Scale scores and produced the highest ratings of treatment satisfaction. Sleep latencies, gross sleep architecture, and overnight oxygenation were unchanged from baseline in any treatment group.[26] While the mechanism of action of THC in OSA is unknown, some preclinical evidence suggests it may work by suppressing excessive vagal activity via peripheral CB1 activation;[27] anecdotal evidence suggests relaxation of tense masseters and mitigation of bruxism may also play a role.

Not surprisingly, several studies have found that cannabinoid therapies improve sleep in patients with chronic pain, including nabilone in patients with diabetic peripheral neuropathic pain,[28] dronabinol in chronic noncancer pain,[29] and smoked THC-dominant cannabis in chronic neuropathic pain.[30]

A crossover trial in 29 patients with fibromyalgia, comparing nabilone (0.5 mg) with amitriptyline (10 mg), found greater improvements in insomnia and sleep restfulness scores in the nabilone group after 2 weeks.[31]

Several nabiximols RCTs have shown sleep improvement in patients with multiple sclerosis, peripheral neuropathic pain, intractable cancer pain, and rheumatoid arthritis, as reviewed in Russo et al., 2007.[32] This likely constitutes the largest data set of placebo-controlled evidence on the effect of THC + CBD on sleep, with 2,000 subjects in phase II and III trials and 1,000 patient-years of data demonstrating marked improvement in subjective sleep parameters and retention of efficacy without need for dose escalation.

A cross-sectional study in 129 Israeli patients ≥50 years of age with chronic pain evaluated the association between sleep problems and medical cannabis use for at least 1 year. After adjusting for age, sex, pain level, and use of sleep and antidepressant medications, cannabis use was associated with fewer nighttime awakenings. No differences between cannabis users and nonusers were found for problems with falling asleep or inability to fall back asleep after waking up early.[33]

A case series of 27 adults with poor sleep who were treated with a CBD-dominant product, usually 25 mg after dinner, found mild benefits on sleep at best; sleep scores improved in the first month in some patients but generally fluctuated over time.[34]

As described in Chapter 21, trauma-related sleep disturbance often responds well to cannabis. In an open-label trial of nabilone in 47 patients with PTSD-related treatment-resistant nightmares, 60% experienced complete resolution of nightmares and another 13% had a satisfactory reduction in symptoms. The dose remained stable over 4–12 months, though most patients had a recurrence of symptoms after discontinuing treatment.[35] Another open-label trial of dronabinol in 10 patients with PTSD also found improvements in sleep quality and nightmares.[36]

As will be described in Chapter 24, patients with dementia have been shown to experience improvements in sleep with low doses of THC.[37,38]

In a case series of three patients with severe intractable cholestatic-related pruritis who had failed to respond to numerous pharmacological agents and UV therapy, all experienced decreased pruritus, marked improvement in sleep, and eventually were able to return to work with the use of dronabinol (5 mg) at bedtime.[39]

In a case report of six patients with restless legs syndrome (RLS) refractory to numerous medications, five smoked cannabis and one used a sublingual CBD product; no other information on dosing or product was provided. All six reported total relief of RLS symptoms and complete improvement in sleep quality. Anecdotally, I have treated numerous patients with RLS who experienced profound improvements with cannabis.

In a case report of four patients with Parkinson's disease and REM sleep behavior disorder, a parasomnia involving the loss of muscle atonia that produces active behavior during dreaming and nightmares, 75 mg of CBD produced complete resolution of symptoms in three patients, and a 300-mg dose resulted in marked improvement in the fourth patient.[40]

Surveys of cannabis users also suggest a beneficial effect on sleep. Among 409 individuals with self-reported insomnia who logged data related to 1,056 medical cannabis administration sessions in a mobile app, there was an average 4.5/10 rating of improvement in perceived insomnia levels related to treatment with cannabis.[41] In a survey of 259 individuals who reported using cannabis for insomnia with knowledge of THC and CBD concentrations in the products they used, increased THC content and decreased time between consumption and bed were indicators of improved sleep quality.[42]

Among 1,000 adult-use-only (nonmedical) customers of cannabis dispensaries in Colorado, 74% reported using cannabis to improve sleep; 84% found it very or extremely helpful, and most of those taking over-the-counter (87%) or prescription sleep aids (83%) reported reducing or stopping these medications.[43] Notably, sleep disorders are not included in criteria for medical cannabis certification in most U.S. states, so access to adult-use markets is important for the large population of individuals with poor sleep.

By comparing cash register data from Colorado before and after the existence of adult-use dispensaries, researchers demonstrated a 236% decrease in a previously growing market share of over-the-counter sleep aids (particularly diphenhydramine- and doxylamine-based products) associated with the opening of cannabis dispensaries.[44]

Preclinical Evidence

Preclinical studies describe a circadian rhythm in circulating endocannabinoid concentrations, with plasma 2-arachidonoylglycerol levels increasing from mid-sleep to early afternoon associated with wakefulness. Conversely, anandamide is associated with sleep-promoting effects, including promotion of slow-wave sleep, possibly via increases in extracellular adenosine concentrations. CB1 agonism has shown favorable results in preclinical models of obstructive sleep apnea and sleep disturbances associated with maternal separation. CBD partially blocked excessive sleepiness in an animal model of narcolepsy, adding to a larger body of evidence supporting the potential wakefulness-promoting properties of CBD.[45]

Treatment Strategies for Clinicians

- I almost always recommend THC-dominant cannabis before bed in patients with primary or secondary sleep disorders. I have seen mixed results with CBD-dominant products on sleep, and I estimate that low and moderate doses of CBD disturb sleep in 10%–20% of my patients who try it. Some patients, however, do report improvement in sleep with CBD taken before bed.

- Inhaled cannabis 15–30 min before bedtime is most effective for addressing sleep latency and RLS.
- Oral or oromucosal delivery is best for promoting sleep maintenance due to its delayed onset and longer duration of action. If liquid products fail to last the whole night, a capsule may provide somewhat longer delayed onset or duration.
- I usually start cannabis-naïve patients at 2 mg of THC before bed and titrate up by 1 mg every 1–2 nights until they reach a mutually agreed-upon goal of sleep duration and number of awakenings.
- If a patient experiences difficulty waking or grogginess in the morning, reduce the dose of THC slightly.
- For patients who wake in the middle of the night and cannot fall back asleep, despite appropriately dosed oral cannabis before bed, inhaled cannabis can be an effective solution to help fall back asleep.
- Chemovar selection is crucial, especially for inhaled cannabis. While some may succeed by shopping for so-called indica varieties, selecting for specific terpene profiles with higher levels of myrcene, linalool, and nerolidol may produce better results, though terpene content is likely not the only factor in the sedating versus stimulating properties of cannabis. I find the best strategy for chemovar selection is to ask the grower or retailer which varieties are most effective for helping with sleep in their other customers.
- In patients who do not respond fully to the aforementioned strategies, I often add a sleep-promoting herbal combination containing hops, lemon balm, valerian, and skullcap. These herbs seem to work well in combination with cannabis. In patients with circadian rhythm disturbance, I add melatonin, typically a 1-mg oral dissolving tablet just before bed.
- The nonpharmacological treatment I most often recommend in combination with cannabis for sleep promotion is the gratitude journal. I keep the instructions simple: write down at least three headlines about something in your day that brought you gratitude, then put down the pen and spend 30–60 s focusing on each entry while feeling like you received a gift.
- The 4-7-8 breathing practice popularized by Andrew Weil, MD, is another simple and effective adjunct: inhale through the nose for a count of four, hold the breath for a count of seven, and exhale through gently pursed lips for a count of eight. Practicing this routine for 5 min can produce a profound sense of calm and balance.

Cautions

- Some varieties of THC-dominant cannabis are clearly stimulating and disturb sleep.
- Cannabis can increase the sedative effects of benzodiazepines and other hypnotic agents and thus increase the risk of falls and other adverse effects. Nevertheless, patients are usually able to first titrate THC up to a dose that produces improvements in sleep or the emergence of mild morning grogginess and then taper the benzodiazepine successfully.
- Patients who use only inhaled cannabis to treat a sleep disturbance often note benefits during the first portion of the night and disturbed sleep later. In an effort to improve their results, many increase the dose of inhaled cannabis, which often leads to tolerance-building and loss of efficacy. These patients should be advised to combine lower doses of inhaled and oral cannabis for benefits of both short and longer duration.
- Sleep disturbance is one of the most common symptoms of cannabis withdrawal; rebound exacerbations in sleep problems may occur after discontinuing cannabis in those who have developed tolerance. Conversely, many patients are able to use appropriately dosed cannabis for a period of time, establish regular sleep patterns, and then successfully taper off the cannabis.

Chapter 23

Cancer

WHILE SUBSTANTIAL EVIDENCE supports the use of cannabis or cannabinoids in treating chemotherapy-induced nausea and vomiting, this is just one fraction of the many potential therapeutic benefits in patients with cancer. On the basis of my clinical experience, nearly any patient with cancer can benefit from appropriately dosed cannabis: it is invaluable in treating cancer-related symptoms, mitigating adverse effects of conventional treatments, supporting emotional and spiritual adjustment to the diagnosis and clinical course, and, when needed, supporting end-of-life care. In the words of integrative oncology expert Donald Abrams, MD:

> To be able to suggest a single agent that could hold benefit in the treatment of nausea, anorexia, pain, insomnia, and anxiety instead of writing prescriptions for 5 or 6 medications that might interact with each other or with cancer-directed therapies seems advantageous.[1]

Additionally, as reviewed in Chapter 8, the endocannabinoid system (ECS) plays a fundamental role in our innate resistance against cancer. Given our knowledge of cannabinoid (CB) receptor activity, as well as several non-CB-receptor-dependent mechanisms of action, it is not a surprise that substantial preclinical in vitro and in vivo evidence shows that exogenous cannabinoids can inhibit cancer growth, trigger apoptosis, prevent metastasis, and reduce tumor angiogenesis.[2] Some studies demonstrate synergistic and protective effects with conventional chemotherapy and radiotherapy. A large body of human anecdotal evidence suggests that many patients experience improved anticancer efficacy when they add cannabis to conventional treatment, and several cases of clear anticancer effects of cannabis monotherapy have also been reported.

The low toxicity and palliative and potential protective effects of cannabis make it a good candidate for adjunctive anticancer therapy, but similar to hundreds of anticancer therapies that fail to translate from rodents to humans, we are far from knowing how to apply these preliminary findings to clinical practice. Complex interactions between cannabinoids, the ECS, and the immune system; the presence or absence of cannabinoid receptors and other targets in cancer cells; the diverse phytoconstituent profiles of cannabis preparations; and the wide range of tolerated and potentially effective doses preclude concrete clinical recommendations on how to best use cannabis to treat cancer. This complexity also challenges future clinical trial design. Nevertheless, informed by a recognition of how little we know, clinicians can effectively guide patients in the use of cannabis for both palliation and potential anticancer effects.

I see a wide variety of patients with cancer in my practice. I treat all ages including pediatrics, those early in the course of their illness, and those close to death. Some patients are referred by their oncologists with specific palliative goals, often related to nausea, anorexia, and pain. Some well-informed patients hope for both palliative and potential anticancer effects in conjunction with conventional treatment. Others have elected to forgo conventional treatment, are on a decidedly alternative treatment path, and are searching for advice on how to use cannabis to "kill cancer."

Among the latter group, I observe a wide range of insight into their medical situation. Few have gracefully accepted their mortality and wish to let nature take its course, yet they remain open to a "miracle." Others lack a clear understanding of their diagnosis and prognosis with or without conventional treatment, which they have typically declined based on prior observations of a friend or family member who experienced a devastating impact on quality of life while undergoing conventional treatment. They often have significant death anxiety that impairs their medical decision-making; many have been misled by exaggerated internet claims of the anticancer effects of cannabis, and, having rejected follow-up with oncology, I am often the only medical professional involved in their care. Donald Abrams aptly describes his experience with this challenging trend:

> One of the more distressing situations that oncologists increasingly face is trying to counsel the patient who has a curable diagnosis, but who seeks to forego conventional cancer treatment in favor of depending on cannabis oil to eradicate their malignancy because of the large number of online testimonials from people claiming such results. Given my long practice in San Francisco, I can assume that a large proportion of my patients have used cannabis during their journey. If cannabis cured cancer, I would have a lot more survivors in my practice today.[3]

Though it is difficult, the art of a successful clinical encounter requires us to synchronize with and validate patients as they present, attend to family members' questions and concerns, provide education on the potential benefits of cannabis, and set concrete treatment goals. In those with uncontrolled death anxiety and uninformed medical decision-making, mitigating anxiety (and sleep disruption) is always my first therapeutic goal, typically accomplished with low-dose cannabis and fostering a therapeutic relationship. I have found that, often, waiting until a follow-up visit to bring up topics like prognosis and the potential risks and benefits of an oncology referral is much more effective than frightening patients who are already distressed in their initial visit.

Among the cases claiming spontaneous remission or arrested progression related to cannabis monotherapy, most patients have used very high doses of cannabinoids, in the range 5–20 mg·kg^{-1}·day^{-1}. By titrating up slowly, patients can often tolerate these high doses, and some also experience progressive improvement in symptoms and quality of life as they reach higher doses. More often, however, I see patients who received excellent palliative effects at low and moderate doses subsequently build tolerance to these symptomatic benefits at the higher doses. Without any certainty that the higher doses are effectively fighting cancer, this trade-off is not, in my opinion, worthwhile, especially when the financial expense of high-dose treatment is considered. Furthermore, I have clearly observed a few cases of an impressive response to low- and moderate-dose cannabis combined with other integrative strategies that typically include diet change and high-dose melatonin.

There is also some potential for high-dose cannabinoid monotherapy to promote cancer progression, particularly if the cancer cells lack CB1 receptors and other cannabinoid targets. In this situation, high doses of Δ^9-tetrahydrocannabinol (THC) may be somewhat immunosuppressive without exerting anticancer effects. Unfortunately, at the time of writing, no commercial testing is available to determine if tumor biopsies express CB1 or CB2. When this becomes available, I will likely avoid high-dose THC treatment in those with CB1/CB2-negative cancers.

For most of my patients with cancer, our shared goal is to mitigate symptoms and allow them to complete a full course of conventional therapy while maintaining a high quality of life. Titrating and fine-tuning cannabis dosing to achieve this goal is straightforward after reviewing Chapters 16 and 17. I believe that, in most cases, the dose of cannabis that supports quality of life, sleep, emotional and spiritual health, and function would be the same dose that conveys any potential anticancer effects. This, however, may not always be the case, and sometimes patients wish to modify their cannabis regimen after learning of cancer progression and lack of response to current therapies.

To help guide my decisions, I look at trends in blood markers of cancer status. While some cancers can be tracked by using specific or semispecific cancer markers (e.g., prostate-specific antigen in prostate cancer, cancer antigen 19-9 in pancreatic cancer, or β-human chorionic gonadotropin in testicular cancer), many cancers lack such indices. Unbeknownst to many clinicians, and infrequently ordered by oncologists, there are several nonspecific markers of cancer progression and response to treatment that can be tracked over time. I find these trends helpful in guiding decisions to continue versus modifying one's experimental treatment regimen.

The neutrophil-to-lymphocyte ratio (NLR) is perhaps the least expensive and most useful test for monitoring therapeutic response in cancers that lack specific markers. A large body of evidence demonstrates higher baseline values are associated with worse prognosis in a wide range of cancers at various stages,[4] though less evidence supports the NLR as a measure of treatment response. How can two values from a complete blood count tell us so much? Neutrophils produce chemokines and cytokines, including transforming growth factor β (TGF-β), that suppress the activity of lymphocytes and natural killer cells; in a feedforward cycle, the interaction of cancer cells with neutrophils has been shown to increase TGF-β, leading to proliferation, infiltration, and metastasis.[5] While TGF-β functions as a potent tumor suppressor in premalignant cells, mutations that eliminate the TGF-β pathway or decouple it from apoptosis not only convert these cells into a full-blown malignant state but also allow them to use TGF-β to create an immunosuppressive tumor microenvironment.[6]

Cutoff values for the prognostic significance of NLR vary by cancer type and stage, but in general, a ratio around 2 is a good sign and a ratio greater than 4 indicates poor prognosis. I find a trend in the NLR over time to be helpful in determining if integrative anticancer strategies are helping or should be adjusted. Similarly, platelet-to-lymphocyte ratio (PLR) is prognostic in many cancer types due to the capacity of platelets to release angiogenic and tumor growth factors, including TGF-β, platelet factor 4, and platelet-derived growth factor; an elevated ratio indicates worse prognosis.[7]

Lactate dehydrogenase (LDH) is another nonspecific blood marker of cancer prognosis and perhaps progression and response to treatment. LDH catalyzes the conversion of pyruvate to lactate and is a key checkpoint of anaerobic glycolysis; it is elevated in many types of cancers and has been linked to tumor growth, maintenance, and invasion.[8]

Clinical Evidence

Cancer patients have long used cannabis as a treatment; the 2,500-year-old mummy known as the "Siberian Ice Maiden," discovered in 1993, is perhaps the earliest evidence. She is believed to have died in her 20s, and magnetic resonance imaging revealed that she had a primary tumor of the right breast and metastatic disease. Her subterranean burial chamber included a pouch of cannabis among other archaeological findings, and while we cannot be certain, many have hypothesized that she used the cannabis to treat cancer-related symptoms or perhaps the cancer itself.[9]

The utility of cannabinoids in addressing chemotherapy-induced nausea and vomiting, especially in patients who fail to respond to conventional antiemetics, is well established. Primarily on the basis of trial data for dronabinol and nabilone, a 2017 National Academies of Sciences report rated the existing evidence of efficacy as "conclusive."[10] Similarly, substantial evidence supports the use of cannabis or cannabinoids in treating pain, including cancer-related pain (see Chapter 20 for more details). Not all data are congruent with this trend, however: three recent phase III randomized controlled trials (RCTs) of patients with advanced cancer pain refractory to opioids, comparing nabiximols to placebo, did not meet the primary end point of significant improvements in pain, though methodological challenges like high withdrawal and mortality rates in the cohorts of these studies may have confounded results.[11,12] Steele et al. recently published a comprehensive review of cannabinoid clinic trials in cancer patients since 2000.[13]

Less is known about the potential benefits of cannabis in patients undergoing radiotherapy than chemotherapy and about the use of cannabis to manage postradiotherapy symptoms. A review of five trials using THC found it effective at reducing anxiety in patients preparing to start radiotherapy and at reducing nausea and vomiting.[14] A placebo-controlled study found that, for patients with head and neck cancers undergoing radiotherapy, quality of life was not improved by the use of nabilone at a maximum dose of 1 mg twice daily.[15] In a survey study of 15 patients with previously treated head and neck cancers, all respondents endorsed the benefits of cannabis in the treatment of long-term residual effects of radiation, including low appetite, pain, and, somewhat surprisingly, xerostomia and sticky saliva.[16]

Though artisanal cannabis has seldom been studied in controlled trials of patients with cancer, emerging observational data are very supportive. In the first 4 months of a medical cannabis program in Minnesota, 743 patients with cancer were surveyed at baseline and within the 4-month period after their first medical cannabis purchase regarding eight symptoms: anxiety, lack of appetite, depression, disturbed sleep, fatigue, nausea, pain, and vomiting. The patients used a variety of cannabis formulations and routes of delivery. Compared to baseline, the outcomes improved for every symptom. Adverse effects were infrequent and mild: drowsiness (2.5%) and dry mouth (2.2%) were the most common.[17]

Among 2,970 cancer patients treated with medical cannabis in Israel between 2015 and 2017, after 6 months of treatment, 902 patients (24.9%) had died and 682 (18.8%)

stopped the cannabis treatment. Of the remaining patients, 1,211 (60.6%) responded to a survey, in which 95.9% reported an improvement in their condition, 3.7% reported no change, and only four patients (0.3%) reported deterioration in their medical condition.[18] The before-and-after ratings of pain intensity and quality of life are illustrated in Figures 23.1 and 23.2, respectively.

FIGURE 23.1

Assessment of Pain Intensity Before and After 6 Months of Cannabis Therapy

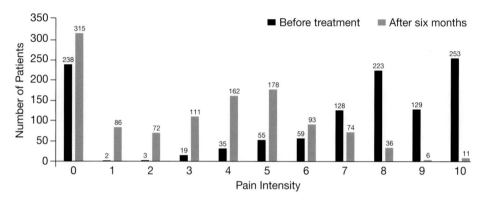

Note. From "Prospective analysis of safety and efficacy of medical cannabis in large unselected population of patients with cancer," by L. B.-L. Schleider, R. Mechoulam, V. Lederman, M. Hilou, O. Lencovsky, O. Betzalel, L. Shbiro, and V. Novack, 2018, European Journal of Internal Medicine, 49, pp. 37–43 (https://doi.org/10.1016/j .ejim.2018.01.023). Copyright © 2018 by European Federation of Internal Medicine. Reprinted with permission.

FIGURE 23.2

Quality of Life Assessment Prior to and
6 Months After Initiation of Cannabis Treatment

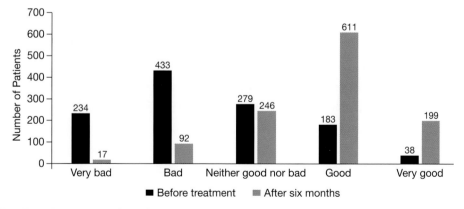

Note. From "Prospective analysis of safety and efficacy of medical cannabis in large unselected population of patients with cancer," by L. B.-L. Schleider, R. Mechoulam, V. Lederman, M. Hilou, O. Lencovsky, O. Betzalel, L. Shbiro, and V. Novack, 2018, European Journal of Internal Medicine, 49, pp. 37–43 (https://doi.org/10.1016/j .ejim.2018.01.023). Copyright © 2018 by European Federation of Internal Medicine. Reprinted with permission.

In a recent RCT, perhaps the only study that has evaluated naturalistic cannabis use in patients with cancer, 30 participants with advanced cancers in Minnesota were randomized to receive "early" medical cannabis treatment (3 months of treatment provided at no charge) versus "delayed" medical cannabis treatment (standard oncology care for 3 months prior to treatment with cannabis). The cannabis dosing, formulation, and routes of administration were determined by a pharmacist at one of two dispensaries. The early treatment group did not require opioid dose escalation, and compared to the delayed group, they had lower mean pain and similar quality of life. Estimated mean daily THC and cannabidiol (CBD) doses at 3 months were 76 mg (range 5–186 mg) and 36 mg (range <1–516 mg), respectively. On a 1–7 scale (where 1 = no benefit or no negative effects and 7 = a great deal of benefit or a great deal of negative effects), the mean perceived benefit of cannabis was 5.1 and mean perceived negative impact was 2.7.[19]

Regarding the anticancer effects of cannabis in humans, peer-reviewed data are limited, and some of the peer-reviewed publications offer poor-quality evidence. Nevertheless, the existing data strongly warrant further investigation.

A phase 1 pilot study of nine patients with recurrent glioblastoma underwent intracranial THC administration. Although the small cohort precluded statistically significant outcomes, the treatment was safe, and some patients seemed to have responded in terms of reduced tumor growth rate as evaluated by magnetic resonance imaging and decreased markers of malignancy in tumor specimens.[20]

One case report of terminal, highly aggressive acute lymphoblastic leukemia in a 14-year-old demonstrated a dose-dependent response to cannabis concentrate, readily measured by blast count. Variations in formulation, dose, and frequency directly correlated with measured disease severity. Authors noted that "where our most advanced chemotherapeutic agents had failed to control the blast counts and had devastating side effects that ultimately resulted in the death of the patient, the cannabinoid therapy had no toxic side effects and only psychosomatic properties, with an increase in the patient's vitality."[21]

A phase 2 RCT of nabiximols added as an adjunct to temozolomide in 21 patients with recurrent glioblastoma, published only as an abstract to date, concluded that nabiximols offers some efficacy as an adjunct to chemotherapy. The 1-year survival rate was 83% with nabiximols, compared to 56% with placebo (*p* = .042). The median survival exceeded 550 days with nabiximols versus 369 days in the placebo recipients.[22]

Two cases were reported of high-grade glioma treated with subtotal resection, chemoradiation, and subsequent procarbazine, lomustine, and vincristine plus CBD (100–450 mg/day). Both patients' responses were, according to the authors, "not commonly observed in patients only treated with conventional modalities." Both had a positive response to the treatment, with no evidence of disease progression for at least for 2 years (one had a recurrence at 2.5 years). Impressively, both patients experienced no adverse effects of aggressive chemotherapy, did not require the typical use of cortico-steroids, and were able to maintain their usual work and sports activities.[23]

In a case series of 119 patients with various cancers, synthetic CBD was adminis-tered twice daily in a 3-days-on, 3-days-off regimen, with an average dose of 10 mg twice daily and a maximum dose (titrated up in the case of increasing tumor mass) of 30 mg twice daily. CBD was the sole treatment for 28 of the subjects. "Clinical responses" were seen in 92% of the 119 cases, including a reduction in circulating tumor cells in many cases and a reduction in tumor size in others, as shown by repeat scans. Unfortu-nately, detailed information was provided for only two cases with rare brain tumors.[24]

A case series of nine patients with grade IV glioblastoma multiforme, who received 400 mg of CBD daily in addition to radiochemotherapy, experienced unusually good sur-vival and quality of life. At the time of publication, eight patients were alive with a mean survival time of 22.3 months (range 7–47 months).[25]

Finally, a single case report of an 81-year-old man with lung adenocarcinoma who declined chemotherapy and radiation (he did not want any treatment that could adversely affect his quality of life) demonstrated a clear response to low-dose CBD (<20 mg daily), based on published radiographic evidence.[26] Additionally, Justin Kander's non-peer-reviewed compendium of successful cases of cannabis adjunctive therapy and mono-therapy is compelling, though limited by selection bias for efficacious reports.[27] The overall response rate of cannabis monotherapy is unknown, as most treatment failures are not reported in online forums or elsewhere, but I suspect it is low. In my practice, no case is true monotherapy because the cannabis is used in conjunction with treatments like diet and lifestyle change, medicinal mushrooms and herbs, high-dose melatonin, inositol hexaphosphate, modified citrus pectin, and others.

Preclinical Evidence

Alterations in the ECS, including endocannabinoid levels, receptor expression and oligomerization, and ECS enzyme activity, have been demonstrated in several cancers. Whether these alterations contribute to or are a response to malignant transformation is complex and poorly understood. For example, anandamide levels have been found to be 2–3 times higher in colorectal cancers than normal tissues.[28] CB2 receptors appear at higher levels in some colon cancers cells than normal epithelial cells.[29] Both CB1 and CB2 are upregulated in hepatocellular carcinoma, and the extent of their overexpression is correlated with improved prognosis.[30]

A large body of evidence demonstrates the anticancer effects of endogenous cannabinoids, synthetic cannabinoids, and phytocannabinoids in multiple cancer types, both in vitro and in vivo. Both THC, typically via direct CB1 and CB2 mechanisms, and CBD, usually via CB-receptor-independent and indirect mechanisms, have been shown to trigger apoptosis, decrease proliferation, decrease invasiveness, decrease angiogenesis, and more. Cannabinol (CBN), cannabigerol (CBG), cannabichromene (CBC), and Δ^9-tetrahydrocannabinolic acid (THCA) have also demonstrated anticancer effects in preclinical models.[31]

The distinct anticancer effects of CBD, THC, and other phytocannabinoids appear to be complementary or synergistic, as demonstrated in several in vivo models. For example, in a glioblastoma mouse xenograft model,* treatment with 7.5 mg/kg THC + 7.5 mg/kg CBD was more effective in reducing tumor growth than the same dose of either agent alone and had similar efficacy to 15 mg/kg THC;[32] in melanoma cells, a combination of 1.0 μM THC + 1.0 μM CBD had similar effects on apoptosis as 5.0 μM doses of either agent alone.[33]

The synergistic anticancer effects of botanical cannabis preparations are much more complex than the interactions of these two cannabinoids. Several studies have compared the effects of purified cannabinoids with multicompound cannabis extracts containing equivalent potencies of the cannabinoid in question. For example, THC-enriched extracts were nearly twice as efficient as purified THC in treating melanoma xenografts.[34] In two human prostate cancer cell lines, the in vitro anticancer effects of purified THC, CBD, CBN, CBG, CBC, cannabidivarin (CBDV), Δ^9-tetrahydrocannabivarin(THCV), cannabigerovarin(CBGV), Δ^9-tetrahydrocannabivarinic acid (THCVA), and cannabigerolic acid (CBGA) were less powerful than those of botanical cannabis extracts enriched with the corresponding cannabinoids.[35] Complex combinations of neutral and acidic cannabinoids were shown to differentially inhibit the proliferation of colorectal cancer and colon polyp cells in vitro, with pronounced effects involving THCA and CBGA that corresponded with relevant changes in tumor gene expression.[36]

Terpenes may convey part of the anticancer effects of botanical cannabis. For example, limonene has been shown to inhibit the development of chemically induced rodent skin, liver and mammary cancers.[37] One study showed that limonene potentiated the ability of CBN to inhibit breast cancer cell growth via inhibition of breast cancer resistance protein.[38]

---

* Many preclinical in vivo studies utilize the mouse xenograft model, in which a series of immunosuppressed mice are injected with cancer cells and subsequently exposed to different treatment conditions; the rate of tumor growth and other outcomes can be observed over time.

Some studies have shown that the synergistic anticancer properties of botanical cannabis are related to minor constituents not commonly evaluated in commercial cannabis analysis. For example, a botanical preparation was more potent than pure THC in producing antitumor responses in cell culture and animal models of ER+/PR+, HER2+, and triple-negative breast cancer. To determine whether the increased potency was due to THC–terpene interactions, the researchers tested pure THC supplemented with the top five most abundant terpenoids present in the extract (β-caryophyllene, linalool, α-humulene, nerolidol, and β-pinene); the reconstituted preparation did not demonstrate an improved effect like the botanical extract.[39]

Dedi Meiri and colleagues at Technion–Israel Institute of Technology analyzed 89 phytocannabinoids in 124 different "natural" (unheated) and decarboxylated cannabis extracts, and they subsequently evaluated 12 extracts representing five major categories of cannabinoid dominance (THC, THCA, CBD, cannabidiolic acid, and CBG) against 12 different cancer cell lines in vitro. The results were striking, with certain cancers inhibited by select cannabis extracts and unaffected by others. The cancer cell lines that were most resilient to all the cannabis extracts had low or undetectable expression of CB1, GPR55, and TPRM8 receptors.[40]

In another experiment published in the same paper, 14 distinct THC-dominant preparations were shown to have vastly different inhibitory effects on lung adenocarcinoma cells in comparison with each other and with purified THC. The anticancer effects were, to some extent, correlated with the presence of low levels of more well-known phytocannabinoids like CBG and CBC but also with the presence of rarely analyzed cannabinoids like CBT-3, 329-11d, and 373-15c. Decarboxylation was also shown to have a pronounced effect on anticancer effects, with one line of prostate cancer (lacking CB1 and GPR55 receptors) much more sensitive to natural extracts, and another line of prostate cancer expressing these receptor proteins more sensitive to decarboxylated extracts.[41] More than any other paper, these data emphasize how little we know and how far we are from identifying which cannabis preparations are best for treating which types of cancer.

Cannabinoids have been shown to be synergistic with chemotherapy agents, including gemcitabine, temozolomide (TMZ), paclitaxel, and 5-fluorouracil, in cell culture models of pancreatic,[42] glioma, gastric,[43] lung,[44] breast,[45] and colon cancers.[46] Not surprisingly, some studies have shown discordant results depending on the concentration of cannabinoids: low doses stimulated cancer proliferation, while higher doses had antineoplastic activity.[47]

In vivo, some notable results of cannabinoid–chemotherapy synergy are seen in rodent glioma studies. In one glioma xenograft model, THC was shown to significantly potentiate the antitumor effects of TMZ, the first-line chemotherapy agent for glioblastoma multiforme, and combination treatment of a nabiximols-like botanical preparation + TMZ produced a strong antitumoral action in both TMZ-sensitive and, notably, in TMZ-resistant tumors.[48] Another study found that THC + CBD sensitized glioma cells and tumors to the effects of radiation. The combination of cannabinoids was more powerful than either cannabinoid alone in vitro, and in vivo work showed dramatic reductions in tumor volumes when both cannabinoids were combined with radiation, all in suboptimal doses.[49]

Finally, chemotherapy-induced peripheral neuropathy (CIPN) is an adverse effect experienced by 40%–80% of patients 3–6 months into their chemotherapeutic treatment, and may present as loss of sensation, hyperalgesia, and/or allodynia. Symptoms may not abate after discontinuing chemotherapy, with 30%–40% of patients experiencing symptoms 6 months or longer after treatment, sometimes leading to debilitating chronic pain. Thus far, efforts to prevent and treat CIPN have been disappointing and limited, respectively. Increasing preclinical data suggest that cannabinoids and ECS modulators may be useful in treating CIPN related to the platinum, taxane, and vinca alkaloid classes of chemotherapeutics.[50] Furthermore, some studies indicate that cannabinoids and ECS modulators may be able to prevent the development of CIPN, which is not surprising when the neuroprotective effects of these compounds are considered.[51]

Treatment Strategies for Clinicians

- Identify clear treatment goals related to symptoms and quality of life, which can typically be achieved with low and moderate doses of cannabis described in Chapters 16 and 17. See Chapters 20, 21, and 27 for more information about using cannabis to treat pain, anxiety, and anorexia, respectively.
- The appetitive and antiemetic effects are often best with inhaled delivery; sipping on cannabis tea can also be very effective for nausea.
- Use cannabis to potentiate or spare other drugs associated with increased morbidity and mortality, such as opioids.
- Beyond symptom management, the psychoactive effects of THC, with appropriate set and setting and sometimes in combination with nonpharmacological modalities, can assist patients in accepting mortality and improve other aspects of their spiritual and social life.
- In patients with a high likelihood of response but who decline conventional treatment, address death anxiety and sleep disturbance as primary treatment goals, foster a therapeutic relationship, and revisit prognosis and potential oncology referral at a follow-up visit.

- I support my patients' personal preference in their medical care, including decisions that may hasten death. I do, however, insist that such decisions are made after carefully considering all the relevant information.
- I have found that patients are best able to prevent chemotherapy- and radiotherapy-related adverse effects, including CIPN, if they take more liberal doses of cannabis on treatment days a few hours prior to treatment.
- Remember that a patient's spouse and family members may be highly critical of cannabis therapy, due to its stigma, and may require extra reassurance and education to enable them to support the patient in the acquisition and administration of sometimes complex treatment plans. Also recognize that the level of distress among spouses and family members is reciprocally related to the patient's quality of life and acceptance of mortality; you may consider consulting with a distressed family member or caretaker to educate them on how they can also use cannabis to help during such a challenging time.

To take advantage of potential anticancer effects of cannabis:
- Use cannabis in combination with conventional treatment, preventing and mitigating adverse effects, with a goal of enabling the patient to complete a full course of chemotherapy or radiotherapy. My patients often describe looking around the oncology office, infusion room, or support group and seeing a collection of peers who look and feel much more sick than themselves, with a few exceptions who are also using cannabis.
- Explain that we are years or decades away from understanding how any individual can best use cannabis to fight a particular type of cancer, but an understanding of the current unknowns can guide clinical recommendations.
- Utilize a wide variety of cannabis chemovars in both raw and decarboxylated forms to include the broadest range of phytoconstituents that may provide synergistic anticancer effects.
- When patients show evidence of disease progression with low to moderate doses of cannabis, if aligned with patient preference and available resources, consider a trial of titrating up to oral doses of 5–20 $mg·kg^{-1}·day^{-1}$ total cannabinoids. CBD-dominant preparations can be taken during the day and rapidly titrated; THC-dominant preparations are taken before bed and titrated more slowly.
- While there is rationale for combining doses of THC and CBD, I find that separating the majority of these agents into day and night during high-dose treatment makes them much more tolerable and conducive to quality of life. While the peak effects of each occur at different times, there will certainly be relevant overlapping concentra-

tions of both in the blood and tissues. It may also be beneficial for THC to exert its maximal effects via CB1 when CBD levels are lower.

- I ask patients to observe their stool for a distinct odor of cannabis; when this occurs, I suspect that additional titration is unlikely to result in greater absorption. If a higher dose is desired, I encourage them to increase the frequency instead of the dose or to take their cannabis with a high-fat meal.

- Caution patients that the palliative effects of cannabis may diminish at higher doses.

- Cannabis concentrates are viscous, sticky, and difficult to work with when undiluted. They are often stored in an oral syringe. I have learned one somewhat-effective technique for measuring these substances: patients can place a small piece of edible rice paper on a digital scale, press the tare button, and then smear the extract on the rice paper until they achieve the desired weight. The paper can then be folded and consumed orally.

- Any high-dose trial should be accompanied by surveillance for potential response, via imaging or cancer-specific markers, when possible, or via trends in NLR, PLR, and LDH. In the absence of evidence of anticancer benefit, do not continue high-dose therapy beyond an agreed-upon time frame, since the immunosuppressive effects of high doses could impair host anticancer activity

- Cancerous and precancerous skin lesions sometimes respond to topical application of cannabis concentrates, but therapy should not be continued in the absence of evidence of a positive response.

Cautions

- In patients taking nivolumab and other cancer immunotherapies, the goal of cannabis use should be to improve one's ability to complete the full treatment course and spare corticosteroids (see Chapter 18 for more information). I recommend avoiding high-dose cannabis in these situations, and I advise patients to avoid any cannabis use several days prior to and following the immunotherapy infusion to avoid limiting the intensity and efficacy of the desired immune response.[52]

- In some but not all reports, prior cannabis use has been associated with an increased incidence of human papillomavirus (HPV)-related (p16-positive) oropharyngeal squamous cell carcinoma (OPSCC), and a potential mechanism involving CB receptor activation of the p38 MAPK pathways has been identified.[53] Understandably, clinicians may hesitate to use cannabis to treat cancer-related symptoms in patients with HPV-related OPSCC. Recent data, however, found no survival difference between cannabis users and nonusers among patients with this diagnosis.[54]

- Some patients wishing to consume high-dose THC, but who cannot tolerate the adverse effects of oral dosing, resort to rectal administration, and they often report minimal psychoactive side effects. I strongly suspect that these patients are wasting their medicine; if it is absorbed, it is going to reach the brain. Cannabis suppositories may be useful in rectal cancers, and certainly they may be helpful during end-of-life care and when other routes of administration are not feasible.
- Patients who experience a presumed anticancer response often ask how long they must continue high-dose therapy, which can be expensive. Because I have observed rapid tumor growth and recurrence after tapering the cannabis dose in a few cases, I am very hesitant to support any dose reduction until the disease has been stable for at least a year, and I typically recommend continuing on the effective dose indefinitely unless adverse effects or cost are prohibitive. I encourage close surveillance after any dosage or formulation change.

Chapter 24

Alzheimer's Disease and Other Forms of Dementia

IN PATIENTS WITH DEMENTIA, cannabis can address a variety of symptoms, including anxiety, agitation, aggression, anorexia, apathy, and sleep disturbance, as well as comorbidities such as chronic pain and gastrointestinal symptoms. On the basis of pre-clinical research, cannabinoids may also exert a neuroprotective effect that could slow disease progression. Given the frequent use of off-label treatments with poor efficacy and high risk in this patient population, cannabis is an appealing treatment alternative.

Despite strong evidence demonstrating increased morbidity and mortality associated with the use of potentially inappropriate medicines (according to Beers Criteria) in older adults,[1] their use continues to be widespread, often due to the lack of alternatives. The prevalence of taking at least one potentially inappropriate medicine in various populations ≥65 years old ranges from 34.2% in U.S. community-dwelling Medicare beneficiaries,[2] to 57.6% in community dwellers in Saudi Arabia,[3] to 72.5% in community dwellers in Argentina,[4] to 88.3% in Belgian nursing home residents.[5] The Beers Criteria include tricyclic antidepressants, antiemetics, antipsychotics, benzodiazepines, non-benzodiazepine hypnotics, nonsteroidal anti-inflammatory drugs, skeletal muscle relaxants, and opioids, all medications that are frequently spared or substituted by cannabis (see Chapter 28 for more details).

Cannabis has been a godsend to many of my patients with dementia and their families. The staff at an assisted living facility where I have had the opportunity to treat patients quickly recognized the benefits and enthusiastically embraced the extra work required to titrate and fine-tune cannabis treatments. Beyond substantially improving the patient's quality of life, often in the context of previous rapidly deteriorating quality, the efficacy of cannabis in reducing or resolving severe agitation, aggression, exit-seeking, and night-time activity has a profound beneficial impact on the entire household or facility.

Clinical Evidence

A placebo-controlled crossover-designed study on 15 patients with probable Alzheimer's disease who were refusing food received 2.5 mg of dronabinol or a placebo every morning and at noon.[6] Body weight of study subjects increased more during the dronabinol treatment than during the placebo periods. Dronabinol treatment decreased the severity of disturbed behavior, as measured by the Cohen-Mansfield Agitation Inventory (CMAI), and interestingly, both behavioral and body mass index improvements persisted during the placebo period in patients who received dronabinol first. Adverse reactions observed more commonly during the dronabinol treatment than during placebo periods included euphoria, somnolence, and tiredness, but these did not require discontinuation of therapy.

In a retrospective systematic chart review, 40 inpatients from the McLean Hospital Geriatric Neuropsychiatry Inpatient Unit diagnosed with dementia demonstrated significant decreases in all domains of the Pittsburgh Agitation Scale and significant improvements in Clinical Global Impression (CGI) scores, sleep duration, and percentage of meals consumed during treatment with dronabinol. The average dose was 7 mg/day. Adverse effects were mild and did not result in discontinuation of treatment.[7]

A similar beneficial effect on nocturnal agitation was reported in an open-label pilot study on six patients treated with 2.5 mg of dronabinol nightly for 2 weeks.[8]

Contrary to the results mentioned above, a randomized, double-blind, placebo-controlled study failed to achieve significant change in the Neuropsychiatric Inventory (NPI) scores of 22 patients following treatment with Δ^9-tetrahydrocannabinol (THC).[9] The lack of efficacy may be related to the low doses of THC, 0.75 mg twice daily and 1.5 mg twice daily, given for 3 consecutive days followed by a 4-day washout.

In an Israeli open-label pilot study, 11 patients with Alzheimer's disease and severe agitation or aggressive behavior were given medical cannabis oil containing 2.5 mg of THC twice daily, titrated up to a maximum of 7.5 mg of THC twice daily (seven of the patients remained at the 2.5 mg dose), and followed for 4 weeks. On average, the 10 patients who completed the study experienced a significant reduction in CGI severity score (from 6.5 to 5.7; $p < .01$) and NPI score (from 44.4 to 12.8; $p < .01$). The NPI domains of significant improvement were delusions, agitation or aggression, irritability, apathy, sleep, and caregiver distress. Adverse effects were minimal: one patient discontinued cannabis oil after 3 days due to dysphagia that was thought to be unrelated to the cannabis oil; one patient who had recurrent falls prior to admission fell again during the study; one patient experienced increased confusion after increasing to 5 mg twice daily, which resolved after returning to 2.5 mg twice daily.[10]

In another prospective observational pilot study, 10 female patients with dementia and severe behavioral symptoms in a nursing home in Geneva were treated with a canna-bis tincture (or oil for three patients with mouth ulcers) with THC:CBD ratio 0.45:1 three times daily, administered with a small piece of chocolate cake. The average daily dose was titrated up to 9 mg of THC and 18 mg of cannabidiol (CBD) over 2 months. The aver-age NPI score decreased from 71.1 to 38.3 after 2 months, the CMAI score decreased from 74.5 to 47.5, and scores on the Unified Parkinson's Disease Rating Scale, a mea-sure of rigidity, decreased from 3.4 to 1.7. The Barthel index for activities of daily living improved in seven patients and decreased in two. Scores on the visual analogue scale for the most invalidating behaviors (screaming, aggressive behavior, tearing clothes) decreased from 9 to 5. Beyond improvement in standardized measures, the qualitative dimension of cannabis therapy in dementia deserves emphasis, as reported in the paper:

> The nurses, several of whom were quite reluctant to the study in the begin-ning, observed in almost all patients less overall rigidity, with more relaxed faces, necks, shoulders, and limbs, making daily washing and transfers easier and more comfortable. They described the patients as calmer, more relaxed, less irritable, and smiling more. Two women with persistent screaming almost stopped doing so, which was a major relief for other patients and the staff. One patient stopped frequent vomiting. Two patients could stop all morphine within 3 months and 1 patient decreased by two-thirds in 2 months. These 3 patients had no more consti-pation, which was noted as an important time gain for the staff, beyond the benefit for the patients. One patient decreased benzodiazepine use by three-fourths after 3 months and 1 patient stopped two antipsychotic medications after 1 month. The feedback from the families was astonishingly positive overall.[11]

In a case report, an 85-year-old Colombian man with history of multiple chronic brain injuries (alcohol-use disorder, hemorrhagic stroke, brain trauma, and chronic use of ben-zodiazepines) developed a major neurocognitive disorder. He had minimal response to antidepressants, antipsychotics, benzodiazepines, and cholinergic medications. After 4 months of cannabis tincture (dosage not published), he showed a significant improve-ment in major behavioral symptoms (irritability and agitation) and in cognitive and motor abilities. He significantly recovered his autonomy, only requiring punctual help for daily life activities. He was able again to spontaneously initiate conversations and recall fam-ily or social recent events. Aggression episodes disappeared, numerous medications were tapered, and scores for Memory Failures of Everyday, Mini-Mental State Exam-ination, and the Barthel index for for activities of daily living all improved markedly.[12] I have observed similar cases in my practice. It is hard to know if the cannabis treatment is actually reversing the cognitive impairment or if tapering the other medications previously needed to control agitation (antipsychotics and benzodiazepines) simply reveals the true baseline function.

Finally, a randomized placebo-controlled crossover trial of nabilone for agitation in Alzheimer's disease was performed with 39 patients in Toronto. Nabilone was titrated up to a maximum of 2 mg daily over 4 weeks, starting at 0.25 mg every night at bedtime. Nine patients did not complete the study due to adverse effects, five during nabilone treatment and four during placebo, and one other patient discontinued during the placebo run-in week due to delusions. Nabilone treatment was associated with a significant reduction in agitation over 6 weeks, with an estimated treatment difference of CMAI improving by –4.0 (95% confidence interval –6.5 to –1.5, p = .003). The authors point out this is a greater difference than that in similar randomized controlled trials conducted with atypical antipsychotics and antidepressants, which have reported improvements in CMAI scores of –2.38 points or less. NPI scores, caregiver burden, and nutritional status also improved with nabilone.[13]

Preclinical Evidence

The activity of the endocannabinoid system declines during aging, as CB1 receptor expression[14] and 2-arachidonoylglycerol levels[15] decrease in the brain tissues of older animals.

Numerous in vitro and in vivo studies have demonstrated that CB1 and CB2 activation, at nonpsychoactive doses, have beneficial effects in experimental models of Alzheimer's disease by reducing the harmful amyloid-β peptide action and tau phosphorylation, as well as by promoting the intrinsic repair mechanisms of the brain. Modulation of neuroinflammation, excitotoxicity, mitochondrial dysfunction, and oxidative stress by the endocannabinoid system is likely involved.[16] This substantial body of preclinical evidence is promising for translation.

Beyond the behavioral benefits demonstrated in the clinical studies summarized above, an important question remains: Can cannabis reverse or prevent progression of cognitive decline? One rodent study demonstrated that THC (3 mg·kg^{-1}·day^{-1}) reversed age-related cognitive decline in mice, aged 12 and 18 months, after a 28-day treatment period. Hippocampal spine density increased, and hippocampal gene transcription patterns of THC-treated 12-month-old mice closely resembled those of untreated 2-month-old mice.[17] Fascinatingly, a similar study using a single ultralow dose of THC (0.002 mg/kg) in female 24-month-old mice improved performance in six different behavioral assays of memory and learning. The treated mice scored similarly to naïve 2-month-old mice, and the beneficial effects of the single dose lasted for at least 7 weeks.[18]

Treatment Strategies for Clinicians

- Consider cannabis as an alternative to Beer's Criteria medications such as antipsychotics, benzodiazepines, hypnotics, muscle relaxants, and opioids, which are known to increase morbidity and mortality in this patient population.[19]
- THC is most effectively used to mitigate symptoms and improve quality of life. The oral or oromucosal dosing range is typically 1–10 mg two to three times daily.
- Combined THC/CBD formulations, for example, a 1:1 ratio, are useful to improve tolerability of THC and likely provide additional neuroprotective benefits.
- CBD-dominant, low-THC formulations may be effective for apathy and fatigue and may have procognitive effects, but they are less likely to be effective for severe agitation unless used in high doses (e.g., 200–800 mg/day), as seen in a head-to-head trial with an atypical antipsychotic in the treatment of schizophrenia.[20] These doses are likely cost-prohibitive for most patients.
- CBD has been shown to reduce appetite and feeding in rodents,[21] and appetite loss is one of the most common CBD-related adverse effects I have observed in this patient population. Use caution in patients with preexisting anorexia and/or low body mass index.
- In my clinical experience, I have found that formulations containing low to moderate levels of Δ^9-tetrahydrocannabinolic acid and cannabidiolic acid have improved efficacy.
- An early afternoon dose of THC can be effective for preventing sundowning symptoms.
- Low-dose THC can be effectively used as needed for breakthrough or episodic symptoms.
- Dronabinol (capsule or liquid formulations) can be effectively used off-label in institutions that prohibit herbal cannabis.
- Formulations of herbal cannabis that enable some oromucosal absorption and have a pleasant taste, such as chocolates or lozenges, may be better tolerated than tinctures or oils (poor palatability) and capsules (erratic absorption and onset).
- Provide orders that enable the nursing staff to titrate the medication as needed.

How to implement:

1. For patients with night symptoms or sleep disturbance, begin with evening or bedtime dosing. For example, an order can read: THC 2 mg PO QHS. Increase by THC 1 mg every third night until the patient experiences satisfactory sleep or adverse

effects such as morning grogginess or increased agitation. If adverse effects occur, lower the dose by 1 mg of THC. Maximum dose is 10 mg at bedtime.

2. After titrating to an effective nighttime dose, which may take 1–2 weeks, evaluate to determine if daytime symptoms are still problematic; in many patients, the day symptoms also improve with nighttime dosing. If symptoms persist, begin daytime treatment with THC/CBD; start with 25% of the nighttime dose of THC and increase slowly. For example, if night symptoms improve with 4 mg of THC, start daytime treatment with 1 mg of THC + 1 mg of CBD and slowly titrate up.

3. For patients who do well with a bedtime dose of THC that produces mild morning grogginess, a morning dose of 10–50 mg of CBD often resolves the grogginess and improves alertness.

Cautions

- There may be an increased fall risk.
  - Preclinical studies have demonstrated that CB1 agonism can produce motor discoordination,[22] and the common adverse effects of cannabis—including dizziness, sedation, and orthostatic hypotension—may result in increased fall risk, already significant in dementia patients.[23] As for many medications used in this patient population, altered gait and other signs of discoordination should be assessed as a potential adverse effect.
  - Patients are more likely to build tolerance to the adverse motor effects of THC faster than the therapeutic effects. Slow titration may therefore allow a widening of the therapeutic window and mitigate potentially increased fall risk.
  - A randomized crossover trial evaluated the effects of 1.5 mg of THC twice daily on balance and gait in 18 community-dwelling dementia patients. Compared to placebo, treatment with THC was associated with a trend toward increase in gait velocity and increase in dynamic sway during preferred speed walking, but the magnitude of these changes was considered not to be clinically significant. There was no difference in the occurrence of adverse effects between 1.5 of mg THC and placebo treatments, and the low-dose THC was well tolerated.[24]

- THC may produce increased adverse effects when combined with anticholinergic medications, including tricyclic antidepressants.[25]

Chapter 25

Seizure Disorders

EPILEPSY IS THE FOURTH MOST COMMON neurological condition, affecting an estimated 50 million people globally.[1] Around 70% of patients achieve seizure control by use of antiepileptic drugs (AEDs), while around 30% continue to have breakthrough seizures despite treatment with two or more AEDs.[2] In patients with drug-resistant epilepsy, the likelihood of a complete clinical response with an additional AED is estimated to be 5%–10%. These patients have increased risk for developmental delay, psychosocial problems, injury, and premature death.[3] The burden on patients' parents and families can be immense.

Polypharmacy is common in patients with drug-resistant epilepsy, with a rationale of addressing the seizures via multiple pharmacological targets. While this approach can improve response in some patients, the trade-off can be severe, as many AEDs have significant adverse effects and toxicity profiles. Tapering and discontinuing AEDs can also be challenging in refractory cases, and some patients end up taking numerous medications without clear evidence of benefit. Although over 20 new seizure medications have been developed over the past several decades, the percentage of patients with medically intractable seizures has not changed dramatically.[4]

The endocannabinoid system is an important and effective target in epilepsy, with both antiepileptic and neuroprotective properties. This concept is far from new, as several ancient cultures describe cannabis as a treatment for seizures. If the descriptions in ancient Assyrian sources referring to "hand of ghost" correlate with seizures, this practice spans 4 millennia. Nineteenth-century physicians, including William O'Shaughnessy and the eminent Sir John Russell Reynolds, one of the greatest 19th-century authorities on clinical cannabis and personal physician to Queen Victoria, published case reports on the effective use of cannabis for epilepsy.[5]

While some preclinical and clinical research on the antiepileptic effects of cannabinoids was undertaken in the 1970s, with promising results, the rapidly growing interest in, and now widespread practice of, using cannabis to treat seizure disorders was ignited by internet communication among parents of children with intractable epilepsy around 2011 and exploded after the airing of the CNN documentary *Weed* in 2013. Patients and their families around the world watched the story of a 4-year-old girl with Dravet syndrome whose seizures were relieved by a cannabidiol (CBD)-dominant variety of cannabis. While I had successfully treated a small number of patients with intractable epilepsy prior to the CNN broadcast, my practice rapidly transformed thereafter, with dozens of the most challenging cases of epilepsy in my state establishing care at my clinic.

Though I had previously observed antiepileptic responses to Δ^9-tetrahydrocannabinol (THC), everyone's focus was suddenly on CBD, and product availability, quality, and consistency were extremely problematic. I established a cannabis analytic laboratory in my clinic to help overcome these challenges and to guide the cannabis breeders and producers working to help my patients. This led to several interesting discoveries. One day, a young woman returned for follow-up with near-resolution of daily seizures; her mother had a minimally-labeled bottle of CBD oil in hand. We ran the sample on high-performance liquid chromatography and discovered it had no detectable CBD or THC; it was a low-potency Δ^9-tetrahydrocannabinolic acid (THCA) glycerin solution. I did not believe the results at first, even though I had previously read rumors on the internet of THCA helping with seizures. After a few other patients returned with the same product and a similar response, I became convinced of the clinical utility of THCA in epilepsy, now confirmed after several years of clinical use. At least, I think it is THCA that is helping, but there may be other components at work. First, any THCA product contains at least trace amounts of THC, which may have therapeutic effects in the ultra-low-dose range. Trace quantities of other phytoconstituents may also contribute to my observed responses.

Whatever the mechanism, it is clear to me that some patients experience seizure reduction with THCA-dominant formulas. Interestingly, rodent data suggest that THCA does not cross the blood–brain barrier (BBB).[6] While it is unknown whether these findings translate to humans, patients with frequent seizures (and other neurological conditions) are likely to have altered function of the BBB,[7] potentially allowing the THCA to act centrally.

We currently have a large body of gold-standard clinical evidence that supports the use of CBD or CBD-dominant preparations in intractable epilepsy, and a growing body of observational data supports treatment with THC and other cannabinoids. Cannabis clinicians willing to treat severely ill pediatric patients receive referrals from pediatric neurologists, who are now very acclimated to the cannabis-related questions that inevitably come up during discussions about a subsequent AED trial. The FDA-approved CBD oral solution Epidiolex, the first cannabis-based medication in the United States, is a testament to the positive results of clinical trials.

Treating seizures with cannabis is both challenging and rewarding; patients and parents require frequent communication and follow-up as they navigate the broad dosing ranges and unusual dose–response effects of cannabis. Coordinating care with neurologists is essential. The clinical course of so many of these refractory cases is devastating with or without cannabis. Nevertheless, the odds of providing some benefit to patients with drug-resistant epilepsy is around 85%, with around 10% experiencing a complete clinical response, and most patients or families report helpful rather than adverse side effects.

Clinical Evidence

The only randomized controlled trials evaluating cannabinoids for seizure disorders have used CBD oral solution (Epidiolex) in patients with Lennox-Gastaut syndrome and Dravet syndrome, two highly refractory and difficult-to-treat seizure disorders.[8,9,10,11] A meta-analysis of these four trials (N = 550) found that the average difference in seizure frequency improvement with CBD at doses of 10 and 20 mg·kg^{-1}·day^{-1}, compared with placebo, was 19.5% (p = .001) and 19.9% (p < .001), respectively. A 50% reduction in all seizure types occurred in 37.2% of patients receiving 20 mg·kg^{-1}·day^{-1} CBD and 21.2% of patients receiving placebo, which was statistically significant, but this demonstrates the high placebo effect associated with subjective (usually parent-reported) outcomes.[12]

Among patients with Lennox-Gastaut syndrome, 5.5% randomized to CBD had complete resolution of drop seizures, versus 0.6% in the placebo group, and 5% of those with Dravet syndrome randomized to CBD experienced complete resolution of convulsive seizures, versus none in the placebo group. The adverse effects significantly associated with CBD compared to placebo in the overall analysis were somnolence (24.5% vs. 8.4%), decreased appetite (20.1% vs. 4.8%), diarrhea (18.2% vs. 8.6%), and increased levels of transaminases (16.1% vs. 0.9%).[13]

An extended access study evaluated the effects of CBD oral solution in 26 children (age range 4–11) over an average of 21 months (range 4–53 months). At 24 months, the number of patients continuing cannabidiol as adjunctive therapy was only nine of the original 26 (34.6%); seven (26.9%) had a sustained >50% reduction in motor seizures, including three (11.5%) who remained seizure-free. Fifteen patients (57.7%) discontinued cannabidiol for lack of efficacy, one because of status epilepticus, and one for severe weight loss. Decreased appetite (38.4%), diarrhea (34.6%) and weight loss (30.7%) were common and in many cases became evident only later in the treatment.[14] The adverse effect profile of high-dose CBD and loss of efficacy over time are common challenges in this population.

Several observational studies on both CBD oral solution and a wide variety of artisanal cannabis preparations have been published. One systematic review found that, among 17 observational studies, an estimated 48.5% of 970 patients achieved 50% or greater reduction in seizures. Among 14 observational studies, 8.5% of 977 subjects achieve complete seizure freedom, notably more than the randomized clinical trials described above.[15]

Given our understanding of phytoconstituent synergy, it is not surprising that artisanal cannabis products containing trace or more substantial amounts of cannabis constituents other than CBD may provide better results. A meta-analysis of observational data published in 2018 compared the safety and efficacy of CBD-rich cannabis extracts with purified CBD in treatment-resistant epilepsy patients (Table 25.1). The strict inclusion criteria, requiring objective measurements of seizures, included 11 publications with 670 total subjects (447 taking CBD extract, 223 taking pure CBD).[16,17]

TABLE 25.1

Comparison of CBD-Rich Cannabis Extract With Purified CBD in Treatment-Resistant Epilepsy Patients

Result	CBD-rich cannabis extract	Purified CBD
Reports of improvement ($p < .0001$)	71%	36%
Reports of >50% seizure reduction ($p = .52$)	37%	42%
Average daily dose (mg/kg/day)	6.0	25.3
Adverse events ($p < .0001$)		
Mild	33%	76%
Severe	7%	26%

These data are significant, though preliminary. The lower average dose, which was probably influenced by affordability in the cannabis extract studies, is likely responsible for the markedly fewer adverse effects. The overall higher likelihood of response with increased safety supports CBD-rich cannabis extract as a potentially preferred alternative to CBD oral solution, as long as families can find a product with appropriate quality control.

It is important to note that seizure reduction is not the only important outcome for these patients and their families. In the preceding analysis, patients in the CBD-rich cannabis extract pool (no data were available for the purified CBD pool) reported numerous secondary improvements including improved awareness (52%), quality of sleep (31%), mood (30%), behavior or aggression (20%), language or cognition (7%), and motor skills (7%). Most AEDs tend to adversely impact these aspects of quality of life.[18] In a study of 53 adults with treatment-resistant epilepsy, treatment with purified CBD, starting at 5 $mg \cdot kg^{-1} \cdot day^{-1}$ and titrated to 50 $mg \cdot kg^{-1} \cdot day^{-1}$, was associated with a clinically significant improvement in quality of life (~10 points on the Quality of Life in Epilepsy-89 measure) after 1 year. Interestingly, the quality of life improvements correlated with improvement in mood but not with a change in seizure frequency or severity.[19] I have also seen this clinically, albeit at much lower doses. Some patients who do not experience reductions in seizures continue to use cannabis due to substantial improvements in these secondary outcomes.

As described in Chapter 18, CBD may interact with AEDs, especially when used in high doses. Higher serum levels of topiramate, rufinamide, N-desmethylclobazam (an active metabolite of clobazam), zonisamide, and eslicarbazepine, may occur with increasing CBD dose. Except for clobazam and N-desmethylclobazam, all mean level changes were within the accepted therapeutic range. Sedation was more frequent with higher N-desmethylclobazam levels in adults, and aspartate aminotransferase/alanine aminotransferase levels were significantly higher in participants taking valproate.[20] I find the interactions of CBD with clobazam and valproate clinically significant, and I monitor labs and adverse effects more closely in patients taking these medications with CBD.

Clinicians should be aware that cannabis and cannabinoids have the potential to exacerbate seizures, on average in 5% of patients in most reports,[21,22,23] though one observational study using THC/CBD 1:20 extract ranging from 1 to 20 $mg \cdot kg^{-1} \cdot day^{-1}$ reported 18% seizure exacerbations.[24] As demonstrated in cases reported in my 2017 paper in the journal *Epilepsy & Behavior*, some patients who experience exacerbations related to a formula dominant in one cannabinoid may respond favorably to another. For example, I described the case of a girl with Dravet syndrome who experienced improvements in cognition and quality of life with CBD at 0.05 $mg \cdot kg^{-1} \cdot day^{-1}$ but increased myoclonic seizures with more CBD. The same patient experienced a 90% reduction in seizures after working up to 2 mg·kg^{-1}·day^{-1} THCA.* Her breakthrough generalized tonic–clonic seizures could be aborted by oromucosal or rectal THC (10 mg) given at seizure onset and repeated after 1 min if needed, which was demonstrated in the inpatient setting via electroencephalographic monitoring.[25] Several other patients have been able to abort seizures, avoid rectal diazepam, and speed postictal recovery by using THC at the seizure onset.†

While most recent epilepsy papers focus on CBD, some observational studies and case reports confirm my clinical success using THC to prevent seizures, usually below 20 mg total daily.[26] In 292 patients with seizures (190 with epilepsy, 64 with psychogenic nonepileptic seizures, and 26 with both types of seizures), 36% were actively using presumed THC-dominant cannabis in the last year. An improvement in seizures related to cannabis use was reported by 84% of those with epilepsy and 72.7% of those with psychogenic nonepileptic seizures; both groups also reported improvements in sleep, stress, and AED-related adverse effects. The mean dose was 1 g/day, mainly via smoking (87%). Other forms of administration included vaporizer (37%), ingestion in food (14.6%), and in capsule form (4.9%).[27]

When the risks and benefits of a cannabis trial are evaluated, especially in pediatric patients, the nonmedical risks must also be considered. Availability of a consistent supply of the medication is frequently interrupted due to horticultural, manufacturing, and economic factors. Higher dosing ranges are financially unfeasible for many patients unless they grow and produce their own medicine, a complex process that presents many potential interruptions in treatment. Sudden loss of access to cannabis may result in rebound seizures. Hospital admissions present challenges, and patients or their guardians often must choose between interrupting cannabis treatment and violating hospital policies that forbid self-administration of medications, especially those with schedule I status. The potential for disruption of medical treatment or family structure related to child protective services and other legal agencies, even when the patient and medical provider operate within local laws, must also be carefully considered on a case-by-case basis.[28]

Finally, we must address the elephant in the room: should cannabis be considered as a first-line therapy in patients with epilepsy? This line of thinking has not yet been

---

* Cannabis allowed this child to leave her wheelchair, play on a playground, and enjoy a good quality of life after years of severe disability. Her family had to make many sacrifices to achieve this, including moving to Maine from out of state. Her mother became an effective political activist, subsequently improving medical cannabis laws in both Maine and her home state.

† A short video of this patient having a generalized tonic–clonic seizure and responding to THC can be seen at https://youtu.be/vwWvi1a85jU or by searching for "Cyndimae - Let me Have My Medicine."

explored in human studies, though the high rate of efficacy in some of the most refractory and challenging cases is promising for equal or greater efficacy in patients with newly diagnosed epilepsy. Furthermore, the significantly better adverse effect profile of cannabis compared to most AEDs makes this an appealing option, especially when lost time in early childhood development is considered. The toxicity of AEDs is the most common impediment to achieving fully effective dosing, with adverse effects ranging from tiredness to memory problems and even death.[29] In my practice, I have ventured to take this approach only in a handful of patients whose parents have a strong personal preference to avoid AEDs but are willing to continue following up with pediatric neurology; thus far, I have seen beneficial effects in all cases.

Preclinical Evidence

Early studies in preclinical models of seizures focused on cannabis extracts, THC, and, later, synthetic CB1 agonists, with mixed results. In some models, THC reduced seizure frequency or severity, while in other studies there was no effect or even a proconvulsive effect. Similarly, synthetic CB1 agonists have shown variable effects in seizure models. Some studies found dose-limiting tolerance to the antiseizure effects of THC.[30]

The anticonvulsant effects of several cannabinoids were compared using a variety of standard seizure models by Karler and Turkanis in 1979.[31] Anticonvulsant effects against the minimal electric shock test in mice were seen at the following doses: CBD (120 mg/kg), THC (100 mg/kg), 11-OH-THC (14 mg/kg), THCA (200–400 mg/kg), Δ^8-THC (80 mg/kg), and cannabinol (230 mg/kg).

CBD has been tested in several animal seizure models, including maximal electroshock, pentylenetetrazole, pilocarpine, penicillin, audiogenic, 6-Hz, subcutaneous metrazole, and cobalt implantation; it was found to have an anticonvulsant effect in all models. In an animal model of Dravet syndrome, CBD was studied in SCN1A knockout mice, showing decreased spontaneous seizure frequency and duration and decreased severity of heat-induced seizures. Interestingly, autisticlike social interaction deficits improved with low-dose CBD but failed to improve with the higher dosages required for seizure control.[32] Cannabidivarin has also shown anticonvulsant properties in vitro and in several in vivo models.[33]

The brain and plasma pharmacokinetic profiles of cannabidiolic acid (CBDA), THCA, cannabichromenic acid, cannabidivarinic acid, cannabigerolic acid (CBGA), and cannabigerovarinic acid (CBGVA) following intraperitoneal administration were recently studied in mice. All were rapidly absorbed and had relatively short half-lives (<4 hr), all shorter than their neutral counterparts except for CBGVA. The brain/plasma ratios for the acids were very low at ≤0.04, indicating poor transport across the BBB. When CBDA was administered in a Tween 80–based vehicle, it had a brain/plasma ratio of 1.9; using this vehicle, CBDA significantly increased the temperature threshold at which the SCN1A knockout mice had a generalized tonic–clonic seizure.[34] As mentioned above, rodent BBB models may not adequately represent BBB function in people with epilepsy and other conditions.

Seizure classification[35]

Focal onset

- aware versus impaired awareness
- motor versus nonmotor
- includes "focal to bilateral tonic–clonic"

Generalized onset

- motor
  - tonic–clonic
  - clonic
  - tonic
  - myoclonic
  - myoclonic–tonic–clonic
  - myoclonic–atonic
  - atonic
  - epileptic spasms

- nonmotor (absence seizures)
  - typical absence
  - atypical absence
  - myoclonic absence
  - eyelid myoclonia

Treatment Strategies for Clinicians

- When initiating treatment, I usually choose among THC-dominant, THCA-dominant, or CBD-dominant formulas based on comorbidities and access. I prefer to first try one of these dominant cannabinoids at a time, rather than a mixed formula, to improve clarity about anti- or proconvulsive responses.

- For patients with pain, gastrointestinal symptoms, behavioral symptoms like self-injury and agitation, sleep disturbance, or who are underweight, I usually start with THC, which is most likely to provide secondary benefits in these symptoms.

- I find that THCA is the least likely to produce beneficial or adverse side effects; its observed efficacy at low doses also makes it appealing for patients or families with limited financial resources. I have seen a high response rate to THCA in patients with absence seizures.

- CBD has a high response rate, though some cases require titration to high doses. I consider CBD in patients with developmental delay, as a remarkable number of patients experience improvements in cognition and communication, often at doses lower than those required to reduce seizures. Some patients and families prefer a treatment with more supporting clinical evidence, and CBD clearly has this backing. I consider starting with THC or THCA, instead of CBD, in patients taking clobazam or valproate, due to potential drug interactions.

- Dosing ranges for the various dominant cannabinoids, based on my clinical experience and that of my colleagues, are somewhat different. I typically begin with twice-daily dosing, and if breakthrough events are observed in the hours prior to a subsequent dose, I increase to three times daily; this most commonly occurs with THCA.

- THC is started at 0.05 $mg \cdot kg^{-1} \cdot day^{-1}$ and titrated up to the maximum tolerated dose (avoiding psychoactive side effects) or 2 $mg \cdot kg^{-1} \cdot day^{-1}$.

- THCA is started at 0.01 $mg \cdot kg^{-1} \cdot day^{-1}$ and titrated up to 2 $mg \cdot kg^{-1} \cdot day^{-1}$ or the maximum tolerated dose of concomitant THC (psychoactive effects).

- CBD is started at 0.1 $mg \cdot kg^{-1} \cdot day^{-1}$ and titrated up to 20 $mg \cdot kg^{-1} \cdot day^{-1}$ or the upper limit of the patient's financial resources.

- The titration method varies with the patient's frequency of seizures.

- The broad effective dosing range can make titration a lengthy process, especially in patients who have infrequent seizures. In these cases, I typically increase the dose by 100% after each subsequent seizure and increase by 50% after observing a sign of early response like longer interval between seizures, decreased length or intensity of seizure, or improved recovery.

- In patients who have daily or near-daily seizures, I typically titrate every 5–10 days depending on the urgency of the situation. If there is no suggestion of a response or adverse effect, I increase the dose by 100%, and if there is some evidence of a response, I increase the dose by 50%.

- Loss of efficacy after increasing the dose can occur, due to tolerance or other factors, and patients should monitor for this. I often observe an especially narrow therapeutic window with THCA, so I titrate by 10%–20% after observing a response.
- For aborting seizures, regardless of my choice for an initial trial, I recommend THC acutely for prolonged seizures or seizure clusters that frequently require benzodiazepine rescue (rectal diazepam or intranasal midazolam). These agents can suppress cardiorespiratory function and increase the risk of hypoxic injury to the brain and heart.
  - Neurologists typically recommend administering the benzodiazepines after 3–5 min of seizure activity or a certain number of seizures in a cluster, but the THC can be given immediately; if THC is not effective, it is still safe to administer the benzodiazepine after the recommended time frame.
  - The potential of THC to mitigate excitotoxicity and inflammation makes this an appealing intervention, and many patients report faster recovery after receiving this treatment.
  - I start with 0.1 mg/kg THC in a concentrated oil vigorously rubbed into the gums or, less frequently, administered rectally. If there is no response in 1–2 min, the dose can be repeated. If 0.1 mg/kg is ineffective, I titrate up to 0.3 mg/kg before concluding that THC is ineffective for aborting seizures. Parents typically carry an oral syringe with a premeasured dosage of THC oil in their first aid kit.
- In patients who experience partial efficacy with one cannabis formula, an additional formula can be added. For example, in a patient with a maximal 75% seizure reduction with a methodical THCA titration trial, a subsequent trial of adding CBD may improve results.
- Some patients require a temporary dose increase or addition of THC during acute illnesses or other conditions that can impact seizure threshold.
- CBDA, CBG, and CBGA may provide antiepileptic effects, but I only have a little clinical experience with these agents at the time of writing and I cannot comment on effective dosing ranges or other aspects of their utility. Trace quantities of these phytoconstituents in broad-spectrum CBD products may improve efficacy.

Cautions

- Cannabis exacerbates seizures in around 5% of patients, based on my experience and observational studies. A seizure exacerbation with one dominant cannabinoid does not preclude a subsequent trial with a different dominant cannabinoid.

- Some patients have a very narrow therapeutic window, especially with THCA. Careful titration and journaling of seizures and other symptoms are essential.

- Artisanal products have variable composition and efficacy from batch to batch, and mislabeling is prevalent. If a certain product produces good results, I always encourage patients or their parents to have the product analyzed by a third-party laboratory. This information is useful in case a subsequent batch is less effective.

- Be cautious of drug interactions, especially relevant for moderate- or high-dose CBD combined with valproate or clobazam.

- When administration occurs via an oral syringe, I have found that patients or parents often make mistakes with volumes <0.1 ml. For example, if I recommend 0.02 ml (often the smallest increment on a 1 ml oral syringe), many parents administer 0.2 ml because the 0.02-ml dose seems unbelievably small.

- Many patients wish to taper AEDs after experiencing benefits with cannabis. This must be done slowly in collaboration with the neurologist, and cannabinoid dosing may need to be adjusted to address breakthrough seizures.

- Some patients build tolerance to the benefits of cannabis, particularly with THC and high-dose CBD.
  - While a 48-hr tolerance break followed by restarting at a 25% lower dose has been effective in some of my patients (similar to other conditions and popular among internet support groups), I do not recommend this approach in patients with seizures, due to the possibility of rebound or withdrawal seizures.
  - If it appears the patient has developed tolerance based on slowly progressive loss of efficacy, slowly tapering the dose can be effective, even though it seems counterintuitive (see Chapter 17 for more details). Consider tapering especially if there has been a trend of titrating associated with temporary improvement followed by recurrence.

- Abrupt discontinuation of cannabis can provoke seizures, and patients with epilepsy who use cannabis for nonmedical purposes may experience seizures during cannabis withdrawal.[36]

Integrative Strategies

- **Vitamin D:**
  - Vitamin D deficiency and hypocalcemia can decrease seizure threshold.
  - Phenytoin, phenobarbital, and carbamazepine interfere with vitamin D metabolism by inducing hepatic microsomal enzymes that metabolize vitamin D and 25-OH-D and impairing calcium absorption from the intestine and mobilization from the bone.
  - Patients with severe epilepsy may be at higher risk for vitamin D and calcium dysregulation due to polypharmacy, poor diet, and reduced exposure to sunlight.
  - Small trials have reported decreased seizure activity with vitamin D supplementation.[37,38]
  - Vitamin D deficiency is a major cause of hypocalcemic seizures in infants. Infants born to vitamin D–deficient mothers are at significantly higher risk to develop hypocalcemic seizures.[39]
  - I recommend supplementing with vitamin D3 (70 $iu \cdot kg^{-1} \cdot day^{-1}$) and testing 25-OH-D once or twice annually, aiming for levels in the 50–70 ng/dl range.

- **Magnesium:**
  - Magnesium is involved in repolarization and hyperpolarization of all nerve cells, and adequate intracellular magnesium is basic to maintaining a healthy seizure threshold.
  - Magnesium is an essential cofactor in vitamin D activation and function,[40] and should be given as a supplement with vitamin D, as taking large doses of vitamin D can induce severe depletion of magnesium, especially when dietary sources are lacking.[41]
  - Magnesium status is more difficult to test because serum levels remain normal in most cases of deficiency, unless severe. The most informative measure may be the intracellular or red blood cell Mg level.
  - Supplementation with chelated Mg can be started at the recommended dietary allowance of 5 $mg \cdot kg^{-1} \cdot day^{-1}$ and titrated to bowel tolerance.
  - I have observed that many patients with epilepsy experience exacerbation of seizures when constipated. I frequently use magnesium as a preferred osmotic laxative. Neurological and neuropsychiatric adverse effects have been reported by gastroenterologists and parents of children treated with poly(ethylene glycol) laxatives,[42] and magnesium can serve dual roles in patients with epilepsy and constipation.

- **Omega-3 fatty acids:**
    - Children with epilepsy have been found to have lower omega-3/omega-6 ratios.[43]
    - Omega-3 fatty acids activate signaling pathways that induce an anti-inflammatory and antioxidant environment.
    - Recent data suggest that omega-3 fatty acids may have neuroprotective and anticonvulsant effects. Animal models demonstrate anticonvulsant effects of omega-3 fatty acids by increasing latency to seizure or raising seizure threshold. Human trials are very limited, with some showing antiepileptic effects of omega-3 supplementation.[44]
    - Most of my epilepsy patients consume very little dietary omega-3 fatty acids. Supplemental omega-3 has very little risk but can potentially benefit seizures, behavior, cognition, and cardiovascular health.

Chapter 26

Autism Spectrum Disorders

AUTISM SPECTRUM DISORDERS (ASDs) are a group of complex neurode-velopment disorders that involve repetitive and characteristic patterns of behavior and challenges with social communication and interaction. The term "spectrum" acknowledges the heterogeneity in symptoms, skills, and levels of disability that can occur in people with ASD. Among 8-year-old children, as many as 1 in 59 (1.7%) receive an ASD diagnosis,[1] with 4 times more males than females. Siblings of children already diagnosed with ASD have a significantly higher incidence of the same disorder, ranging from 15% to 25% depending on sex and clinical severity.[2]

While ASDs are clearly multifactorial conditions, an emerging body of evidence implicates dysfunction in the endocannabinoid system, a regulator of emotional responses, behavioral reactivity to context, social interaction, sensory signaling, seizure susceptibility, and circadian rhythm.

DSM-5 Diagnostic Criteria for ASD (abbreviated):[3]

- Persistent deficits in social communication and social interaction occur across multiple contexts.
- Restricted, repetitive patterns of behavior, interests, or activities are exhibited.
- Symptoms are present in the early developmental period (but they may not become fully manifest until social demands exceed limited capacities, or they may be masked by learned strategies in later life).
- Symptoms cause clinically significant impairment in social, occupational, or other important areas of current functioning.

- These disturbances are not better explained by intellectual disability (intellectual developmental disorder) or global developmental delay.

The DSM-5 has also identified three severity levels of ASD:

level 1, "requiring support"

level 2, "requiring substantial support"

level 3, "requiring very substantial support"

Clinical Evidence

Children with ASD have been found to have lower levels of the circulating endocannabinoids anandamide (AEA), oleoylethanolamine (OEA), and palmitoylethanolamine (PEA), compared with a matched neurotypical control group (Figure 26.1). Serum levels of 2-arachidonoylglycerol were not significantly different.[4] While AEA has a function similar to that of Δ^9-tetrahydrocannabinol (THC), OEA and PEA have low affinity for CB1 and CB2 receptors and may exert their effects on the central nervous system by activation of peroxisome proliferator-activated receptors and the TRPV1 receptor, which is similar to the mechanism of action of cannabidiol (CBD).

FIGURE 26.1
Lower Serum Endocannabinoid Levels in Children with ASD

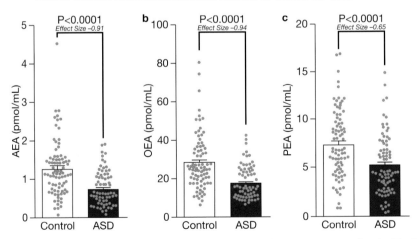

Note. From "Lower circulating endocannabinoid levels in children with autism spectrum disorder," by A. Aran, M. Eylon, M. Harel, L. Polianski, A. Nemirovski, S. Tepper, A. Schnapp, H. Cassuto, N. Wattad, and J. Tam, 2019, *Molecular Autism, 10,* Article 2 (https://doi.org/10.1186/s13229-019-0256-6). Copyright © 2019 by the authors. Open Access under Creative Commons Attribution 4.0 International License (http://creativecommons.org/licenses/by/4.0/).

The first published report of cannabinoid therapeutics in ASD was a case study of a 6-year-old by with early infant autism, who was treated with dronabinol (total daily dose 3.6 mg: 2 drops in the morning, 1 drop midday, 3 drops in the evening). On the Aberrant Behavior Checklist, hyperactivity decreased by 27 points, lethargy by 25 points, irritability by 12 points, stereotypic behavior by 7 points, and inappropriate speech by 6 points. No adverse effects were reported.[5]

Observational data from Chile were reported on 20 children and one adult with ASD, with a roughly equal distribution of the three severity levels. Two-thirds of the patients were unsuccessfully treated with risperidone, aripiprazole, quetiapine, and/or methylphenidate. Seventy-one percent of patients received balanced THC/CBD extracts; 19.0% received CBD-dominant extracts, and 9.5% received THC-dominant extracts. According to the Clinical Global Impression (CGI) scale, 67% of patients had significant improvement (very much improved, 19.0%; much improved, 47.6%). Adverse events included more agitation ($n = 2$), more irritability ($n = 1$), somnolence ($n = 1$), insomnia ($n = 1$), and seizure aggravation ($n = 1$), all of which were successfully addressed by changing the cannabis formula.[6]

Observational data from Israel were reported for the use of CBD-rich cannabis oil as adjuvant therapy in 60 children with ASD and severe behavioral problems (77% low-functioning, 83% boys). The cannabis oil was given sublingually 2–3 times daily, with doses titrated up over 2–4 weeks to effect and tolerability; the starting CBD dose was 1 $mg \cdot kg^{-1} \cdot day^{-1}$ and the maximum dose was 10 $mg \cdot kg^{-1} \cdot day^{-1}$. According to the CGI scale, 61% of patients had significant improvement in behavior problems (much improved or very much improved). In 29 patients with an insufficient response to the original 1:20 formulation, higher THC:CBD ratios were tried (up to 1:6). The higher THC:CBD ratio was reported to be much better in 13 patients, slightly better in seven, equivalent in six, and worse in three. Communication and anxiety were the strongest domains of improvement, and the most common adverse effects were sleep disturbances (14%), restlessness (9%), nervousness (9%), loss of appetite (9%), and gastrointestinal disturbances (7%). One girl who received a higher THC:CBD ratio (maximum THC dose 0.72 $mg \cdot kg^{-1} \cdot day^{-1}$) had a transient serious psychotic event that required treatment with antipsychotic medication.[7]

A different Israeli group also reported observational data on 188 patients with ASD, 90% with restlessness, 80% with rage attacks, and 79% with agitation. The children were primarily treated with THC/CBD oil, 1:20 ratio, with an average dose of 4.0 ± 3.0 mg of THC and 79.5 ± 61.5 mg of CBD given three times daily. Insomnia, reported in 46 patients (24.4%), was treated with an evening does of THC oil, average 5.0 ± 4.5 mg. Thirty percent of patients reported significant improvement, 54% reported moderate improvement,

7% had slight improvement and 9% had no change in their condition (Figure 26.2). Of the 55 patients taking antipsychotic medications, 11 discontinued them and three reduced the dose. The most common side effect was restlessness (6 patients), and of the 17 patients who discontinued the treatment but responded to the follow-up questionnaire, 12 described no therapeutic effect and five discontinued treatment due to side effects.[8]

FIGURE 26.2
Quality of Life Reported by Patients Before and After 6 Months of Cannabis Treatment

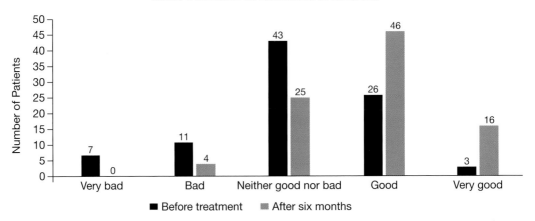

Note. From "Real life experience of medical cannabis treatment in autism: Analysis of safety and efficacy," by L. B.-L. Schleider, R. Mechoulam, N. Saban, G. Meiri, and V. Novack, 2019, *Scientific Reports*, *9*(1), Article 200 (https://doi.org/10.1038/s41598-018-37570-y). Copyright © 2019 by the authors. Open Access under Creative Commons Attribution 4.0 International License (http://creativecommons.org/licenses/by/4.0/).

A third Israeli group also reported similar findings: 53 children received 1:20 CBD-rich oil up to 0.8 mg/kg THC and 16 mg/kg CBD. Self-injury and rage attacks (*n* = 34) improved in 67.6% and worsened in 8.8% of subjects. Hyperactivity symptoms (*n* = 38) improved in 68.4%, did not change in 28.9%, and worsened in 2.6%. Sleep problems (*n* = 21) improved in 71.4% and worsened in 4.7%. Anxiety (*n* = 17) improved in 47.1% and worsened in 23.5%. Adverse effects were mild; distinct from the other two cohorts described earlier, the most common adverse event was somnolence (23%), followed by decreased appetite (11%).[9]

A functional magnetic resonance imaging study of 34 healthy men (half with ASD) was performed following oral administration of 600 mg of CBD or matched placebo. The subjects with ASD, but not the neurotypical subjects, showed significant changes in crucial properties of brain function in key regions commonly implicated in ASD: increased low-frequency fluctuations in the cerebellar vermis and the right fusiform gyrus and altered vermal functional connectivity with several of its subcortical (striatal) and cortical targets.[10]

ASD-related neurobiopsychological disturbances are correlated with at least three major deficiencies: pineal hypofunction with decreased melatonin, diminished or altered activity of the brain endocannabinoid system, and abnormally low levels of oxytocin. Researchers in Italy tested a combined approach to these deficiencies in 30 subjects with ASD. Twelve received melatonin-only treatment (10 mg, 30 min before sleep, titrated up to 100 mg), 12 received melatonin plus CBD (2 mg, titrated up to 10 mg twice daily), and six received melatonin, CBD, and oxytocin (1,850 IU po twice daily). There was no control group. Subjects were followed for at least 6 months. As illustrated in Figure 26.3, melatonin correlated most with sleep improvement, CBD with reduced anxiety, and oxytocin with improved social and affective relationships.[11]

FIGURE 26.3
Percent of Subjects with Improvement in Sleep, Anxiety, and Social and Affective Relationships

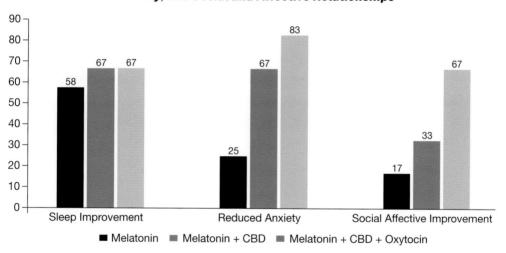

Note. Figure created by Dustin Sulak with data from "A neuroendocrine therapeutic approach with the pineal hormone melatonin, cannabidiol and oxytocin (MCO regimen) in the treatment of the autism spectrum disorders," by A. Caddeo, R. Trampetti, G. Messina, E. Porta, G. Di Fede, R. Tartarelli, O. Tartarelli, A. Monzon, G. Porro, and P. Lissoni, 2020, *Journal of Immunology and Allergy, 1*(2), 1–7. Copyright © 2020 by the authors.

Preclinical Evidence

Reduced endocannabinoid system activity has been demonstrated in several animal models of ASD, including mouse fragile X, mouse neuroligin 3, BTBR mice, and rat valproic acid, with involvement in specific and relevant brain regions. Activation of the endocannabinoid system in these models of ASD reversed the autistic symptoms, including aversive memory and anxietylike behaviors, social impairments, cognitive deficits, and communication abnormalities.[12]

Oxytocin is a neuropeptide crucial in many aspects of social behavior, including affiliation and reward, and as mentioned earlier, increasing data indicate dysfunction of the oxytocin system in ASD. In male mice, oxytocin has been shown to drive anandamide-mediated endocannabinoid signaling to control social reward,[13] highlighting the importance of both systems as potential targets in treating ASD.

Treatment Strategies for Clinicians

- Most of my clinical experience with ASD has been in severe cases requiring urgent solutions for self-injurious and violent behavior or comorbid ASD with epilepsy. In cases of violent and self-injurious behavior, I have observed cannabis succeed where antipsychotic, benzodiazepine, and sympatholytic medications have failed.
- For severe behavior issues, I have found THC-dominant formulations to be more effective than CBD-dominant ones, though few of my patients are able to afford doses of CBD as high as those described in the observational studies summarized above. Note that, even at a 1:20 THC:CBD ratio, the doses of THC administered in those cases were significant, and increasing the THC content in one study resulted in a much better response in almost half the patients that did not benefit from the 1:20 formula.
- Those who respond to THC often do so in the 0.2–2 mg·kg^{-1}·day^{-1} range. As always, start low, go slow, and do not be afraid to go all the way.
- Including Δ^9-tetrahydrocannabinolic acid and cannabidiolic acid has improved the response in several of my patients.
- In my experience with less severe cases of ASD comorbid with epilepsy, I have observed that low doses of CBD often result in improved communication and interaction, a benefit that typically emerges prior to titrating to an effective anticonvulsant dose of CBD.
- In patients living in a facility that will not administer herbal cannabis, off-label use of dronabinol is often an effective treatment.
- For low-severity patients wishing to improve communication and social engagement, reduce anxiety, and improve focus and capacity to participate at school, consider a trial of CBD (0.2–2 mg·kg^{-1}·day^{-1}, divided two to three times daily).
- Cannabigerol (CBG) may be helpful for mood, speech, anxiety, and other symp-

toms.[14] My early clinical impression is that CBG can produce anxiolytic effects at lower doses than CBD and is more likely to help with hyperactivity.

Cautions

- I have observed several cases with excellent responses to THC lose benefits over time, likely due to tolerance-building. Most cases recover efficacy after a 2-day tolerance break followed by a 25% dose reduction, with subsequent titration if needed. If rebound agitation or violent behavior occurs during the tolerance break, consider treatment with a sympatholytic medication like clonidine.
- To avoid tolerance, titrate THC slowly to find the lowest effective dose.
- In hyperactive patients with low appetite, consider a trial of balanced THC/CBD or THC-dominant formulas to avoid potential exacerbation of those symptoms.
- While CBD may cause or worsen hyperactivity and restlessness at low doses, higher doses may be successfully used to overcome this paradoxical effect.
- CBD may cause or exacerbate sleep disturbance, as mentioned in one Israeli study. Giving the second daily dose of CBD earlier in the afternoon and a low dose of THC before bed is often effective.

Chapter 27

Anorexia and Cachexia

ANOREXIA (APPETITE LOSS) and cachexia (depletion of metabolically active lean body mass) are common complications of many chronic malignant and nonmalignant medical conditions. Cachexia is associated with worse prognosis in several conditions, including chronic airway disease, chronic heart failure, renal failure, acquired immune deficiency syndrome (AIDS), dementia, chronic liver disease, and cancer, often independent of other prognostic factors. The anorexia–cachexia syndrome is one of the most common causes of death among cancer patients and is present in 80% of these patients at death.[1] Cancer cachexia is defined as weight loss >5% over the past 6 months (in the absence of simple starvation), body mass index <20 and any degree of weight loss >2%, or sarcopenia.[2]

Anorexia nervosa is a distinctive and serious psychiatric disorder characterized by an intense fear of weight gain, disturbed body image, and severe dietary restriction or other weight-loss behaviors such as excessive exercise. Cognitive and emotional dysfunction, medical morbidity, and psychiatric comorbidity are common. The condition often has a relapsing or protracted course and can lead to disability and death. In high-income countries, the lifetime prevalence of anorexia nervosa in the general population is reported to be around 1% in women and less than 0.5% in men. Common comorbidities include anxiety disorders, obsessive-compulsive disorder, osteoporosis, dehydration, and cardiovascular symptoms such as bradycardia.[3]

While increased appetite and food consumption have long been described as side effects of recreational cannabis use (i.e., the munchies), the orexigenic (appetite-stimulating) effects of cannabis can be a useful side benefit or primary goal of treatment for many patients. Importantly, appetite and food intake are only one aspect of body weight and nutritional status; digestion, absorption, metabolism, inflammation, autonomic function, endocrine function, and mental health all play a role. Several of these components can also be strategically addressed with cannabis.

The endocannabinoid system has been shown to play a crucial role in food intake and metabolism via modulation of ghrelin, leptin, orexin, and adiponectin signaling pathways. The orexigenic effect of cannabinoids is mediated via CB1 receptor signaling, particularly in hypothalamic and mesolimbic regions of the brain.[4] Thus, Δ^9-tetrahydrocannabinol (THC) is the primary phytocannabinoid used clinically to stimulate appetite. Interestingly, as described in Chapter 29, chronic cannabis use is inversely associated with obesity and cardiometabolic risk factors,[5,6] which may suggest that the prometabolic effects of cannabis offset the potential increase in consumption.

Clinical Evidence

The clinical evidence for using cannabinoids to stimulate appetite and weight gain is unimpressive, perhaps in part because most studies evaluated low-dose oral THC or, in a few cases, low-quality inhaled cannabis from the National Institute on Drug Abuse, with THC potency in the range of 4%.

AIDS-Associated Anorexia and Weight Loss

Several trials have evaluated cannabis or dronabinol in the treatment of AIDS wasting syndrome or AIDS-associated anorexia, summarized in two systematic reviews. While the prevalence of AIDS wasting syndrome has been reduced dramatically since the introduction of antiretroviral therapies in the mid-1990s, this syndrome likely has overlapping pathophysiology with other forms of cachexia and can inform our understanding of the efficacy of cannabinoids in patients with weight loss.

One review covered four randomized trials involving 255 patients: two trials comparing dronabinol to placebo, one comparing dronabinol to placebo and smoked cannabis, and one comparing dronabinol to megestrol acetate. This review found that dronabinol or cannabis treatment was associated with greater weight gain than placebo, with limited evidence suggesting a concurrent improvement in functional status. The comparison trial found that megestrol acetate was associated with greater weight gain than dronabinol and that combining dronabinol with megestrol acetate did not lead to additional weight gain.[7]

A second review on AIDS wasting syndrome evaluated seven randomized controlled trials that compared dronabinol and inhaled cannabis with placebo and with each other. In one study, the individuals' weights increased significantly more ($p < .01$) on higher doses of cannabis and dronabinol (10 mg) than on lower doses. In a second trial, median weight increased by 3.0 kg with inhaled cannabis (p=.021) and by 3.2 kg with 2.5 mg of dronabinol (p=.004) when compared with a placebo group, which had a 1.1-kg increase over 21 days. Overall, the authors concluded that evidence for the efficacy and safety of cannabis and cannabinoids was lacking to support their utility in treating AIDS-associated anorexia.[8] Despite its poor efficacy, the FDA-labeled indication of dronabinol was expanded to include treatment of anorexia associated with weight loss in patients with AIDS in 1992, and it retains that indication at the time of writing.

Cancer-Related Cachexia

Clinical research on cancer-related anorexia-cachexia syndrome is limited. One study compared 2.5-mg THC capsules versus cannabis extract containing 2.5 mg of THC + 1 mg of cannabidiol (CBD) versus placebo, administered twice daily. Only 164 of 243 subjects completed the trial, a notable confounder. Increased appetite was reported by 73% of those who took cannabis extract, 58% of those who took the THC, and 69% of patients receiving placebo.[9]

Another trial of 469 advanced cancer patients using 2.5 mg of dronabinol twice daily, 800 mg of megestrol acetate once daily, or a combination of the two found improvement in appetite in 49% of those receiving dronabinol, 75% of those receiving megestrol, and 66% in combination treatment. A weight gain of ≥10% over baseline was reported by 11% of those in the megestrol group, compared with 3% in the dronabinol group and 8% in the combination group.[10]

Anorexia Nervosa

An early 4-week double-blind crossover study of 11 female patients with primary anorexia nervosa that compared THC (up to 10 mg three times daily) with diazepam (up to 5 mg three times daily, used as an active placebo) failed to show any difference in weight gain or caloric intake between the two groups. The THC group demonstrated more somatization, interpersonal sensitivity, and sleep disturbance.[11] I suspect the dose of THC was excessive and resulted in adverse and paradoxical effects.

In a prospective double-blind crossover trial in 24 women with anorexia nervosa, 2.5 mg of dronabinol or placebo was given twice daily for 4 weeks, in addition to standard psychotherapy and nutritional interventions. The participants had a significant weight gain of 1.00 kg (95% CI 0.40 to 1.62) during dronabinol therapy and 0.34 kg (95% CI −0.14 to 0.82) during placebo therapy (p = .03). No statistically significant differences in Eating Disorder Inventory-2 scores were observed. The authors concluded that low-dose dronabinol was a safe adjuvant palliative therapy in a highly selected subgroup of chronically undernourished women with anorexia nervosa.[12]

Endocannabinoid system alterations have been identified in patients with anorexia nervosa. Mutations in endocannabinoid system genes that code for CB1 receptor and the enzyme fatty acid amide hydrolase,[13] as well as CB2 receptor,[14] have been associated with anorexia nervosa. Compared to healthy controls, patients with anorexia nervosa have increased blood levels of anandamide,[15] increased blood markers of CB1 expression (inversely associated with disease severity),[16] and increased CB1 receptor availability in positron emission tomographic imaging of cortical and subcortical brain areas involved in integration of interoceptive information, gustatory information, reward, and emotion processing.[17] These findings may indicate endocannabinoid system dysfunction and compensatory responses.

Preclinical Evidence

A large body of preclinical work has informed a detailed understating of the role of the endocannabinoid system in hunger, feeding, orosensory reward, metabolism, and body weight, with CB1 emerging as a primary target for orexigenic effects. Preclinical studies on CBD in relation to appetite and body weight have been inconclusive and indicate a potential dose-dependent bidirectional effect. CBD has been shown to inhibit the orexigenic effects of CB1 agonists. Cannabinol has been shown to induce food intake in rats, while cannabigerol did not alter food intake. An excellent review of these preclinical studies can be found in Roger Pertwee's *Handbook of Cannabis*.[18]

Treatment Strategies for Clinicians

- Low-dose, inhaled THC-dominant cannabis 10–15 min before meals produces the best orexigenic effects in my patients. Specific cannabis chemovars seem to have better results, and patients can be encouraged to compare several varieties to find what works best for them. The orexigenic effects are sometimes diminished at higher doses of inhaled cannabis, so use careful titration starting at one inhalation.
- On the basis of the available literature and my clinical experience, cannabis is less likely to have a profound impact on cachexia, though it is often useful for other symptoms (e.g., sleep or pain) in patients with this condition. I suggest oromucosal or oral dosing tailored to improve other symptoms, with inhaled cannabis utilized to improve appetite and enjoyment of food.

- Primary anorexia may be less likely to respond to cannabis than secondary anorexia related to nausea, anxiety, or pain.
- In patients with anorexia nervosa, use caution, precision dosing, and close observation. While THC is most likely to be helpful, I have observed a greater likelihood of bidirectional and adverse effects, especially anxiogenesis, in this patient population.
- For anorexia nervosa, I recommend that clinicians avoid titrating cannabis with the goal of increasing food consumption; this behavior is already overemphasized in the patient's thoughts, and additional attention can be counterproductive. Rather, titrate cannabis slowly to achieve improvements in anxiety, obsessive-compulsive symptoms, gastrointestinal symptoms, and sleep. Setting concrete goals with outcomes other than eating can be helpful, and these are likely best achieved with oromucosal dosing. After these goals are achieved, add inhaled cannabis if needed.
- Consider cannabis as a tool to augment concurrent cognitive and behavioral treatments, especially those related to transforming ego-syntonic beliefs and building self-esteem. Cannabis can relax rigid thought patterns and promote cognitive flexibility and capacity for change.

Cautions

- Inhaled THC-dominant cannabis should be avoided or used very cautiously in patients with anorexia nervosa and hypotension or orthostatic symptoms.
- Building tolerance to THC should be avoided, as this could interfere with CB1 activity and diminish appetite.
- Avoid chemovars containing significant levels of Δ^9-tetrahydrocannabivarin, which can suppress appetite at low levels.
- Use CBD sparingly, with a goal of mitigating THC-related side effects, as it can diminish the appetite-stimulating effects of THC in humans.[19]

Chapter 28

Drug Substitution and Harm Reduction

PATIENTS COMMONLY PRESENT to my practice with a goal of using cannabis to help discontinue or spare the use of other medications perceived to be more dangerous. A growing body of evidence supports this as a realistic outcome, especially with opioids and other classes of medications recognized for dangerous overuse. Other data suggest that patients are able to use cannabis as a substitute for alcohol, tobacco, and illicit drugs. Cannabis clinicians can reduce harm and improve outcomes by providing guidance for patients with this intention and by suggesting substitution when appropriate.

Though I have observed frequent drug substitution in my clinic over the last decade, I am still impressed by the frequency of patients reporting discontinuation of opioids, benzodiazepines, and other classes of drugs that are traditionally difficult to taper. Clinicians without previous experience using cannabis as a therapeutic agent, residents, and medical students who shadow me in the clinic are often astounded by the number of patient reports of drug substitution in a single day.

Drug Substitution: Observational Data

Numerous observational studies indicate that drug substitution is a common practice among cannabis users. In 2009, Amanda Reiman published a survey of 350 medical cannabis users at a dispensary in Berkeley, California. Sixty-six percent of respondents had used cannabis as a substitute for prescription drugs, 40% as a substitute for alcohol, and 26% as a substitute for illicit drugs. The most common reasons given for substituting were fewer adverse effects (65%), better symptom management (57%), and less withdrawal potential (34%) with cannabis.[1]

In a survey of 473 Canadian adult users of cannabis for therapeutic purposes, administered in 2011–2012, substitution of cannabis for alcohol, illicit drugs, or prescription drugs was reported by 87% of respondents; 80.3% reported substitution for prescription drugs, 51.7% for alcohol, and 32.6% for illicit substances. Patients with gastrointestinal symptoms were the most likely to substitute prescription drugs (94%).[2]

A survey of 2,774 self-selected individuals who had used cannabis at least once in the previous 90 days, administered between 2013 and 2016, found that 46% of respondents reported using cannabis as a substitute for prescription drugs, with an average of two drug substitutions reported per affirmative responder. All 50 U.S. states and 42 countries were represented in the survey; only a slightly higher percentage of those who reported substituting resided in states where medical cannabis was legal at the time of the survey. The most common class of medication substitution was narcotics and opiates (36%), followed by anxiolytics and benzodiazepines (14%), antidepressants (13%), and nonsteroidal anti-inflammatory drugs and nonopioid analgesics (10%). This illustrates the common practice of substituting multiple medications with cannabis, as well as the legal risk patients are willing to take to use a treatment that is potentially safer and more effective than what is prescribed by their clinicians, especially in the case of opioids.[3]

A survey of 1,513 members of medical cannabis dispensaries in New England found that among the 215 who regularly used opioids, 76.7% had reduced their use since they began medical cannabis; 40.9% reported reducing their dose "a lot" and 35.8% reported reducing their dose "slightly." Many patients also reported substituting anxiety, migraine, sleep, and antidepressant medications, as well as alcohol, with cannabis. Patients were more likely to tell their family members and friends than their primary care providers about their medical cannabis use.[4]

In a survey of 271 Canadian medical cannabis patients administered in 2015, 63% reported using cannabis as a substitute for prescription drugs, particularly opioids (30%), benzodiazepines (16%), and antidepressants (12%). Patients also reported substituting cannabis for alcohol (25%), cigarettes and tobacco (12%), and illicit drugs (3%). At least once daily use was reported by 88% of patients; vaporization was the most preferred delivery method, and the most common amount of cannabis flower used per day was 1–2 g, with 29% using a larger amount. The classes of medication substitution, in patients with pain versus mental health diagnoses, are illustrated in Figure 28.1.[5]

In a 2016 qualitative study, medical cannabis users in Rhode Island believed that cannabis is superior to and has fewer side effects than prescription medications and that it globally improves quality of life. Factors interfering with cannabis use included stigma, cost, inability for health-care providers to relay instructions regarding dosing and method of use, lack of patient education at dispensaries, and inability to legally travel with cannabis across state lines.[6]

Few studies have evaluated the use of cannabinoids in patients undergoing standard substance abuse treatments. In an observational study of 63 patients with opioid use disorder undergoing naltrexone therapy, intermittent cannabis users stayed in the treatment program for an average of 113 days, whereas consistent cannabis users lasted an average of 68 days, and those who did not use cannabis at all lasted only 47 days. Investigators also found that intensive behavioral therapy helped the consistent cannabis users but did not help the nonusers.[7] I hypothesize that the improved response to behavioral therapy is related to the proneuroplastic, anxiolytic, and improved self-efficacy effects of cannabis.

One placebo-controlled trial ($n = 60$) found that dronabinol reduced withdrawal symptoms during acute opioid detoxification and that cannabis use was associated with greater extended-release naltrexone treatment retention.[8] This corroborates the common practice among opioid users who use cannabis to mitigate opioid withdrawal symptoms.

FIGURE 28.1
Medical Cannabis Substitution by Condition

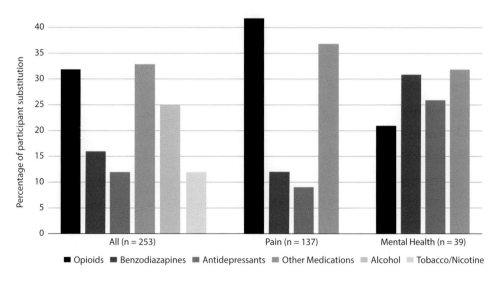

Note. Chart created by Dustin Sulak, with data from "Medical cannabis access, use, and substitution for prescription opioids and other substances: A survey of authorized medical cannabis patients," by P. Lucas and Z. Walsh, 2017, *The International Journal on Drug Policy, 42*, pp. 30–35 (https://doi.org/10.1016/j.drugpo.2017.01.011). Copyright © 2017 by Elsevier. Reprinted with permission.

A cross-sectional study of 100 randomly selected adult male patients attending a community drug treatment clinic in Delhi, India, who were stabilized on buprenorphine for >3 months, found that the 35 patients with recent cannabis use were on significantly lower doses of buprenorphine, yet they did not experience more opioid craving or withdrawals compared to their non-cannabis-using peers. Recent cannabis use did not impact illicit opioid use, productivity, or quality of life.[9] This suggests that cannabis use is safe in patients with opioid use disorder who are taking opioid agonist medications and that cannabis likely potentiates the treatment.

Cannabidiol in Substance Abuse Treatment

There is a strong rationale for using cannabidiol (CBD) in the treatment of substance use disorders, given its excellent safety profile, low abuse liability, nonrewarding effects on numerous receptor systems, and ability to mitigate anxiety, a core feature of substance abuse that often triggers craving and promotes relapse. Again, clinical evidence is limited.

A pilot clinical study produced findings consistent with preclinical evidence, demonstrating that CBD reduced craving induced by heroin-related cues in heroin abusers. Similar to the protracted effects seen in animals, the attenuation of general craving by CBD lasted a full week after its last administration.[10] In a follow-up double-blind randomized controlled trial, 42 drug-abstinent patients with heroin use disorder were randomized to receive 400 or 800 mg of CBD or a placebo once daily for 3 days. The researchers evaluated acute (1–24 hr), short-term (during 3 days of treatment), and protracted (7 days after the last dose) effects on anxiety and craving after patients viewed either a neutral video (nature scenes) or a drug cue (video showing heroin use). Both CBD doses attenuated the anxiety and craving triggered by the drug cue, with remarkable protracted benefits 7 days later. CBD also reduced the increases in heart rate and salivary cortisol induced by the drug cue.[11]

Several of my patients have reported using oral or inhaled CBD-dominant cannabis as an aid in tobacco cessation, an observation supported by a small amount of clinical evidence. In a randomized controlled trial of 24 tobacco smokers, those who received a CBD inhaler reduced the number of smoked cigarettes by 40% over the course of 1 week, while those who received a placebo inhaler did not change their tobacco consumption.[12] In another study, a single oral dose of 800 mg of CBD after overnight abstinence in 30 tobacco smokers did not change craving or withdrawal symptoms, but it did reduce the salience of cigarette cues relative to placebo,[13] suggesting that the benefits of CBD for tobacco reduction require ongoing use as a substitute substance.

Cocaine Abuse

While many of the recent data on cannabis-related drug substitution have focused on opioids and other prescription drugs, earlier research suggested benefits in patients who abuse stimulants. In a study published in 1999, researchers in Brazil followed 25 male patients strongly addicted to crack cocaine who reported self-medicating with cannabis to combat withdrawal symptoms over 9 months. Seventeen (68%) were able to stop using crack after an average of 5.2 weeks, consuming 3–4 cannabis cigarettes daily during the first 3 months. They reported decreased anxiety, weight gain, improved sleep, and decreased cravings for crack. In the subsequent 6 months, cannabis use was only occasional, but the participants reported significant changes in habits and attitudes associated with the cultural differences between crack- and cannabis-using social groups.[14]

In a 2002 ethnographic study of 33 Jamaican women who were dependent on crack cocaine and were followed for 9 months, 14 succeeded in stopping crack use, with 13 attributing their success to *ganja*.* Among the others who continued to use crack, those who combined it with cannabis in *seasoned cigarettes* were at least able to maintain their weight, care for their children, and reduce the adverse effects of the crack.[15]

More recent work exploring the interface between cannabis and crack cocaine confirmed these findings. A 2015 qualitative study on 27 crack users in Brazil (young men of low socioeconomic status, with little schooling, who were living on the street) revealed that combination with cannabis reduced the undesirable effects of crack, including craving, paranoia, and aggression, and improved sleep, appetite, weight gain, and sexual function. A few participants did not perceive the combination as beneficial, reporting decreased intensity of the pleasurable stimulating effects of crack when combined with cannabis and undesirable depressive effects of cannabis.[16] A longitudinal analysis of 122 subjects in Vancouver, Canada, found that intentional use of cannabis was positively associated with decreased frequency of crack cocaine use.[17]

Conversely, other studies suggest that long-term cannabis dependence might increase cocaine craving and risk of relapse among individuals with polydrug substance use disorders.[18,19] This suggests that patterns of cannabis use, including intention and mindfulness, phytoconstituent composition, dosage, route of administration, and social changes, likely influence patients' outcomes. The qualitative data from Jamaica and Brazil are illustrative and worth reading to gain insight into these desperate situations; for example,

---

* *Ganja* is a Jamaican term for cannabis.

"The pure rock makes me aggressive because I want to smoke more, and if someone stops me from doing this, I become violent, even if it is a family member. With marijuana, I control this situation because I am more relaxed, less anxious."[20]

Reports from successful patients can inform clinicians on the front lines of treating substance abuse, who will inevitably work with others intending to use cannabis to reduce their use of more harmful substances. I believe that if cannabis is used under medical supervision as an adjunct to nonpharmacological therapy, with appropriate education on the safest and most effective use patterns, with legal access to cannabis and avoidance of the underground drug market, the potential benefits of cannabis for patients with stimulant addiction could be enhanced.

Alcohol Withdrawal and Substitution

At the turn of the 19th century in the United States, cannabis was listed as a treatment for delirium tremens in standard medical texts[21,22] and manuals.[23,24] Psychiatrist and addictionologist Tod Mikuriya, MD, who is considered the grandfather of medical cannabis in the United States, reported qualitative data and provided a compelling discussion related to 92 patients from his practice who used cannabis as a substitute for alcohol:[25]

"Even if use is daily, cannabis replacing alcohol (or other addictive, toxic drugs) reduces harm because of its relatively benign side-effect profile. Cannabis-only usage is not associated with car crashes; it does not damage the liver, the esophagus, the spleen or the digestive tract.

The chronic alcohol-inebriation-withdrawal cycle ceases with successful cannabis substitution. Sleep and appetite are restored, ability to focus and concentrate is enhanced, energy and activity levels are improved, and pain and muscle spasms are relieved. Family and social relationships can be sustained as pursuit of long-term goals ends the cycle of crisis and apology."

Aside from the aforementioned observational data demonstrating the practice of substituting cannabis for alcohol in several studies, no prospective clinical evidence exists. Considering the immense morbidity and prevalence of alcohol misuse, more studies are indicated, as described in a recent review.[26]

Preclinical Evidence in Substance Abuse

The endocannabinoid system (ECS) plays a key role in the pathogenesis of substance abuse disorders. The rewarding effect of abused substances is thought to be primarily mediated by the mesolimbic dopamine pathway, which contains particularly high densities of CB1 receptors (ventral tegmental area and nucleus accumbens). In animal models, acute exposure to CB1 agonists augments dopamine transmission, lowers the brain reward threshold, and establishes persistent self-administration of substances of abuse. CB1 agonists also produce per se rewarding effects. CB1 antagonists decrease the reinforcing effects of substances of abuse.[27] Not surprisingly, Δ^9-tetrahydrocannabinol (THC) has demonstrated biphasic effects in the brain stimulation reward model of addiction liability, with low doses decreasing the reward threshold and high doses increasing the threshold; high doses may act similarly to antagonists by downregulating CB1 activity.[28] Compared to other classes of abused drugs, cannabinoid modulation in animal models of stimulant abuse is minimal.[29]

Substance reward is only one part of substance dependence, which involves learned behaviors like compulsive substance intake, loss of control, and persistent intake despite the adverse effects of the substance and tolerance to its pleasurable responses; the ECS also modulates these neuroplastic events. Animal models reveal that the ECS modulates the ability of drugs and drug-associated cues to reinstate drug-seeking behavior in animal models of relapse: CB1 agonism can elicit relapse to cannabinoid-, heroin-, and nicotine-seeking behavior. Chronic exposure to drugs of abuse generally results in impaired CB1 function and loss of endocannabinoid-mediated synaptic plasticity in addiction-related neural circuits.[30] Animal evidence confirms that cannabinoid therapies have a potential role in treating substance abuse disorders, but they are likely a double-edged sword that can both help and harm.

Adolescent Cannabis Use

I have observed a trend in my practice of increasing adolescent and young adult patients who clearly use cannabis in problematic ways and are brought to my clinic by family members in need of help. These patients often have untreated behavioral health issues beyond problematic substance use.

I take the perspective that the substance misuse is not the problem but rather an ineffective solution to an underlying problem. After I explain this concept and invite the patient to explore the nature of the underlying problem, we frequently identify anxiety, sleep disturbance, social isolation, social media addiction, untreated trauma, and other challenges. By providing certification to legally use cannabis under medical supervision, access to cannabis in a legal marketplace (requiring parental cooperation in those under 18 years of age), and an ongoing therapeutic relationship, I can reduce the potential harm of their cannabis use. Many of these patients had not considered that cannabis could be used in ways that support their health because the only exposure they have had comes from peers, who often strive for pronounced psychoactive effects; they have experienced no modeling of healthy adult or therapeutic cannabis use.

Conclusions

Clearly, patients are already using cannabis as a substitute for drugs with a higher risk profile, including prescriptions, illicit substances, alcohol, and tobacco. But can cannabis be recommended by clinicians as a harm reduction tool in the treatment of substance abuse disorders? While the current clinical evidence is sparse, it is important to recognize that this usage is already happening, though mostly patient-directed and unmonitored by clinicians. Can clinicians improve outcomes through education and monitoring?

Cannabis is safer than many other substances of abuse, less likely to cause dependence, and clearly has a better safety profile than currently approved harm-reduction agents like methadone and buprenorphine. And cannabis does more than simply replace a substance: it helps patients reflect on their lives, find a point of internal balance, and restore their sense of self.[31] Cannabis can mitigate underlying physical and mental symptoms like pain, insomnia, anxiety, and depression that lead to problematic substance use, while likely providing protective effects against the adverse physiological effects of alcohol[32] and other drugs via its neuroprotective and anti-inflammatory properties. Furthermore, the cultural qualities of cannabis-endorsing social groups are likely more supportive to health than those of other substances.

I have certainly observed cannabis worsening the clinical course of some patients with substance abuse disorders. This is most likely to occur, in my experience, in patients with comorbid psychotic, bipolar, and personality disorders. In these cases, patients can lose control of their cannabis use, and high doses of inhaled THC precipitate further deterioration of their condition.

Not all of my patients follow my guidance on cannabis use patterns, and some clearly demonstrate problematic use. Even in the most challenging of these cases, however, I often find myself thankful it is cannabis and not some other substance that is being misused.

The concept of harm reduction as an alternative to abstinence is now well-established in addiction medicine. Unfortunately, my patients still frequently report discrimination against cannabis use from both clinicians and their peers in the recovery community. The shaming and hiding of cannabis use in 12-step and other peer support programs is detrimental and ironic, especially amid the liberal use of caffeine, tobacco, and sugar often present in these settings. Some of my patients who have successfully used cannabis to reduce or eliminate problematic use of other substances, frustrated by their inability to benefit from much-needed peer support, have successfully started "green" support groups that embrace cannabis as a tool in recovery.

Patient Narrative

I AM 38 YEARS OLD and I struggled with opiate and alcohol addiction for about 15 years. Long hours as a chef and a couple of minor surgeries where I was prescribed opiates led me to become dependent on them to get through my day. Pretty soon I was fully consumed by addiction.

Even after going to 2 detoxes and a 28-day rehab in 2010, I still struggled to stay clean for the next 2 years. The 12 step meetings that I was going to several times a week discouraged cannabis use, so I tried to do it their way and didn't use any. That didn't work and led to several relapses. In 2012, I decided to start using a little bit of cannabis before bed to help me get a good night's sleep, and when I was getting stressed, angry, etc. It was very effective in keeping me centered and on the path to recovery, although I didn't feel comfortable (and still don't) sharing this with fellow addicts at meetings.

I had been a cannabis smoker on and off since I was 18, and always enjoyed the effects. In the throes of my opiate addiction, however, I got out of the routine of regular cannabis using. I believe that this is because cannabis use tends to magnify my own problems and shortcomings in my mind when I use it, and no drug addict wants to take such an honest look at themselves.

As of right now I have been free of active addiction since January 2012. I have also been a patient of Integr8 Health since 2012. Cannabis is the only thing that I am currently prescribed, and the only substance that I use for pain, stress, etc. I don't know if I would be here today, and sober, if it wasn't for cannabis. I use cannabis throughout the day and before bed, and live a happy, healthy, productive life with my wife and 2 daughters.

Treatment Strategies for Clinicians

- With almost any drug that can potentially be reduced or replaced by cannabis, initiation and titration of cannabis can precede tapering of the drug. This provides an easier course for patients, who are often able to enjoy a period of stability and decreased symptoms before a taper that may result in rebound or reemergence of symptoms.

- Titrate cannabis as needed to address breakthrough symptoms during a drug taper. Inhaled delivery is often the most effective for acute cravings and attentional fixation on the drug.

- When opioids and benzodiazepines are being substituted, I recommend titrating the cannabis until the patient experiences minor adverse effects like impairment or sedation, which are potential signs of reaching a dose producing clinically relevant synergistic or additive effects, prior to tapering the drug. I learned this from numerous patients who reported reaching a dose of cannabis that "made the pills feel too strong, so I started cutting them in half."

- I encourage my patients to take a dose of cannabis with every dose of an opioid or benzodiazepine.

- Cannabis can ameliorate most acute opioid withdrawal symptoms, but if breakthrough symptoms occur, I recommend loperamide for diarrhea, promethazine for nausea and vomiting, clonidine for agitation and cardiovascular symptoms, and cyclobenzaprine for spasms. The combination of cannabis with low doses of all these agents has produced excellent relief in several patients struggling with opioid withdrawal symptoms; the combined sedative effects often allow patients to sleep through the worst of the withdrawal.

- I often effectively prescribe 50–100 mg of 5-hydroxytryptophan, 1–3 times daily, for patients experiencing withdrawal symptoms related to selective serotonin reuptake inhibitors.

- For patients with substance abuse disorder, using cannabis containing both THC and CBD may decrease the risk of problematic use and improve benefits.

Cautions

- Patients who use cannabis for harm reduction have a higher risk of problematic use and require closer monitoring and longer visits that promote the therapeutic relationship.

- THC-dominant inhaled cannabis, and especially inhaled concentrates, produce the strongest rewarding effects, and therefore have the greatest risk of triggering cravings for other, more rewarding substances and increasing the risk of relapse. While inhaled cannabis can be very effective for acute cravings, those in remission may do better with oral and oromucosal delivery.

- Some clinicians may still abruptly discontinue medications or generally refuse to continue treating a patient after they establish care with a cannabis clinician. Always take the time to correspond with the rest of the health-care team to avoid these disruptions in care and take advantage of the opportunity to educate and build relationships with your colleagues.

- Some patients are so enthusiastic about their success with cannabis that they elect to abruptly discontinue medications without discussion with any health-care provider, including drugs that are dangerous to stop without a taper (such as benzodiazepines and gabapentinoids). I usually proactively discuss these risks at an initial visit, which also serves to give the patient hope for eventually reaching their goals.

- For patients who wish to use cannabis as a substitute for drug abuse, be sure to define success in the context of harm reduction. Complete abstinence may be unattainable for many patients, but goals related to reduced frequency of drug use and risky behavior, improved lifestyle and social factors, and attendance at follow-up visits likely are attainable for most.

Chapter 29

Cannabis for Health Promotion and Disease Prevention

IN THE LAST DECADE, I have seen cannabis provide symptom relief and disease management in countless highly refractory cases. We understand that its distinct efficacy is due, at least in part, to its ability to interact with the endocannabinoid system (ECS) and its network pharmacological effects of synergistic phytoconstituents acting on multiple physiological targets. I cannot help but ask, if this medicine can be so effective in challenging-to-treat conditions, could it potentially be used to prevent them?

Why prevention? As of 2014, 60% of adult Americans had at least one chronic condition,* 42% had more than one, and 12% had five or more (Figure 29.1).[1] According to

FIGURE 29.1

Prevalence of Chronic Diseases in the United States, 2014

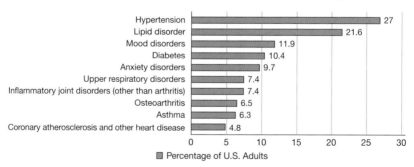

Source: Adapted from "Multiple chronic conditions in the United States," by C. Buttorff, T. Ruder, and M. Bauman, 2017 (https://www.rand.org/content/dam/rand/pubs/tools/TL200/TL221/RAND_TL221.pdf). Copyright © 2017 by RAND Corporation. Adapted with permission.

---

* A chronic condition is defined as a physical or mental health condition that lasts more than 1 year and causes functional restrictions or requires ongoing monitoring or treatment.

the U.S. Centers for Disease Control and Prevention, most chronic diseases can be prevented by eating well, being physically active, avoiding tobacco and excessive drinking, and getting regular health screenings.[2] Of the $3.5 trillion in U.S. annual health-care expenditures, 90% is for people with chronic conditions.[3]

Our current health-care system disproportionately emphasizes disease management over disease prevention, and other industries essential for an effective disease prevention system (e.g., agriculture, food systems, and environmental protection) lack collaborative capacity, equity, leadership, and resources. While effective solutions to this huge problem are beyond my expertise, I believe that one plant species, and the physiological insight it has stimulated, can help.

Support for this theory comes primarily from epidemiological data on health outcomes in cannabis users versus nonusers and from preclinical data that suggest mechanisms which may be responsible for the observed differences. While these data are suggestive, we are far from concluding that an increased prevalence of cannabis use will prevent disease and promote health. Cannabis use is not a singular factor; it is clear that the way in which one uses cannabis determines its impact on health. We do know that the ECS is intimately involved in our homeostatic response to illness and injury, making it an excellent target for health promotion and disease prevention.

Sleep

As detailed in Chapter 22, insufficient sleep, reported in 30%–35% of the general population, is strongly associated with higher rates of chronic illness, including obesity, diabetes, hypertension, coronary artery disease, stroke, asthma, and arthritis, as well as frequent mental distress.[4] Sleep also impacts our productivity, cognition, mood, and social interactions. Though the connection is obvious to clinicians, public health interventions often fail to address the profound potential to reduce morbidity, mortality, and health-care costs by improving sleep in the general population.

Could cannabis be used as a home remedy alternative to over-the-counter and prescription sleep aids? With the right formulation and education on dose and delivery method, I am convinced the answer is yes, supported by the data reviewed in Chapter 22 and my clinical experience. Beyond the benefit of improved sleep, it is likely that periodic or nightly cannabis use would provide additional health-promoting benefits, as described below.

Obesity and Type 2 Diabetes

The prevalence of obesity and diabetes, distinct but overlapping metabolic disorders, continues to increase despite public health efforts. In the United States, 40% of the adult population is obese and another 32% is overweight;[5] 10.5% of the population has diabetes and 34.5% has prediabetes.[6] Among individuals with diabetes, approximately 95% have type 2, a condition largely related to lifestyle choices but influenced by genetics and other factors. Sadly, as the United States exports its food systems and eating habits around the world, global obesity rates are catching up, with worldwide 13% prevalence of obesity (2016)[7] and 8.5% diabetes (2014).[8]

In 2017, the U.S. total estimated cost of diagnosed diabetes was $327 billion,[9] over 9% of total health-care costs, and this does not begin to describe the cost of diabetes related to human suffering and functional impairment. Paradoxically, after decades of steady decline, global hunger has slowly been on the rise since 2015, with 821 million reported undernourished (2017).[10] According to the United Nations, global undernourishment could be resolved by 2030 if the global community invested $267 billion per year.[11] I do not know how we can correct the dysfunctional resource distribution and consumption, primarily related to carbohydrate-rich food, impacting billions of individuals globally.

Could cannabis prevent obesity and diabetes? Several cross-sectional studies have identified a lower prevalence of both diseases in cannabis users compared to nonusers. For example, among 43,093 participants in the National Epidemiologic Survey on Alcohol and Related Conditions (2001–2002), the obesity prevalence of those who reported cannabis use ≥3 times weekly was 14.3%, compared to 22% in nonusers. Among the 9,282 subjects in the National Comorbidity Survey-Replication (2001–2003), the obesity prevalence of those who reported cannabis use ≥3 times weekly was 17.2%, compared to 25.3% in nonusers.[12]

A cross-sectional meta-analysis of eight independent large samples from the National Health and Nutrition Examination Survey (NHANES) (2005–2012) and National Survey on Drug Use and Health (2005–2012) found that recent cannabis smoking and diabetes mellitus were inversely associated; the meta-analytic summary *OR* was 0.7 (95% confidence interval [CI] 0.6–0.8).[13]

In data from NHANES (2009–2016), among 129,509 adults aged 18–59 years, cannabis use was associated with lower fasting insulin and homeostatic model assessment of insulin resistance in obese adults but not in nonobese adults, even at a low frequency of less than four uses per month. Interestingly, former cannabis users with high lifetime use had significantly lower fasting insulin levels that persisted, independent of the duration of time since last use.[14]

These results are compelling, but most cross-sectional studies rely on self-reporting of cannabis use and health outcomes and often rely on vague measures of cannabis use (e.g., current use, former use, or never use). Longitudinal studies with observational biomarker data, however, confirm the findings.

For example, in the Pittsburgh Youth Study, 253 men from the youngest cohort were followed prospectively from approximately age 7 to 32. Frequency of cannabis use was assessed yearly from approximate ages 12 to 20 and again at approximate ages 26, 29, and 32; a variety of cardiometabolic risk factors were also assessed at approximately age 32. Greater cannabis use was associated with lower body mass index (BMI), smaller waist-to-hip ratio, better high- and low-density lipoprotein cholesterol levels, lower triglyceride levels, lower fasting glucose and homeostatic model assessment of insulin resistance, lower systolic and diastolic blood pressure, and fewer metabolic syndrome criteria. The relatively lower BMI of cannabis users compared to nonusers mediated most of the effects on other cardiovascular risks.[15]

In a 2-year longitudinal study of 401 adolescents, age 14–17 at baseline, increases in cannabis use were accompanied by statistically significant greater decreases in BMI over time. Findings remained unchanged after adjustment for sex, ethnicity, depression, alcohol, and nicotine.[16]

The aforementioned observational data cannot confirm a direction of causality; perhaps there is some other common factor associated with both cannabis use and improved metabolic status. It seems paradoxical that cannabis, which can increase appetite, may prevent weight gain and metabolic dysfunction. Indeed, cannabis users may eat more. Fifteen years of longitudinal data from 3,617 young adults participating in the Coronary Artery Risk Development in Young Adults (CARDIA) study demonstrated that those who had consumed cannabis for more than 1,800 days over 15 years consumed on average 619 more calories per day than nonusers, yet they showed no difference in BMI.[17] Cross-sectional NHANES data also demonstrated lower BMI in cannabis users (24.7 ± 0.3) compared to nonusers (26.6 ± 0.1), despite users consuming 564 additional calories daily ($p < .0001$).[18]

Rodent data support the possibility of a causal relationship, potentially mediated via the interaction of Δ^9-tetrahydrocannabinol (THC), the gut microbiome, and metabolism. Gut microbiota are involved in the regulation of adipose tissue physiology, including adipogenesis, through endocannabinoid signaling; changes in microbiota (i.e., prebiotic treatment, antibiotics, and germ-free conditions) can reverse obesity-induced changes in endocannabinoid tone in adipose tissue.[19] Adult male mice fed an obesity-inducing diet experienced reduced weight and fat mass gain, and reduced energy intake, when they were treated with 2 mg/kg THC daily for 3 weeks and 4 mg/kg THC for 1 additional week, administered ip. The treatment did not impact the weight or fat mass of lean mice. Interestingly, the alterations in gut microbiota caused by the obesity-inducing diet were prevented by the THC treatment.[20] Whether THC caused modifications in gut microbiota leading to the prevention of weight gain in high-fat feeding, or whether the altered microbiota were a consequence of THC-induced prevention of weight gain, or both, remains to be elucidated.

As discussed in Chapter 8, obese individuals experience elevated circulating postprandial anandamide levels. Insulin and leptin resistance, a common feature in obesity, likely leads to endocannabinoid overproduction in adipose tissue, downregulates fatty acid amide hydrolase and CB1 expression in adipose tissue, and stimulates CB1-mediated lipogenesis in the liver. This feedforward dysfunction promotes fat accumulation and further contributes to metabolic syndrome.[21] As a partial agonist at CB1, THC may mitigate the excessive peripheral CB1 activity and restore balance to ECS dysregulation in obesity and metabolic syndrome.

Other phytocannabinoids, such as Δ^9-tetrahydrocannabivarin (THCV) and cannabidiol (CBD), also hold promise for preventing and treating metabolic dysfunction. THCV was evaluated in a double-blind, placebo-controlled clinical trial in which 62 subjects with type 2 diabetes were randomized to five treatment arms: THCV in its pure form (5 mg) twice a day, CBD (100 mg) twice a day, two combinations of THCV and CBD, and placebo. THCV decreased fasting glucose by 12.6 mg/dL ($p < .05$), increased adiponectin ($p < .01$), and improved beta-cell function with only mild to moderate adverse events. Interestingly, these positive effects of THCV were lost when it was combined with CBD.[22] THCV, a neutral antagonist at CB1 (brings receptor activity to baseline level), certainly has potential for the treatment of obesity and insulin resistance without the adverse effect profile of rimonabant, the CB1 inverse agonist (which reduces activity below baseline level; see Chapter 15 for more details).

When I started recommending cannabis to my patients, I was very cautious with my patients who had obesity or type 2 diabetes, who I thought might experience increased appetite and weight gain as an adverse effect. While I have infrequently observed this in my patients, the far more common outcome is an improvement in metabolic status, lower insulin requirements, and weight loss. Whether this is due to improved sleep, decreased distress and circulating cortisol, decreased pain with increased activity levels, substitution for alcohol, alterations in gut microbiota, or direct effects on metabolism and adipose tissue physiology, I cannot be sure. Whatever the mechanism, the existing data support the concept of appropriate cannabis use as a potential preventative measure and treatment for obesity and diabetes.

Coronary Artery Disease

Heart disease is the leading cause of death in the United States, accounting for around 1 in 4 deaths, and it costs the United States $219 billion each year in health-care services, medicines, and lost future productivity due to premature mortality.[23] Coronary artery disease (CAD) is the most common type of heart disease, accounting for over half of heart-disease related deaths.

Some observational data suggest that cannabis use may provide a protective effect in CAD, beyond its potential preventative benefit via enhancing sleep, potentially preventing obesity and diabetes, and other indirect actions. In a hospital record review of 1,273,897 patients in eight states, 3,854 patients reported cannabis use on admission. The incidence of acute myocardial infarction (AMI) in those <50 years of age was higher among cannabis users compared to nonusers but was lower among cannabis users ≥50 years (Figure 29.2). Among those <70 years old without reported alcohol, cocaine, or methamphetamine use, after controls for age, race, payer, and known cardiac risk factors, the cannabis users were significantly less likely to die (OR 0.79, p = .016), experience shock (OR 0.74, p = .001), or require an intra-aortic balloon pump (OR 0.80, p = .03) after AMI than patients with no reported cannabis use. However, cannabis users were more likely to require mechanical ventilation (OR 1.19, p = .004), perhaps related to the pulmonary effects of cannabis smoking (Figure 29.3).[24]

FIGURE 29.2

Incidence of Acute Myocardial Infarction Stratified by Age and Cannabis Use

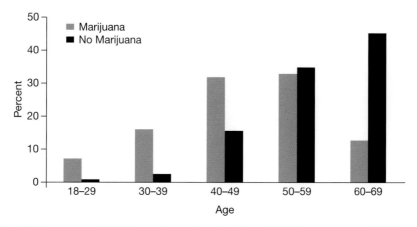

Note. From "Marijuana use and short-term outcomes in patients hospitalized for acute myocardial infarction," by C. P. Johnson-Sasso, C. Tompkins, D. P. Kao, & L. A. Walker, 2018, *PLOS ONE, 13*(7), Article e0199705 (https://doi.org/10.1371/journal.pone.0199705). Copyright © 2018 by the authors.

FIGURE 29.3

Multivariable Odds Ratios of Each Outcome Associated with Cannabis in Final Study Population

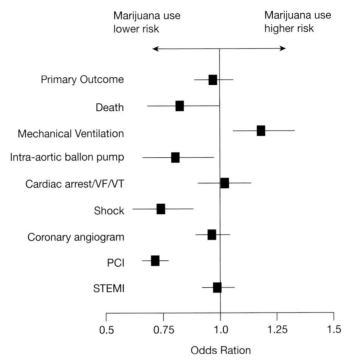

Note. VF, ventricular fibrillation; VT, ventricular tachycardia; PCI, percutaneous coronary intervention; STEMI, ST-elevation myocardial infarction. From "Marijuana use and short-term outcomes in patients hospitalized for acute myocardial infarction," by C. P. Johnson-Sasso, C. Tompkins, D. P. Kao, & L. A. Walker, 2018, *PLOS ONE*, *13*(7), Article e0199705 (https://doi.org/10.1371/journal.pone.0199705). Copyright © 2018 by the authors.

A slightly higher prevalence of AMI with markedly reduced mortality has been reported elsewhere. In retrospective data from the 2010–2014 National Inpatient Sample (NIS) for AMI patients age 11–70 years, cannabis use increased the risk of AMI by 3% after adjustment for age, gender, race, payer status, smoking, cocaine abuse, amphetamine abuse, and alcohol abuse (adjusted *OR* 1.031, 95% CI 1.018–1.045, *p* < .001). Similar to the data presented earlier, cannabis users had lower mortality (adjusted *OR* 0.742, 95% CI 0.693–0.795, *p* < .001), mean length of hospital stay (4.7 ± 5.9 days vs. 5.6 ± 8.0 days), and total hospital charges ($76,272.23 vs. $85,702.22, *p* < .001).[25]

Two other cross-sectional studies failed to show a statistically significant difference in AMI-related mortality between those who reported cannabis use and those who did not.[26,27] In another cross-sectional study from the NIS that evaluated the relationship between cannabis use and percutaneous coronary intervention, there were no differences in in-hospital mortality, bleeding, stroke, or transient ischemic attack between cannabis users and nonusers, but cannabis users had significantly lower odds of in-hospital vascular complications (*OR* 0.73, 95% CI 0.58–0.90, *p* = .004).[28]

A systematic analysis of the association between cannabis use and acute coronary syndrome found that 28 of 33 studies suggested an increased risk of both acute coronary syndrome and chronic cardiovascular disease with cannabis use, though a high risk of bias was acknowledged.[29] The acute cardiovascular adverse effects of inhaled cannabis, and the toxic components of cannabis smoke, could explain this trend. But why might cannabis users be less likely to die after AMI?

CB2 activation triggers prohomeostatic and protective intracellular pathways in cardiac, immune, and vascular cells in both human and animal models of atherosclerosis, resulting in reduced atherosclerosis and ischemic damage.[30] The bulk of the preclinical evidence suggests a role for cannabinoids in preventing damage from ischemia or reperfusion injuries, supporting the findings of reduced mortality after AMI described above.[31] For example, a mouse study found that 0.002 mg/kg THC, administered ip 2 hr prior to AMI, improved fractional shortening, troponin leakage, infarct size, and accumulation of neutrophils to the infarct area.[32] This ultralow effective dose could represent circulating THC and 11-OH-THC activity in cannabis users even hours or days after their last use.

Increasing evidence also suggests that cannabinoids could be used for CAD prevention. For example, one study of atherosclerosis in mice found that oral THC at 1 mg·kg^{-1}·day^{-1} (a surprisingly low dose for mice, below the psychotropic threshold) significantly inhibited disease progression; the effects were reversed with a CB2 inhibitor.[33]

While epidemiological data from people who self-reported smoking cannabis for nontherapeutic purposes suggested a slightly higher rate of cardiovascular disease in this group, the largest prospective study to date, the CARDIA study, failed to show an association between lifetime or recent cannabis use and cardiovascular events.[34] Data from the CARDIA study failed to show any association between cannabis use and levels of C-reactive protein and interleukin-6 but did show slightly increased levels of fibrinogen in cannabis users.[35]

As described above, emerging evidence supports the possibility that therapeutic use patterns, including very low doses, could have a protective effect both indirectly, via mitigating risk factors like sleep disturbance and obesity, and directly, by preventing atherosclerosis and ischemic injury. Use of nonsmoked delivery methods likely eliminates any potential for increased cardiovascular risk.

Stroke and Other Brain Injuries

Stroke is the fifth leading cause of death in the United States and a major cause of serious disability, costing the United States $34 billion annually in medical care and lost productivity.[36] Intravenous thrombolysis with tissue plasminogen activator and thrombectomy are still the only approved treatments for acute ischemic stroke, but these treatments are limited to patients who present within a narrow time frame. Furthermore, immediate reperfusion therapy does not directly address the secondary neurological sequelae that lead to continued brain injury after stroke: excitotoxicity, oxidative stress, pathological ion gradients, inflammation, and increased permeability of the blood–brain barrier. Cells in the ischemic penumbra can progress to permanent damage,[37] and stroke researchers are desperate to identify effective neuroprotective treatments. In the last few decades, more than 1,000 acute stroke treatments have been tested in the laboratory. While 69% of the preclinical studies have had a positive outcome, only 6% of the 50 interventions that made it to phase III clinical trials have been positive. This large disparity is explained by different primary end points and time to treatment, publication bias, neglected quality criteria, and low power.[38]

The neuroprotective effects of endo- and phytocannabinoids are well established and are reviewed in Chapters 8 and 13. Clearly, the animal data on the use of cannabinoids to limit infarct size after experimental stroke are well established, as summarized in Table 29.1.

TABLE 29.1
Cannabinoid Reduction of Lesion Volume in Preclinical Models of Stroke[39]

Cannabinoid treatment	No. of experiments	No. of animals	Standardized mean difference in lesion volume after treatment [95% CI]	p value
Endocannabinoids	25	268	–1.72 [–2.62, –0.82]	.0002
THC	13	115	–1.43 [–2.01, –0.86]	<.00001
CBD	21	188	–1.20 [–1.63, –0.77]	<.00001

Source: Dustin Sulak. From data in England, Timothy J., et al. (2015). "Cannabinoids in experimental stroke: a systematic review and meta-analysis." Journal of Cerebral Blood Flow & Metabolism, *35*(3), 348–358.

How well might these preclinical data translate? The pleiotropic effects of cannabinoids on the ischemic penumbra and cerebral vasculature after stroke, combined with their excellent safety and tolerability, make them promising candidates for human research. The U.S. Department of Health and Human Services was issued a patent titled *Cannabinoids as antioxidants and neuroprotectants* in 2003, which details the use of cannabis-related compounds in the treatment of "acute ischemic neurological insults" among other neurological disorders.[40] Perhaps due, in part, to the issuing of this patent, no clinical trials have been published on the use of phytocannabinoids for acute stroke. One multicenter, placebo-controlled, phase III trial of dexanabinol, a noncompetitive *N*-methyl-D-aspartate receptor antagonist that is considered a cannabinoid because of its chemical structure (it is an inactive enantiomer of HU-210) but has no CB1 or CB2 activity, was performed in patients with traumatic brain injury (TBI).[41] Dexanabinol was safe but not effective for treating TBI. I hope to see similar trials of THC and CBD for patients with stroke and TBI.

In the meanwhile, we are left with some promising observational data. Among 446 cases of TBI at a level 1 trauma center in California, 18.4% (82) were positive for THC on a toxicology screen. The overall mortality rate was 9.9%; it was 11.5% in the THC-negative group and 2.4% in the THC-positive group. After use of regression analysis to account for age, alcohol, head Abbreviated Injury Scale Score, Injury Severity Score, mechanism of injury, gender, and ethnicity, a positive THC screen was found to be a strong independent predictor of survival (mortality *OR* 0.224, 95% CI 0.051–0.991; p = .049).[42]

The neuroprotective potential of cannabis also shows up in patients with spontaneous intracerebral hemorrhage (ICH). Among 725 cases from an international multicenter cohort, the 8.6% (62) with positive urine drug screens for THC had a milder presentation (p = .017) and better outcomes (modified Rankin Scale, adjusted *OR* 0.544, 95% CI 0.330–0.895), though there was no significant difference in hematoma volume or location between the groups. Nineteen percent of the THC-positive subjects had no disability, while only 3% of the THC-negative subjects had no disability.[43]

Similarly, a cross-sectional study that used data from the NIS (2004–2011, n = 2,496,165 cannabis users and n = 116,163,454 nonusers, age 15–54) found that cannabis use was not an independent predictor of ICH after adjustment for other illicit drug use and ICH risk factors (*OR* 1.063, 95% CI 0.963–1.173). The cannabis users had fewer adverse discharge dispositions (*OR* 0.78, 95% CI 0.72–0.86), reduced length of hospitalization (*OR* 0.54, 95% CI 0.48–0.61), and lower hospitalization cost (*OR* 0.72, 95% CI 0.64–0.81), but interestingly, they had higher in-hospital mortality (*OR* 1.26, 95% CI 1.12–1.41).[44]

It appears that cannabis may have a protective effect in the setting of acute brain injury, but it may slightly increase the risk of cerebrovascular events. Keep in mind that the aforementioned observational data reflect the outcomes of people mostly using cannabis for nontherapeutic purposes, likely mostly via smoking and using higher doses than clinicians would recommend to their patients. We clearly need more studies, especially on the use of cannabinoids in the acute and recovery phases of brain trauma. In the meanwhile, I strongly suspect that low-dose cannabis, used to promote sleep and resilience to stress, would convey a protective effect to those who experience brain injury.

Cancer

As of 2016, the lifetime risk of developing cancer other than skin cancer was 40.1% for men and 38.7% for women in the United States. While the human and economic burden of cancer is immense, public health and clinical strategies to prevent cancer are profoundly inadequate, and the allocation of resources to cancer prevention is disproportionately low compared to that of cancer treatment. The strong evidence for a supporting role of the ECS in our natural resistance against cancer and the preclinical antineoplastic effects of phytocannabinoids raise the question: Can cannabis be used to prevent cancer?

The answer seems to be yes in preclinical studies. As described in Chapter 18, the 2-year toxicology studies in rats and mice found significantly lower incidences of several cancer types in the animals dosed with THC.[45] Does this protective effect translate to people?

Again, we must rely on the observational data from cannabis smokers to begin to answer this important question. It is clear that heavy cannabis smokers are exposed to substantial amounts of carcinogens; we would suspect this population to have higher incidents of lung cancer, but this is not the case, perhaps due to an antineoplastic effect of the active compounds delivered along with the toxins in the smoke.

In one of the best-designed studies on this topic, researchers investigated the association between cannabis use and lung cancer in a large Southern Californian case–control study with 611 lung cancer cases and 1,040 controls, with a large prevalence of high-dose cannabis smokers. After adjustment for several confounders, including cigarette smoking and alcohol consumption, there was no significant association between joint-years (where 1 joint-year is equivalent to smoking one joint per day for 1 year) and upper or lower respiratory cancers. Indeed, among those with ≥60 joint-years versus 0 joint-years, the data trended toward lower rates of lung cancer (adjusted OR 0.62, 95% CI 0.32–1.2).[46]

Similarly, researchers from the International Lung Cancer Consortium conducted a pooled case–control study based on data from six studies in the United States, United Kingdom, and New Zealand. One advantage of this project was its ability to analyze the relationship between cannabis use and lung cancer in a large subgroup of non–tobacco smokers. Compared with nonhabitual or never cannabis users, the pooled *OR* of lung cancer in habitual cannabis smokers was 0.96 (95% CI 0.66–1.38); for those with ≥10 joint-years, the pooled *OR* was 0.94 (95% CI 0.67–1.32). Both results are not statistically significant, indicating no increase or decreased incidence of lung cancer in heavy cannabis users. In the subgroup of cannabis users who did not use tobacco, results were similar.[47]

While an absence of neoplastic effects in the lungs of heavy users is promising, do any data indicate a protective effect against other cancers? In one case, yes, and in another, the opposite. Overall, the association between cannabis use and cancer in the general population is minimal to nil.

In the California Men's Health Study, 84,170 participants aged 45–69 years were followed over 11 years. After adjustment for age, race or ethnicity, and BMI, cannabis use (without concurrent tobacco use) was associated with a 45% reduction in bladder cancer incidence (hazard regression 0.55, 95% CI 0.31–1.00). Using tobacco but not cannabis was associated with an increased risk of bladder cancer (hazard regression 1.52, 95% CI 1.12–2.07), and for those using both cannabis and tobacco, there was no statistically significant association.[48] Perhaps this particular cancer type is especially sensitive to cannabis, and cannabis use may have the ability to mitigate the strong association between tobacco and bladder cancer, but these observational data do not prove causality. At the time of writing, this study provides the strongest epidemiological data for decreased cancer incidence in cannabis users.

Conversely, three testicular cancer case–control studies were fairly consistent with one another, reporting an increased risk in cannabis users. The strongest association was found for development of non-seminoma tumors: those using cannabis on at least a weekly basis had 2.5 times greater odds of developing a non-seminoma testicular germ cell tumor compared those who never used cannabis (*OR* 2.59, 95% CI 1.60–4.19). There was no clear association between seminoma tumors and cannabis use.[49] There has been no suggested biological mechanism explaining a causal relationship, but I wonder if the young men who are most susceptible to these cancers have a tendency to use cannabis in greater excess, thereby dysregulating their ECS.

The largest number of studies for a cancer site involve head and neck cancer. Among eight case–control studies and two pooled analysis studies on head and neck cancer and cannabis use, one study reported an increased risk, five studies reported no association, and one study reported a decreased risk of head and neck cancer. The three studies that investigated human papillomavirus (HPV), cannabis, and head and neck cancer suggest that HPV may be a modifying factor, with inconsistent evidence suggesting higher rates of HPV-positive oropharyngeal squamous cell carcinoma in cannabis smokers.[50]

A recent review concluded that, for other cancer types, the association between cannabis use and an increased or decreased incidence is also inconclusive.[51] Interactions between the ECS, cannabis, and cancer are certainly complex. I suspect that low-dose cannabis used to optimize the function of the ECS may be protective against some cancers, not just indirectly—via better sleep, less obesity and diabetes, and alcohol and tobacco substitution—but also directly, via its antineoplastic effects.

Substituting Alcohol, Tobacco, and Other Substances

As described in Chapter 28, those using cannabis for both therapeutic and nontherapeutic purposes report a high rate of substitution for tobacco, alcohol, and illicit drugs. Though cannabis legalization has not been associated with decreased tobacco and alcohol sales in the United States, it is not clear that passage of a medical cannabis policy per se results in increased prevalence or frequency of cannabis use, and it is too early to know if adult-use legalization results in increased use in the general population.[52] In other words, most people who substitute cannabis for alcohol, tobacco, and other more dangerous substances are already doing so regardless of its legality. It is clear that the alcohol, tobacco, and illicit drug use have an immense negative impact on public health and that cannabis is frequently used as a safer alternative to these substances.

Most people have an innate drive to experience altered states of consciousness, perhaps analogous or related to our drive for sex.[53] While this can be met with a variety of natural and health-promoting activities, like exercise and meditation, many use plants and drugs to temporarily shift out of their ordinary reality. This is recognized in the field of harm reduction, in which safer substances are used to satisfy the drive for psychoactivity as replacements for those with greater risk. Among all psychoactive substances, cannabis has one of the best safety profiles, lowest rates of dependence and problematic use, and highest likelihood of positive side effects, like those described above. If harm reduction programs embrace cannabis as a tool to support abstinence from more dangerous substances, providing education and guidance on how to use cannabis for best results and minimal potential harm, I suspect we could make greater strides in combatting the immense negative impact of substance abuse on public health.

Cannabis as a Crutch, Cannabis as a Tonic

I am frequently asked if my cannabis-using patients are able to eventually stop using cannabis, a relevant question that might demonstrate its effectiveness as a healing intervention. While many are able to stop, most of my patients continue to use cannabis but shift their pattern of use as their health improves. To describe this to my patients, I use the analogy of the crutch and the tonic.

When a person fractures a bone in their leg, a crutch is needed to prevent weight bearing that would interrupt the healing process. Similarly, during an illness a patient may need to "lean on" cannabis more strongly to allow them to both function and heal.

Eventually, however, the person with the broken leg has to put down the crutch, as the force vectors generated by bearing weight stimulate the final healing process of the bone, without which complete healing would not occur. The cannabis user also must rely less on cannabis and more on their internal resources to progress through the latter stages of healing, during which the use patterns typically evolve to those described at the end of this chapter. At some point, patients will notice times when they feel better before they use cannabis, perhaps a sign that their inner pharmacy has regained its capacity to impart the benefits that previously required the intake of cannabis.

After putting down the crutch, the individual can continue using cannabis without medical supervision (in jurisdictions where it is legal to do so) as a tonic to improve stress resilience, as a spiritual and social tool, and as a home remedy for mild symptoms. Our relationship with cannabis can evolve throughout the different chapters of illness, wellness, and aging in our lives.

Social and Spiritual Connection

As I complete this book in the early months of the global COVID-19 crisis, the world is quickly becoming aware, through direct experience, of the importance of social connection and the potential harm of social isolation. Previous research has demonstrated that social network structure and function are strongly intertwined with anxiety and depression symptoms in the general population, perhaps especially in older adults.[54] Several studies have demonstrated that the presence of social connections is associated with important positive health effects including decreased mortality,[55] better immune function,[56] and lower levels of cardiovascular disease progression.[57] Social isolation in children, based on longitudinal data followed into adulthood, has persistent and cumulative detrimental effects on adult health, with isolated children at a significantly higher risk of poor adult health, even after control for other well-established childhood risk factors (low childhood socioeconomic status, low childhood IQ, childhood overweight), health-damaging behaviors (lack of exercise, smoking, alcohol misuse), and exposure to stressful life events.[58] The health effects of social isolation are mediated through both health behaviors and neuroendocrine mechanisms.[59]

Clearly, our potential to improve health and prevent disease, both in the short run and decades hence, is dependent on our social connectivity. In these times of change, this is a more important consideration than ever. I believe that cannabis, especially when used with this intention, has the capacity to promote social connectivity. The mild psychoactive effects of appropriately dosed cannabis often shift our psychological filters toward an increased emphasis of mutual similarities, feeling of openness and a decreased perception of threat and dissimilarity. Older research has demonstrated that cannabis users are more likely to score lower on quarrelsomeness and higher on selflessness;[60] though the association may not be causal, I suspect it is.

Descriptions of feeling more connected to something greater than self after using cannabis, be it family, society, nature, or God, are common among my patients. Patients consistently report that the acute effects of cannabis promote altruism, forgiveness, empathy, a greater willingness to participate in social interactions, and increased capacity to enjoy them. My patients and their spouses frequently comment on the contribution cannabis has made to their relationship in general, and specifically to verbal and physical intimacy.

There are many examples of medical cannabis use leading to improved social connectivity. In the early days of medical cannabis legalization, the health effects of socialization among cannabis users was clear in the social clubs that served as a distribution source for patients. While the acquisition of cannabis for therapeutic purposes, as recommended by their physicians, was the major rationale of patients for seeking membership, almost without exception they expressed greater satisfaction in the social interaction and activities they experienced. The setting itself served therapeutic purposes for them by providing a natural environment in which to socialize with others who not only were struggling with serious disease but also were frequently isolated, frightened, and depressed. Members often stated that the socialization they encountered and the friends they made at the clubs were health producing.[61]

Where I practice, patients are able to not only grow and produce their own cannabis but also, for a modest fee, attain state licensure to be a "cannabis caregiver" and sell and distribute extra medicine to other patients. I have repeatedly observed patients who begin by purchasing from a caregiver, progress to a mentoring relationship in which the patient becomes self-sufficient in producing his or her own medicine, and finally graduate to caregiver status, providing medicine and mentorship to other patients in need. The capacity and opportunity to help others in this way appears to be a powerful therapy unto itself.

While stress is implicated as a cause or contributing factor to most diseases, stress in itself is not necessarily harmful. Our reaction to stress has the capacity to produce detrimental or beneficial health consequences. Stress comes from our inability to adapt to our ever-changing environment. Adaptation is, of course, an essential component of health promotion and disease prevention.

Eustress, defined as a form of stress having a beneficial effect on health, motivation, performance, and emotional well-being, occurs when we embrace both the challenging and supportive aspects of an event or situation. Distress, conversely, leads to feelings of being overwhelmed, anxiety, depression, and decreased performance. It occurs more often when one perceives the challenging aspects of an event or situation without simultaneously perceiving the supportive aspects.

Our perception therefore determines whether we experience distress or eustress; we all have the power to transform distress into eustress, though sometimes our rigid perception limits our capacity to do so. Cannabis, which in even in non-impairing doses can increase psychological flexibility and help users shift their relationship with a stressful situation, can be used strategically to move beyond perceptual limitations fostering distress. Specific recommendations on how to do so are detailed in the summary at the end of this chapter.

While social isolation clearly has its challenges, like all things in life, it also presents opportunities. Solitude is frequently a component of spiritual training in many religions and spiritual practices. For those unable to connect with social networks due to COVID-19 or myriad other factors, deepening one's spiritual connection presents an appealing alternative; again, I believe that appropriately used cannabis can support this process. Innumerable patients have reported this in my practice, describing cannabis-enhanced benefits of prayer, meditation, study of religious texts, attending religious events, and spending time in nature. The use of cannabis and other psychoactive substances to augment spiritual experiences is, of course, nothing new. For example, a recent discovery of cannabis residue on an altar from the "Holy of Holies" inner chamber of the Judahite shrine of Arad (~750 B.C.E.) strongly suggests it was burned in the temple for a deliberate psychoactive effect.

As described in Chapter 17, one of the prominent qualitative effects of medical cannabis on its users is the "restored self," a feeling of having their "lives back" with greater acceptance of their medical condition.[62] In my experience, this pivotal change not only improves quality of life but also promotes self-care and self-efficacy. The neuroendocrine effects of restored self likely promote a physiological environment more conducive to health and healing.

The capacity of cannabis to promote social and spiritual connectivity is frequently underutilized by clinicians. Simply suggesting this potential to your patients can produce profound improvements in health and quality of life, and it may be one of the most important ways in which cannabis can be used to promote health and prevent disease.

Conclusions

Lester Grinspoon, associate professor emeritus of psychiatry at Harvard Medical School and one of the pioneering leaders of the medical cannabis movement, provided consistent support for cannabis reform and health-promoting cannabis use until his recent death at the age of 92. In addition to recreational and medical use, Grinspoon identified a third application of cannabis, "the enhancement of a broad range of human activities."

> Everybody that has used marijuana knows that an ordinary meal can taste like a culinary treat and that it can enhance sexual experiences. But these are enhancements that are right there on the surface. Once one becomes more experienced with cannabis he can experience or appreciate phenomena in another way, for example understand art in a better way, use it for creative purposes or spirituality.[63]

I wish a deeper and more meaningful life to all my patients, students, and readers of this book. We are facing unprecedented challenges to our mental and physical health. To thrive in this rapidly changing environment, we will need tools to improve our resilience to mental and physical stress and stay connected to ourselves, each other, and nature. It is clear to me that cannabis is an excellent tool for this purpose, but *how* to use it is the key.

From Grinspoon's 1971 book *Marihuana Reconsidered*, the following statement from astronomer Carl Sagan is, perhaps, now more relevant than ever:

> The illegality of cannabis is outrageous, an impediment to full utilization of a drug which helps produce the serenity and insight, sensitivity and fellowship so desperately needed in this increasingly mad and dangerous world.[64]

Like Grinspoon, Sagan, and countless others who have observed the incontrovertible benefits of cannabis in both the sick and the well, I am dedicated to the continued liberation of this plant species that has so much to offer humanity. It is clear to me that cannabis works best with education, and decades of prohibition have interrupted the transmission of information on how to best use cannabis to promote health and treat disease. I warmly welcome you, the reader, to take up the task of disseminating this knowledge to help those in need.

How to Advise Patients to Use Cannabis as a Tonic to Promote Health and Prevent Disease

- Use the lowest effective dose and avoid building tolerance.
  - The ECS is a critical component of our ability to maintain health and prevent disease.
  - Building tolerance to THC downregulates CB1 and likely CB2 receptor activity, undermining the homeostatic capacity of the ECS.
  - Intermittent periods of abstinence prevent tolerance building and provide a chance for the ECS to adjust to changes in one's internal and external environment.
- Avoid or limit smoking.
  - Low-dose oromucosal delivery can provide nonimpairing performance enhancement and resilience to stress.
  - Flower vaporization is generally the healthiest way to inhale cannabis.
  - The rapid onset after inhalation can be useful to compartmentalize stress, for example, after finishing the work day and preparing for family time. Inhalation is also useful for augmenting exercise, meditation, prayer, and time in nature.
- Use cannabis to improve response to stress.
  - Low doses of cannabis can promote physiological resilience to stress and reduce emotional reactivity; users often comment that they are able to stay calm in challenging situations and feel less worn out at the end of the day.
  - Most cannabis users can find a personal dose of cannabis that is non-impairing but improves stress resilience and the psychological flexibility needed to transform distress into eustress. This typically involves a low dose of THC, e.g. 1-3mg PO, with an equal or higher dose of CBD, though CBD-dominant preparations sometimes work well.
  - Higher doses of THC, often inhaled, can be used periodically as an adjunct to introspection and mental adaptation. I instruct patients to first identify the fac-

tors causing distress in their life, then use cannabis to acheive mild to moderate psychoactive effects, and then simply reflect on these factors. Journaling greatly enhances the process. Powerful realizations often ensue that transform distress to eustress and persist after the acute effects of cannabis wear off.

- Use cannabis to promote restorative sleep.
  - Adequate restorative sleep is essential in any strategy to maintain health and prevent disease. See Chapter 22 for specific strategies.
- Use cannabis to enhance health-promoting activities like exercise, meditation, prayer, play, creativity, observing art, and savoring.
  - When cannabis is used to enhance the hedonic response and satisfaction associated with healthy behaviors, it increases the likelihood of regularly incorporating these behaviors into one's routine.
  - For those who are wondering where to start, I suggest the Wellness Activities section of my patient education website Healer.com, which includes video instructions for gentle movements, meditations, and breathing practices I find especially compatible with the mild psychoactive effects of cannabis.
  - For those who already regularly engage in a spiritual practice, periodically try the same practice under the gentle influence of cannabis.
- Use cannabis to enhance social connectivity.
  - Intentionally create an internal mindset and external setting that promotes beneficial social interaction. For example, share cannabis before enjoying art, going for a walk in nature, or listening to an album. Avoid activities that preclude interaction like watching television. Articulate the intention to deepen communication, friendship, or intimacy.
  - Cannabis can facilitate difficult conversations like repairing from a rupture in a relationship.
  - Be careful to avoid overconsumption, which can interfere with, rather than enhance, communication. Individuals with different sensitivities to cannabis can consume different amounts, delivery methods, and chemovars.
- Drink cannabis tea.
  - Cannabis tea is one of the most underrated delivery methods, and it is especially applicable for those wishing to experience the nonpsychoactive health benefits of the low- and ultra-low-dose range of cannabis.
  - While many recipes abound and produce different results, I usually recommend the simple method of pouring hot water over a pea-sized piece of cannabis flower, ideally from a type II variety (containing Δ^9-tetrahydrocannabinolic acid and cannabidiolic acid), allowing it to steep for 5 min, and drinking.

- The low solubility of THC in the water prevents any unintended psychoactive effects yet delivers a tiny dose of THC that is likely physiologically active (see Chapter 17 for more information on the ultra-low-dose range). The cannabinoid acids convey anti-inflammatory and other benefits likely useful in health promotion.

My Path to Cannabis Medicine

At age 16, I recognized incongruencies in my public-school education about cannabis, and its illegality, with my firsthand experience. That made me curious to learn more. At age 17, I started reading Dr. Andrew Weil's writings and was surprised to find his first two books were devoted to the health benefits of psychoactive experiences, providing a context for me to use cannabis for my own healing and growth. In 1997, as a freshman undergraduate at Indiana University in Bloomington, I joined a student group called the Citizen's Alliance for the Legalization of Marijuana (CALM), led by longtime cannabis activist Mike Truelove.

I soon became a committed cannabis legalization activist myself, reading scientific papers, creating flyers, setting up tables around campus, and educating those willing to stop by. I spoke at the CALM annual music and education event on the nutritional properties of hemp seeds and the safety of cannabis. I hungrily read the 1997 book *Marijuana myths, marijuana facts: A review of the scientific evidence*[1] and the 1999 Institute of Medicine report on "Marijuana and Medicine".[2] After college, I had the habit of "plugging in" with the local cannabis activism group wherever I went. I felt called to make a difference, but at that time I was more focused on the injustice of prohibition and mass incarceration than the potential to help sick people.

As a second-year medical student, at an American Academy of Osteopathy convocation in 2006, I attended a presentation on Cannabimimetic Effects of Osteopathic Manipulation, by John McPartland, DO. I had no idea that he was so well-recognized for his contributions to both endocannabinoid and hemp botany research, but I certainly felt excited by the interface between the worlds of cannabis and osteopathy. We developed a mentoring relationship, which I highly value to this day, and he invited me to an elective rotation at his rural osteopathic practice in Vermont. I was surprised that, despite his vast expertise in both cannabis and osteopathy, he was not combining them in his clinical practice, in part due to the restrictiveness of medical cannabis laws in Vermont.

During another fourth-year medical school rotation, this time in Maine, I touched base with Jonathan Leavitt, a local activist who was collecting signatures for a ballot initiative to significantly expand the very limited medical cannabis program in Maine. His initiative passed in November 2009, adding dispensaries, smaller cannabis producers called "caregivers," and additional indications, including chronic pain refractory to conventional treatment, Crohn's disease, severe nausea, and others. In an instant, the door opened for thousands of illegal cannabis-using patients in Maine to become legal; all they needed was a physician's recommendation.

Not surprisingly, few physicians were willing to provide that recommendation. One of those few was herbalist and integrative medicine expert John Woytowicz, MD, a faculty member at my residency program who had been recommending cannabis to patients for years under the limited law. His schedule allowed him to do only a few medical cannabis consultations with residents each month. I received great benefit from his example and teaching during my internship year.

Two months after starting my private practice, in the fall of 2009, I received a call from Jonathan Leavitt, asking if I was done with my training and if he could send me a few patients he knew; I accepted. After I certified the first few patients, word got out in the cannabis community that a young integrative doctor was willing to recommend medical cannabis. My practice was soon overrun with demand from a clearly underserved patient population. I hired nurse practitioner Laurel Sheppard, and together we saw over 1,500 cannabis patients in our first year. I am so grateful to still be working with Laurel.

It was, in many ways, the dream of a traditional osteopathic general practitioner. An incredible variety of pathology, most refractory to conventional treatment, walked through my door each day. At first, all were already using cannabis. I quickly recognized two powerful interventions I could offer my patients, beyond listening to their stories and the osteopathic treatment nearly all received. The first was the harm reduction from the risk of arrest and incarceration. The second, less expected, was relieving a burden of guilt. These patients knew that cannabis relieved their symptoms and worked better than other treatments they had tried, but they were ashamed to admit their use, or conflicted about the divergence between their own experience and the government narrative. I was the first medical authority who had acknowledged that their cannabis use could be safe, effective, and healthy, allowing us to quickly build rapport and foster therapeutic relationships.

I learned a tremendous amount from my patients' cannabis histories, trials and errors, and diverse use patterns to address a wide variety of demographics and disease. I observed a medicine with incredibly versatility, absurdly wide dosing range, and remarkable tolerability. Many of my most successful strategies were taught to me by patients in the first few years. They also inspired me to continually scour the primary scientific literature for guidance, at a time when it was rapidly expanding.

In 2010, I met Jeffrey Hergenrather, MD, and Ethan Russo, MD, two other mentors who generously shared and continue to share their years of knowledge and experience with me, and who confirmed many of my hard-to-believe early observations.

During my decade of experience in cannabis medicine, I have recognized two advantages that have helped me pioneer this field: the trained ability to osteopathically palpate patients' responses to changes in dosing and formulation, and an analytic laboratory that lived in my office for nearly four years. The need for the lab emerged from an influx of pediatric seizure patients using unlabeled, untested, artisanal preparations of cannabis. My younger brother Clayton Sulak, who had recently completed an undergraduate degree in pharmacognosy, my brother-in-law and business partner Brad Feuer, and I joined forces to set up a refurbished high-performance liquid chromatograph in 2014 and begin looking inside the medicines my patients were making and purchasing. My orientation to dosing suddenly became based on milligrams instead of drops and puffs, and my capacity to understand what was working for patients, and what was not working, expanded drastically.

Today, my practice is as rewarding as ever. I have the pleasure of working with my wife, Danielle Saad, DO, a skilled osteopath and cannabis clinician, as co–medical director. We still follow many of the patients from that first year. Most of our new patients have little or no prior experience with cannabis and are referred by their primary care provider or a specialist. We are seeing some of the most challenging cases from all disciplines of medicine, and while cannabis is not effective for them all, most find it helps in some way, some find it miraculous, and remarkably few have negative effects. I can barely imagine a general practice without access to cannabis as a tool. I know I would miss witnessing the frequent profoundly life-changing responses, and would have to rely more heavily on less effective and more dangerous treatments.

I wrote this book to empower and facilitate other clinicians to safely and effectively use cannabis as a tool, as my mentors and partners have done for me. It is dedicated to all of our patients.

Disclosure

The following financial and nonfinancial relationships were present during my preparation of this book and may have influenced its content:

- **Healer, Inc.** I am a cofounder, equity owner, and paid employee of this company, which focuses on solving problems in the medical cannabis industry. Healer provides patient education, industry professional education, clinical education, consulting for cannabis producers and dispensaries, research and development on cannabis extraction and formulation, and cannabis products. My work with Healer includes a patent for a concentrated cannabinoid production process.[3]
- **Zelira Therapeutics (formerly Zelda Therapeutics).** This Australian company has focused on preclinical and clinical trials of cannabis and cannabinoids. I serve as a paid member of the scientific advisory board.
- **COR Analytics.** This company provides data collection and analytics for the cannabis industry. I serve as a paid member of the scientific advisory board.
- **Spectrum Therapeutics (Canopy Growth Corporation).** I have received honoraria from this international medical cannabis company for participating in education and research symposia.
- **Society of Cannabis Clinicians.** I serve as a volunteer member of the board of directors for this nonprofit professional membership organization.
- **Patients Out of Time.** I serve as a volunteer member of the board of directors for this nonprofit cannabis education organization.

References

Chapter 2: The History of Cannabinoid Medicine

1. McPartland, J. M. (2018). Cannabis systematics at the levels of family, genus, and species. *Cannabis and Cannabinoid Research, 3*(1), 203–212.
2. McPartland, J. M., & Hegman, W. (2018). Cannabis utilization and diffusion patterns in prehistoric Europe: a critical analysis of archaeological evidence. *Vegetation History and Archaeobotany, 27*(4), 627–634.
3. Russo, E. B. (2014). The pharmacological history of cannabis. In *Handbook of cannabis* (pp. 23–43). Oxford University Press.
4. Yang, S. (1998). *The divine farmer's materia medica: a translation of the Shen Nong Ben Cao Jing.* Blue Poppy Enterprises, Inc.
5. Russo, E. B. (2014). The pharmacological history of cannabis. In *Handbook of cannabis* (pp. 23–43). Oxford University Press.
6. Fankhauser M. (2002). History of cannabis in Western medicine. In F. Grotenhermen & E. Russo (Eds.), *Cannabis and Cannabinoids* (Chapter 4, pp. 37–51). The Haworth Integrative Healing Press.
7. Zuardi, A. W. (2006). History of cannabis as a medicine: a review. *Revista Brasileira de Psiquiatría, 28*(2), 153–157.
8. Du Toit, B. M. (1980). *Cannabis in Africa: a survey of its distribution in Africa, and a study of cannabis use and users in multi-ethnic South Africa.* AA Bolkema.
9. De Pinho, A. R. (1980). Social and medical aspects of the use of cannabis in Brazil. In D. L. Browman & R. A. Schwarz (Eds.), *Spirits, Shamans, and Stars: Perspectives from South America* (p. 85). Mouton Publishers.
10. O'Shaughnessy, W. B. (1838–1840). On the preparations of the Indian hemp, or gunjah (*Cannabis indica*). *Transactions of the Medical and Physical Society of Bengal, 71*(102), 421–461.
11. McMeens, R. R. (1860). Report of the Ohio State Medical Committee on *Cannabis indica*. *Transactions of the Fifteenth Annual Meeting of the Ohio State Medical Society at Ohio White Sulphur Springs, June 12 to 14, 1860* (pp. 75–100). Ohio State Medical Society.
12. Fronmüller, B. (1869). *Klinische Studien über die schlafmachende Wirkung der narkotischen Arzneimittel.* Enke.
13. Clendinning, J. (1843). Observations on the medicinal properties of the *Cannabis sativa* of India. *Medico-Chirurgical Transactions, 26*, 188.
14. Mattison, J. (1891). The treatment of the morphine-disease. *Indian Medical Gazette, 26*(3), 65.
15. Mattison, J. B. (1891). *Cannabis indica* as an anodyne and hypnotic. *St. Louis Medical and Surgical Journal, 61*, 265–271.
16. Fankhauser M. (2002). History of cannabis in Western medicine. In F. Grotenhermen & E. Russo (Eds.), *Cannabis and Cannabinoids* (Chapter 4, pp. 37–51). The Haworth Integrative Healing Press.
17. Maisto, S., Galizio, M., & Connors, G. (2003). *Drug Use and Abuse* (4th ed., pp. 426–428). Wadsworth Publishing.
18. Burnett, M., & Reiman, A. (2014, October 8). How did marijuana become illegal in the first place? *Drug Policy Alliance.* http://www.drugpolicy.org/blog/how-did-marijuana-become-illegal-first-place
19. Schaffer Library of Drug Policy. (1937, May 4). *Statement of Dr. William C. Woodward, The Marihuana Tax Act of 1937.* http://www.druglibrary.org/schaffer/hemp/taxact/woodward.htm
20. Adams, R. (1940). Marihuana. *Science, 92*(2380), 115–119.

21. Gaoni, Y., & Mechoulam, R. (1964). Isolation, structure, and partial synthesis of an active constituent of hashish. *Journal of the American Chemical Society, 86*(8), 1646–1647.

22. LaGuardia, F. (1944). *The Laguardia Committee Report New York, USA (1944)*.

23. Lee, M. A. (2008, July 19). *Synthetic pot as a military weapon? Meet the man who ran the secret program*. AlterNet. https://www.alternet.org/2008/07/synthetic_pot_as_a_military_weapon_meet_the_man_who_ran_the_secret_program/

24. Weil, A. T., Zinberg, N. E., & Nelsen, J. M. (1969). Clinical and psychological effects of marijuana in man. *International Journal of the Addictions, 4*(3), 427–451.

25. Zinberg, N. E., & Weil, A. T. (1970). A comparison of marijuana users and non-users. *Nature, 226*(5241), 119.

26. Weil, A. T. (1970). Adverse reactions to marihuana: Classification and suggested treatment. *New England Journal of Medicine, 282*(18), 997–1000.

27. Nahas, G. G., & Greenwood, A. (1974). The first report of the National Commission on Marihuana (1972): Signal of misunderstanding or exercise in ambiguity. *Bulletin of the New York Academy of Medicine, 50*(1), 55.

28. Russo, E., Mathre, M. L., Byrne, A., Velin, R., Bach, P. J., Sanchez-Ramos, J., & Kirlin, K. A. (2002). Chronic cannabis use in the Compassionate Investigational New Drug Program: An examination of benefits and adverse effects of legal clinical cannabis. *Journal of Cannabis Therapeutics, 2*(1), 3–57.

29. Devane, W. A., Dysarz, F. 3., Johnson, M. R., Melvin, L. S., & Howlett, A. C. (1988). Determination and characterization of a cannabinoid receptor in rat brain. *Molecular pharmacology, 34*(5), 605–613.

30. Munro, S., Thomas, K. L., & Abu-Shaar, M. (1993). Molecular characterization of a peripheral receptor for cannabinoids. *Nature, 365*(6441), 61.

31. Devane, W. A., Hanus, L., Breuer, A., Pertwee, R. G., Stevenson, L. A., Griffin, G., ... & Mechoulam, R. (1992). Isolation and structure of a brain constituent that binds to the cannabinoid receptor. *Science, 258*(5090), 1946–1949.

32. Mechoulam, R., Ben-Shabat, S., Hanus, L., Ligumsky, M., Kaminski, N. E., Schatz, A. R., ... & Pertwee, R. G. (1995). Identification of an endogenous 2-monoglyceride, present in canine gut, that binds to cannabinoid receptors. *Biochemical pharmacology, 50*(1), 83–90.

33. Sugiura, T., Kondo, S., Sukagawa, A., Nakane, S., Shinoda, A., Itoh, K., Yamashita, A., & Waku, K. (1995). 2-Arachidonoylgylcerol: a possible endogenous cannabinoid receptor ligand in brain. *Biochemical and biophysical research communications, 215*(1), 89–97.

34. O'Shaughnessy's. (2008, Fall/Winter). *Tod Mikuriya, MD —Notes for a Biography*. https://beyondthc.com/product/tod-mikuriya-md-notes-for-a-biography/

35. Benson, J. A., Jr., Watson, S. J., Jr., & Joy, J. E. (Eds.). (1999). *Marijuana and medicine: assessing the science base*. National Academies Press.

36. Hampson, A. J., Axelrod, J. & Grimaldi, M. (2003, October 7). *Cannabinoids as antioxidants and neuroprotectants*. (U.S. Patent No. 6,630,507). U.S. Patent and Trademark Office.

37. Russo, E. B. (2016). Current therapeutic cannabis controversies and clinical trial design issues. *Frontiers in Pharmacology, 7*, 309.

38. U.S. Food and Drug Administration. (2018, December 20). *Statement from FDA Commissioner Scott Gottlieb, M.D., on signing of the Agriculture Improvement Act and the agency's regulation of products containing cannabis and cannabis-derived compounds*. https://www.fda.gov/news-events/press-announcements/statement-fda-commissioner-scott-gottlieb-md-signing-agriculture-improvement-act-and-agencys

39. Veiga, A. (2019, March 21). *Cannabis-derived CBD oil finding place in ever more products*. ABC News. https://abcnews.go.com/Business/wireStory/cannabis-derived-cbd-oil-finding-place-products-61835976

40. National Academies of Sciences, Engineering, and Medicine. (2017). *The health effects of cannabis and cannabinoids: The current state of evidence and recommendations for research*. The National Academies Press. https://doi.org/10.17226/24625

Chapter 3: Cannabinoid Medicine as a Solution to the Greatest Challenges in Health Care

1.. National Center for Health Statistics, Centers for Disease Control. (2017). *Health, United States, 2016: In Brief*. Government Printing Office.

2. Davis, K., Stremikis, K., Squires, D., & Schoen, C. (2014). *Mirror, mirror on the wall: How the performance of the U.S. health care system compares internationally*. CommonWealth Fund.

3. National Research Council and Institute on Medicine. (2013). *U.S. health in international perspective: Shorter lives, poorer health*. National Academies Press.

4. Davis, K., Stremikis, K., Squires, D., & Schoen, C. (2014). *Mirror, mirror on the wall: How the performance of the U.S. health care system compares internationally*. CommonWealth Fund.

5. Nahin, R. L. (2015). Estimates of pain prevalence and severity in adults: United States, 2012. *The Journal of Pain, 16*(8), 769–780.

6. Mansfield, K. E., Sim, J., Jordan, J. L., & Jordan, K. P. (2016). A systematic review and meta-analysis of the prevalence of chronic widespread pain in the general population. *Pain, 157*(1), 55.

7. Gatchel, R. J., & Okifuji, A. (2006). Evidence-based scientific data documenting the treatment and cost-effectiveness of comprehensive pain programs for chronic nonmalignant pain. *The Journal of Pain*, 7(11), 779–793.

8. National Academies of Sciences, Engineering, and Medicine. (2017). *The health effects of cannabis and cannabinoids: The current state of evidence and recommendations for research*. National Academies Press.

9. Russo, E. B. (2008). Clinical endocannabinoid deficiency (CECD). *Neuroendocrinology Letters*, 29(2), 192–200.

10. Pacher, P., & Kunos, G. (2013). Modulating the endocannabinoid system in human health and disease–successes and failures. *FEBS Journal*, 280(9), 1918–1943.

11. Kwan, P., & Brodie, M. J. (2000). Early identification of refractory epilepsy. *New England Journal of Medicine*, 342(5), 314–319.

12. Sulak, D., Saneto, R., & Goldstein, B. (2017). The current status of artisanal cannabis for the treatment of epilepsy in the United States. *Epilepsy & Behavior*, 70, 328–333.

Chapter 4: From the Bench to the Bedside and Vice Versa

1. Brodie, J. S., Di Marzo, V., & Guy, G. W. (2015). Polypharmacology shakes hands with complex aetiopathology. *Trends in Pharmacological Sciences*, 36(12), 802–821.

2. Li, X., Wu, L., Liu, W., Jin, Y., Chen, Q., Wang, L., Fan, X., Li, Z., & Cheng, Y. (2014). A network pharmacology study of Chinese medicine QiShenYiQi to reveal its underlying multi-compound, multi-target, multi-pathway mode of action. *PLOS ONE*, 9(5), Article e95004.

Chapter 5: Cannabinoid Receptors

1. Devane, W. A., Dysarz, F. 3., Johnson, M. R., Melvin, L. S., & Howlett, A. C. (1988). Determination and characterization of a cannabinoid receptor in rat brain. *Molecular pharmacology*, 34(5), 605–613.

2. Matsuda, L. A., Lolait, S. J., Brownstein, M. J., Young, A. C., & Bonner, T. I. (1990). Structure of a cannabinoid receptor and functional expression of the cloned cDNA. *Nature*, 346, 561–564.

3. Munro, S., Thomas, K. L., & Abu-Shaar, M. (1993). Molecular characterization of a peripheral receptor for cannabinoids. *Nature*, 365(6441), 61.

4. Maejima, T., Hashimoto, K., Yoshida, T., Aiba, A., & Kano, M. (2001). Presynaptic inhibition caused by retrograde signal from metabotropic glutamate to cannabinoid receptors. *Neuron*, 31(3), 463–475.

5. Howlett, A. C., & Abood, M. E. (2017). CB1 and CB2 receptor pharmacology. *Advances in Pharmacology*, 80, 169–206.

6. Howlett, A. C., & Abood, M. E. (2017). CB1 and CB2 receptor pharmacology. *Advances in Pharmacology*, 80, 169–206.

7. Hebert-Chatelain, E., Marsicano, G., & Desprez, T. (2017). Cannabinoids and mitochondria. In M. Melis (Ed.), *Endocannabinoids and lipid mediators in brain functions* (pp. 211–235). Springer.

8. Glass, M., & Northup, J. K. (1999). Agonist selective regulation of G proteins by cannabinoid CB1 and CB2 receptors. *Molecular Pharmacology*, 56(6), 1362–1369.

9. McPartland, J. M., Matias, I., Di Marzo, V., & Glass, M. (2006). Evolutionary origins of the endocannabinoid system. *Gene*, 370, 64–74.

10. Edwards, J. G. (2014). TRPV1 in the central nervous system: Synaptic plasticity, function, and pharmacological implications. In *Capsaicin as a therapeutic molecule* (pp. 77–104). Springer.

11. Yang, H., Zhou, J., & Lehmann, C. (2016). GPR55—A putative "type 3" cannabinoid receptor in inflammation. *Journal of Basic and Clinical Physiology and Pharmacology*, 27(3), 297–302.

12. Tudurí, E., Imbernon, M., Hernández-Bautista, R. J., Tojo, M., Fernø, J., Diéguez, C., & Nogueiras, R. (2017). GPR55: a new promising target for metabolism?. *Journal of Molecular Endocrinology*, 58(3), R191-R202.

13. Pertwee, R. G. (2007). GPR55: A new member of the cannabinoid receptor clan? *British Journal of Pharmacology*, 152(7), 984–986.

14. Petitet, F., Donlan, M., & Michel, A. (2006). GPR55 as a new cannabinoid receptor: still a long way to prove it. *Chemical Biology & Drug Design*, 67(3), 252–253.

15. Russo, E. Personal communication, April 30, 2020.

16. Tyagi, S., Gupta, P., Saini, A. S., Kaushal, C., & Sharma, S. (2011). The peroxisome proliferator-activated receptor: A family of nuclear receptors role in various diseases. *Journal of advanced pharmaceutical technology & research*, 2(4), 236.

Chapter 6: Endogenous Cannabinoid Ligands: The Endocannabinoids

1. Devane, W. A., Hanus, L., Breuer, A., Pertwee, R. G., Stevenson, L. A., Griffin, G., Gibson, D., Mandelbaum, A., Etinger, A., & Mechoulam, R. (1992). Isolation and brain structure of a brain constituent that binds to the cannabinoid receptor. *Science*, 258, 1946–1949.

2. Mechoulam, R., Ben-Shabat, S., Hanus, L., Ligumsky, M., Kaminski, N. E., Schatz, A. R., ... & Pertwee, R. G. (1995).

Identification of an endogenous 2-monoglyceride, present in canine gut, that binds to cannabinoid receptors. *Biochemical pharmacology*, 50(1), 83–90.

3. Sugiura, T., Kondo, S., Sukagawa, A., Nakane, S., Shinoda, A., Itoh, K., ... & Waku, K. (1995). 2-Arachidonoylgylcerol: a possible endogenous cannabinoid receptor ligand in brain. *Biochemical and biophysical research communications*, 215(1), 89–97.

4. Zygmunt, P. M., Ermund, A., Movahed, P., Andersson, D. A., Simonsen, C., Jönsson, B. A., ... & Mallet, C. (2013). Monoacylglycerols activate TRPV1–a link between phospholipase C and TRPV1. *PLoS One*, 8(12), e81618.

5. Joshi, N., & Onaivi, E. S. (2019). Endocannabinoid system components: Overview and tissue distribution. In *Recent advances in cannabinoid physiology and pathology* (pp. 1–12). Springer.

6. Reviewed in Hillard, C. J. (2018). Circulating endocannabinoids: from whence do they come and where are they going? *Neuropsychopharmacology*, 43(1), 155.

7. Reviewed in Petrosino, S., & Di Marzo, V. (2017). The pharmacology of palmitoylethanolamide and first data on the therapeutic efficacy of some of its new formulations. *British Journal of Pharmacology*, 174(11), 1349–1365.

8. Fu, J., Gaetani, S., Oveisi, F., Verme, J. L., Serrano, A., de Fonseca, F. R., ... & Piomelli, D. (2003). Oleylethanolamide regulates feeding and body weight through activation of the nuclear receptor PPAR-α. *Nature*, 425(6953), 90–93.

9. Laleh, P., Yaser, K., & Alireza, O. (2019). Oleoylethanolamide: A novel pharmaceutical agent in the management of obesity—an updated review. *Journal of Cellular Physiology*, 234(6), 7893–7902.

10. Suardíaz, M., Estivill-Torrús, G., Goicoechea, C., Bilbao, A., & de Fonseca, F. R. (2007). Analgesic properties of oleoylethanolamide (OEA) in visceral and inflammatory pain. *PAIN®*, 133(1–3), 99–110.

11. Rondanelli, M., Opizzi, A., Solerte, S. B., Trotti, R., Klersy, C., & Cazzola, R. (2008). Administration of a dietary supplement (*N*-oleyl-phosphatidylethanolamine and epigallocatechin-3-gallate formula) enhances compliance with diet in healthy overweight subjects: a randomized controlled trial. *British Journal of Nutrition*, 101(3), 457–464.

12. van Kooten, M. J., Veldhuizen, M. G., de Araujo, I. E., O'Malley, S. S., & Small, D. M. (2016). Fatty acid amide supplementation decreases impulsivity in young adult heavy drinkers. *Physiology & behavior*, 155, 131–140.

13. Mangine, G. T., Gonzalez, A. M., Wells, A. J., McCormack, W. P., Fragala, M. S., Stout, J. R., & Hoffman, J. R. (2012). The effect of a dietary supplement (N-oleyl-phosphatidyl-ethanolamine and epigallocatechin gallate) on dietary compliance and body fat loss in adults who are overweight: A double-blind, randomized control trial. *Lipids in health and disease*, 11(1), 1–8.

14. Mechoulam, R., Fride, E., & Di Marzo, V. (1998). Endocannabinoids. *European Journal of Pharmacology*, 359(1), 1–18.

15. Petrosino, S., Schiano Moriello, A., Cerrato, S., Fusco, M., Puigdemont, A., De Petrocellis, L., & Di Marzo, V. (2016). The anti-inflammatory mediator palmitoylethanolamide enhances the levels of 2-arachidonoyl-glycerol and potentiates its actions at TRPV1 cation channels. *British Journal of Pharmacology*, 173(7), 1154–1162.

16. Petrosino, S., Schiano Moriello, A., Cerrato, S., Fusco, M., Puigdemont, A., De Petrocellis, L., & Di Marzo, V. (2016). The anti-inflammatory mediator palmitoylethanolamide enhances the levels of 2-arachidonoyl-glycerol and potentiates its actions at TRPV1 cation channels. *British Journal of Pharmacology*, 173(7), 1154–1162.

Chapter 7: Endocannabinoid Enzymes and Transporters

1. Tsuboi, K., Sun, Y. X., Okamoto, Y., Araki, N., Tonai, T., & Ueda, N. (2005). Molecular characterization of N-acylethanolamine-hydrolyzing acid amidase, a novel member of the choloylglycine hydrolase family with structural and functional similarity to acid ceramidase. *Journal of Biological Chemistry*, 280(12), 11082–11092.

2. Lu, H.-C., & Mackie, K. (2016). An introduction to the endogenous cannabinoid system. *Biological Psychiatry*, 79(7), 516–525.

3. Joshi, N., & Onaivi, E. S. (2019). Endocannabinoid system components: Overview and tissue distribution. In *Recent advances in cannabinoid physiology and pathology* (pp. 1–12). Springer.

4. Jung, K.-M., & Piomelli, D. (2016). Cannabinoids and endocannabinoids. In *Neuroscience in the 21st century: From basic to clinical* (pp. 1811–1841). Springer.

5. Mayo, L. M., Asratian, A., Lindé, J., Morena, M., Haataja, R., Hammar, V. Augier, G., Hill, M. N., & Heilig, M. (2020). Elevated anandamide, enhanced recall of fear extinction, and attenuated stress responses following inhibition of fatty acid amide hydrolase (FAAH): a randomized, controlled experimental medicine trial." *Biological Psychiatry*, 87(6), 538–547.

6. Huggins, J. P., Smart, T. S., Langman, S., Taylor, L., & Young, T. (2012). An efficient randomised, placebo-controlled clinical trial with the irreversible fatty acid amide hydrolase-1 inhibitor PF-04457845, which modulates endocannabinoids but fails to induce effective analgesia in patients with pain due to osteoarthritis of the knee. *PAIN®*, 153(9), 1837–1846.

7. Van Esbroeck, A. C., Janssen, A. P., Cognetta, A. B., Ogasawara, D., Shpak, G., Van Der Kroeg, M., ... & Allarà, M. (2017). Activity-based protein profiling reveals off-target proteins of the FAAH inhibitor BIA 10-2474. *Science*, 356(6342), 1084–1087.

8. Nicolussi, S., & Gertsch, J. (2015). Endocannabinoid transport revisited. In G. Litwack (Ed.), *Vitamins & hormones: Vol. 98. Hormones and transport systems* (pp. 441–485). Academic Press.

9. Di Marzo, V. (2018). New approaches and challenges to targeting the endocannabinoid system. *Nature Reviews Drug Discovery, 17*(9), 623–639.

10. Pertwee, R. G. (Ed.). (2014). *Handbook of cannabis.* Oxford University Press.

Chapter 8: Endocannabinoid Signaling and Homeostatic Function

1. McPartland, J. M. (2008). The endocannabinoid system: an osteopathic perspective. *The Journal of the American Osteopathic Association, 108*(10), 586–600.

2. Glass, M., Dragunow, M., & Faull, R. L. (1997). Cannabinoid receptors in the human brain: a detailed anatomical and quantitative autoradiographic study in the fetal, neonatal and adult human brain. *Neuroscience, 77,* 299–318.

3. Han, J., Kesner, P., Metna-Laurent, M., Duan, T., Xu, L., Georges, F., ... & Liu, Q. (2012). Acute cannabinoids impair working memory through astroglial CB1 receptor modulation of hippocampal LTD. *Cell, 148*(5), 1039–1050.

4. Howlett, A. C., & Abood, M. E. (2017). CB1 and CB2 receptor pharmacology. *Advances in Pharmacology, 80,* 169–206.

5. McPartland, J. M. (2008). The endocannabinoid system: an osteopathic perspective. *The Journal of the American Osteopathic Association, 108*(10), 586–600.

6. Viveros, M.-P., Marco, E.-M., Llorente, R., & López-Gallardo, M. (2007). Endocannabinoid system and synaptic plasticity: implications for emotional responses. *Neural Plasticity, 2007,* Article 52908. https://doi.org/10.1155/2007/52908

7. Chevaleyre, V., Takahashi, K. A., & Castillo, P. E. (2006). Endocannabinoid-mediated synaptic plasticity in the CNS. *Annual Review of Neuroscience, 29,* 37–76.

8. Xu, J.-Y., & Chen, C. (2015). Endocannabinoids in synaptic plasticity and neuroprotection. *The Neuroscientist, 21*(2), 152–168.

9. Mechoulam, R., Spatz, M., & Shohami, E. (2002). Endocannabinoids and neuroprotection. *Science Signaling, 2002*(129), Article re5. https://doi.org/10.1126/stke.2002.129.re5

10. Xu, J.-Y., & Chen, C. (2015). Endocannabinoids in synaptic plasticity and neuroprotection. *The Neuroscientist, 21*(2), 152–168.

11. Heiss, W.-D., & Graf, R. (1994). The ischemic penumbra. *Current Opinion in Neurology, 7*(1), 11–19.

12. Fernández-Ruiz, J., Moro, M. A., & Martínez-Orgado, J. (2015). Cannabinoids in neurodegenerative disorders and stroke/brain trauma: from preclinical models to clinical applications. *Neurotherapeutics, 12*(4), 793–806.

13. Galve-Roperh, I., Aguado, T., Palazuelos, J., & Guzman, M. (2007). The endocannabinoid system and neurogenesis in health and disease. *The Neuroscientist, 13*(2), 109–114.

14. Prenderville, J. A., Kelly, Â. M., & Downer, E. J. (2015). The role of cannabinoids in adult neurogenesis. *British Journal of Pharmacology, 172*(16), 3950–3963.

15. Van Sickle, M. D., Oland, L. D., Mackie, K., Davison, J. S., & Sharkey, K. A. (2003). Δ^9-Tetrahydrocannabinol selectively acts on CB1 receptors in specific regions of dorsal vagal complex to inhibit emesis in ferrets. *American Journal of Physiology-Gastrointestinal and Liver Physiology, 285*(3), G566-G576.

16. Ishac, E. J., Jiang, L., Lake, K. D., Varga, K., Abood, M. E., & Kunos, G. (1996). Inhibition of exocytotic noradrenaline release by presynaptic cannabinoid CB 1 receptors on peripheral sympathetic nerves. *British journal of pharmacology, 118*(8), 2023–2028.

17. Micale, V., & Drago, F. (2018). Endocannabinoid system, stress and HPA axis. *European Journal of Pharmacology, 834,* 230–239.

18. Ziegler, C. G., Mohn, C., Lamounier-Zepter, V., Rettori, V., Bornstein, S. R., Krug, A. W., & Ehrhart-Bornstein, M. (2010). Expression and function of endocannabinoid receptors in the human adrenal cortex. *Hormone and metabolic research, 42*(02), 88–92.

19. Pacher, P., Bátkai, S., & Kunos, G. (2006). The endocannabinoid system as an emerging target of pharmacotherapy. *Pharmacological Reviews, 58*(3), 389–462.

20. Pandey, R., Mousawy, K., Nagarkatti, M., & Nagarkatti, P. (2009). Endocannabinoids and immune regulation. *Pharmacological research, 60*(2), 85–92.

21. Galiègue, S., Mary, S., Marchand, J., Dussossoy, D., Carrière, D., Carayon, P., ... & Casellas, P. (1995). Expression of central and peripheral cannabinoid receptors in human immune tissues and leukocyte subpopulations. *European journal of biochemistry, 232*(1), 54–61.

22. Cabral, G. A., Rogers, T. J., & Lichtman, A. H. (2015). Turning over a new leaf: cannabinoid and endocannabinoid modulation of immune function. *Journal of Neuroimmune Pharmacology, 10*(2), 193–203.

23. Pandey, R., Mousawy, K., Nagarkatti, M., & Nagarkatti, P. (2009). Endocannabinoids and immune regulation. *Pharmacological research, 60*(2), 85–92.

24. Pandey, R., Mousawy, K., Nagarkatti, M., & Nagarkatti, P. (2009). Endocannabinoids and immune regulation. *Pharmacological research, 60*(2), 85–92.

25. Chang, Y.-H., Lee, S. T., & Lin, W.-W. (2001). Effects of cannabinoids on LPS-stimulated inflammatory mediator release from macrophages: involvement of eicosanoids. *Journal of Cellular Biochemistry*, *81*(4), 715–723.

26. Fukuda, S., Kohsaka, H., Takayasu, A., Yokoyama, W., Miyabe, C., Miyabe, Y., ... & Nanki, T. (2014). Cannabinoid receptor 2 as a potential therapeutic target in rheumatoid arthritis. *BMC musculoskeletal disorders*, 15(1), 1–10.

27. Dalgleish, A. G., & O'Byrne, K. J. (2002). Chronic immune activation and inflammation in the pathogenesis of AIDS and cancer. *Advances in Cancer Research*, *84*, 231–276.

28. McKallip, R. J., Nagarkatti, M., & Nagarkatti, P. S. (2005). Δ-9-tetrahydrocannabinol enhances breast cancer growth and metastasis by suppression of the antitumor immune response. *The Journal of Immunology*, *174*(6), 3281–3289.

29. DiPatrizio, N. V. (2016). Endocannabinoids in the Gut. *Cannabis and Cannabinoid Research*, *1*(1), 67–77.

30. Darmani, N. A. (2005). Endocannabinoids and gastrointestinal function. In *Endocannabinoids* (pp. 412–437). CRC Press.

31. DiPatrizio, N. V. (2020, February 13). Personal communication.

32. Lee, Y., Jo, J., Chung, H. Y., Pothoulakis, C., & Im, E. (2016). Endocannabinoids in the gastrointestinal tract. *American Journal of Physiology-Gastrointestinal and Liver Physiology*, *311*(4), G655-G666.

33. Pandey, R., Mousawy, K., Nagarkatti, M., & Nagarkatti, P. (2009). Endocannabinoids and immune regulation. *Pharmacological research*, 60(2), 85–92.

34. Wang, M., Meng, N., Chang, Y., & Tang, W. (2016). Endocannabinoids signaling: molecular mechanisms of liver regulation and diseases. *Front. Biosci.(Landmark Ed)*, *21*, 1488–1501.

35. Mallat, A., Teixeira-Clerc, F., Deveaux, V., Manin, S., & Lotersztajn, S. (2011). The endocannabinoid system as a key mediator during liver diseases: new insights and therapeutic openings. *British journal of pharmacology*, 163(7), 1432–1440.

36. Bazwinsky-Wutschke, I., Zipprich, A., & Dehghani, F. (2019). Endocannabinoid system in hepatic glucose metabolism, fatty liver disease, and cirrhosis. *International Journal of Molecular Sciences*, *20*(10), 2516.

37. Teixeira-Clerc, F., Julien, B., Grenard, P., Van Nhieu, J. T., Deveaux, V., Li, L., ... & Lotersztajn, S. (2006). CB1 cannabinoid receptor antagonism: a new strategy for the treatment of liver fibrosis. *Nature medicine*, 12(6), 671–676.

38. De Ternay, J., Naassila, M., Nourredine, M., Louvet, A., Bailly, F., Sescousse, G., Maurage, P., Cottencin, O., Carrieri, P. M., & Rolland, B. (2019). Therapeutic prospects of cannabidiol for alcohol use disorder and alcohol-related damages on the liver and the brain. *Frontiers in Pharmacology*, *10*, 627. https://doi.org/10.3389/fphar.2019.00627

39. Wang, M., Meng, N., Chang, Y., & Tang, W. (2016). Endocannabinoids signaling: molecular mechanisms of liver regulation and diseases. *Front. Biosci.(Landmark Ed)*, 21, 1488–1501.

40. Bazwinsky-Wutschke, I., Zipprich, A., & Dehghani, F. (2019). Endocannabinoid system in hepatic glucose metabolism, fatty liver disease, and cirrhosis. *International Journal of Molecular Sciences*, *20*(10), 2516.

41. Van Der Poorten, D., Shahidi, M., Tay, E., Sesha, J., Tran, K., McLeod, D., ... & George, J. (2010). Hepatitis C virus induces the cannabinoid receptor 1. *PLoS One*, 5(9), e12841.

42. Hézode, C., Zafrani, E. S., Roudot-Thoraval, F., Costentin, C., Hessami, A., Bouvier-Alias, M., ... & Mallat, A. (2008). Daily cannabis use: a novel risk factor of steatosis severity in patients with chronic hepatitis C. *Gastroenterology*, 134(2), 432–439.

43. Ishida, J. H., Peters, M. G., Jin, C., Louie, K., Tan, V., Bacchetti, P., & Terrault, N. A. (2008). Influence of cannabis use on severity of hepatitis C disease. *Clinical gastroenterology and hepatology*, 6(1), 69–75.

44. Brunet, L., Moodie, E. E., Rollet, K., Cooper, C., Walmsley, S., Potter, M., ... & Canadian Co-infection Cohort Investigators. (2013). Marijuana smoking does not accelerate progression of liver disease in HIV–hepatitis C coinfection: a longitudinal cohort analysis. *Clinical Infectious Diseases*, 57(5), 663–670.

45. Liu, T., Howell, G. T., Turner, L., Corace, K., Garber, G., & Cooper, C. (2014). Marijuana use in hepatitis C infection does not affect liver biopsy histology or treatment outcomes. *Canadian Journal of Gastroenterology and Hepatology*, 28.

46. Kelly, E. M., Dodge, J. L., Sarkar, M., French, A. L., Tien, P. C., Glesby, M. J., ... & Peters, M. G. (2016). Marijuana use is not associated with progression to advanced liver fibrosis in HIV/hepatitis C virus–coinfected women. *Reviews of Infectious Diseases*, 63(4), 512–518.

47. Bermúdez-Silva, F. J., Suárez, J., Baixeras, E., Cobo, N., Bautista, D., Cuesta-Muñoz, A. L., ... & Mechoulam, R. (2008). Presence of functional cannabinoid receptors in human endocrine pancreas. *Diabetologia*, 51(3), 476–487.

48. González-Mariscal, I., & Egan, J. M. (2018). Endocannabinoids in the Islets of Langerhans: the ugly, the bad, and the good facts. *American Journal of Physiology—Endocrinology and Metabolism*, 315(2), E174-E179.

49. González-Mariscal, I., & Egan, J. M. (2018). Endocannabinoids in the Islets of Langerhans: the ugly, the bad, and the good facts. *American Journal of Physiology—Endocrinology and Metabolism*, 315(2), E174-E179.

50. Veilleux, A., Di Marzo, V., & Silvestri, C. (2019). The expanded endocannabinoid system/endocannabinoidome as a potential target for treating diabetes mellitus. *Current Diabetes Reports*, 19(11), 117.

51. Reviewed in Mazier, W., Saucisse, N., Gatta-Cherifi, B., & Cota, D. (2015). The endocannabinoid system: pivotal orchestrator of obesity and metabolic disease. *Trends in Endocrinology & Metabolism*, 26(10), 524–537.

52. Reviewed in Mazier, W., Saucisse, N., Gatta-Cherifi, B., & Cota, D. (2015). The endocannabinoid system: pivotal orchestrator of obesity and metabolic disease. *Trends in Endocrinology & Metabolism*, 26(10), 524–537.

53. Reviewed in van Eenige, R., van der Stelt, M., Rensen, P. C., & Kooijman, S. (2018). Regulation of adipose tissue metabolism by the endocannabinoid system. *Trends in Endocrinology & Metabolism*, 29(5), 326–337.

54. Engeli, S., Böhnke, J., Feldpausch, M., Gorzelniak, K., Janke, J., Bátkai, S., ... & Jordan, J. (2005). Activation of the peripheral endocannabinoid system in human obesity. *Diabetes*, 54(10), 2838–2843.

55. Engeli, S., Böhnke, J., Feldpausch, M., Gorzelniak, K., Janke, J., Bátkai, S., ... & Jordan, J. (2005). Activation of the peripheral endocannabinoid system in human obesity. *Diabetes*, 54(10), 2838–2843.

56. Reviewed in Mazier, W., Saucisse, N., Gatta-Cherifi, B., & Cota, D. (2015). The endocannabinoid system: pivotal orchestrator of obesity and metabolic disease. *Trends in Endocrinology & Metabolism*, 26(10), 524–537.

57. Reviewed in van Eenige, R., van der Stelt, M., Rensen, P. C., & Kooijman, S. (2018). Regulation of adipose tissue metabolism by the endocannabinoid system. *Trends in Endocrinology & Metabolism*, 29(5), 326–337.

58. Doris, J. M., Millar, S. A., Idris, I., & O'Sullivan, S. E. (2019). Genetic polymorphisms of the endocannabinoid system in obesity and diabetes. *Diabetes, Obesity and Metabolism*, 21(2), 382–387.

59. Rossi, F., Bellini, G., Luongo, L., Manzo, I., Tolone, S., Tortora, C., ... & Nobili, B. (2016). Cannabinoid receptor 2 as antiobesity target: Inflammation, fat storage, and browning modulation. *The Journal of Clinical Endocrinology & Metabolism*, 101(9), 3469–3478.

60. McPartland, J. M. (2008). Expression of the endocannabinoid system in fibroblasts and myofascial tissues. *Journal of Bodywork and Movement Therapies*, 12(2), 169–182.

61. McPartland, J. M. (2008). The endocannabinoid system: an osteopathic perspective. *The Journal of the American Osteopathic Association*, 108(10), 586–600.

62. Maccarrone, M., Bab, I., Bíró, T., Cabral, G. A., Dey, S. K., Di Marzo, V., ... & Sharkey, K. A. (2015). Endocannabinoid signaling at the periphery: 50 years after THC. *Trends in pharmacological sciences*, 36(5), 277–296.

63. Maccarrone, M., Bab, I., Bíró, T., Cabral, G. A., Dey, S. K., Di Marzo, V., ... & Sharkey, K. A. (2015). Endocannabinoid signaling at the periphery: 50 years after THC. *Trends in pharmacological sciences*, 36(5), 277–296.

64. Yamada, Y., Ando, F., & Shimokata, H. (2007). Association of candidate gene polymorphisms with bone mineral density in community-dwelling Japanese women and men. *International Journal of Molecular Medicine*, 19(5), 791–801.

65. Tam, J., Trembovler, V., Di Marzo, V., Petrosino, S., Leo, G., Alexandrovich, A., ... & Karsak, M. (2008). The cannabinoid CB1 receptor regulates bone formation by modulating adrenergic signaling. The FASEB journal, 22(1), 285–294.

66. Wasserman, E., Tam, J., Mechoulam, R., Zimmer, A., Maor, G., & Bab, I. (2015). CB1 cannabinoid receptors mediate endochondral skeletal growth attenuation by Δ^9-tetrahydrocannabinol. Annals of the New York Academy of Sciences, 1335(1), 110–119.

67. Turcotte, C., Blanchet, M. R., Laviolette, M., & Flamand, N. (2016). Impact of cannabis, cannabinoids, and endocannabinoids in the lungs. *Frontiers in pharmacology*, 7, 317.

68. Grassin-Delyle, S., Naline, E., Buenestado, A., Faisy, C., Alvarez, J. C., Salvator, H., ... & Devillier, P. (2014). Cannabinoids inhibit cholinergic contraction in human airways through prejunctional CB1 receptors. *British journal of pharmacology*, 171(11), 2767–2777.

69. Pini, A., Mannaioni, G., Pellegrini-Giampietro, D., Beatrice Passani, M., Mastroianni, R., Bani, D., & Masini, E. (2012). The role of cannabinoids in inflammatory modulation of allergic respiratory disorders, inflammatory pain and ischemic stroke. *Current drug targets*, 13(7), 984–993.

70. Shang, V. C. M., O'Sullivan, S. E., Kendall, D. A., & Roberts, R. E. (2016). The endogenous cannabinoid anandamide increases human airway epithelial cell permeability through an arachidonic acid metabolite. *Pharmacological research*, 105, 152–163.

71. Zuardi, A. W. (2006). History of cannabis as a medicine: a review. *Brazilian Journal of Psychiatry*, 28(2), 153–157.

72. Reviewed in Chua, J. T., Argueta, D. A., DiPatrizio, N. V., Kovesdy, C. P., Vaziri, N. D., Kalantar-Zadeh, K., & Moradi, H. (2019). Endocannabinoid system and the kidneys: from renal physiology to injury and disease. *Cannabis and cannabinoid research*, 4(1), 10–20.

73. Reviewed in del Río, C., Millán, E., García, V., Appendino, G., DeMesa, J., & Muñoz, E. (2018). The endocannabinoid system of the skin. A potential approach for the treatment of skin disorders. *Biochemical pharmacology*, 157, 122–133.

74. Reviewed in Fride, E. (2008). Multiple roles for the endocannabinoid system during the earliest stages of life: Pre- and postnatal development. *Journal of Neuroendocrinology*, 20, 75–81.

75. Reviewed in Bukiya, A. N. (2019). Physiology of the endocannabinoid system during development. In *Recent advances in cannabinoid physiology and pathology* (pp. 13–37). Springer.

76. López-Cardona, A. P., Pérez-Cerezales, S., Fernández-González, R., Laguna-Barraza, R., Pericuesta, E., Agirregoitia, N., ... & Agirregoitia, E. (2017). CB1 cannabinoid receptor drives oocyte maturation and embryo development via PI3K/Akt and MAPK pathways. *The FASEB Journal*, 31(8), 3372–3382.

77. Grimaldi, P., Orlando, P., Di Siena, S., Lolicato, F., Petrosino, S., Bisogno, T., ... & Di Marzo, V. (2009). The endocannabinoid system and pivotal role of the CB2 receptor in mouse spermatogenesis. *Proceedings of the National Academy of Sciences*, 106(27), 11131–11136.

78. Rossato, M., Ion Popa, F., Ferigo, M., Clari, G., & Foresta, C. (2005). Human sperm express cannabinoid receptor

Cb1, the activation of which inhibits motility, acrosome reaction, and mitochondrial function. *The Journal of Clinical Endocrinology & Metabolism*, 90(2), 984–991.

79. Fride, E., Ginzburg, Y., Breuer, A., Bisogno, T., Di Marzo, V., & Mechoulam, R. (2001). Critical role of the endogenous cannabinoid system in mouse pup suckling and growth. *European journal of pharmacology*, 419(2-3), 207–214.

80. Reviewed in Velasco, G., Sánchez, C., & Guzmán, M. (2016). Anticancer mechanisms of cannabinoids. *Current Oncology*, *23*(Supplement 2), S23.

81. Costa, L., Amaral, C., Teixeira, N., Correia-da-Silva, G., & Fonseca, B. M. (2016). Cannabinoid-induced autophagy: Protective or death role?. *Prostaglandins & other lipid mediators*, *122*, 54–63.

82. Lissoni, P., Messina, G., Porro, G., Trampetti, R., Lissoni, A., Rovelli, F., Cenay, V., Porta, E., & Di Fede, G. (2018). The modulation of the endocannabinoid system in the treatment of cancer and other systemic human diseases. *Global Drugs and Therapeutics*, *3*, 1–4. https://doi.org/10.15761/GDT.1000163

83. Reviewed in Velasco, G., Sánchez, C., & Guzmán, M. (2016). Anticancer mechanisms of cannabinoids. *Current Oncology*, *23*(Supplement 2), S23.

84. Reviewed in Velasco, G., Sánchez, C., & Guzmán, M. (2016). Anticancer mechanisms of cannabinoids. *Current Oncology*, *23*(Supplement 2), S23.

85. Pyszniak, M., Tabarkiewicz, J., & Łuszczki, J. J. (2016). Endocannabinoid system as a regulator of tumor cell malignancy–biological pathways and clinical significance. *OncoTargets and Therapy, 9,* 4323.

86. Batty, G. D., Russ, T. C., Stamatakis, E., & Kivimäki, M. (2017). Psychological distress in relation to site specific cancer mortality: pooling of unpublished data from 16 prospective cohort studies." *The BMJ*, *356*, Article j108. https://doi.org/10.1136/bmj.j108

87. Lissoni, P., Messina, G., Lissoni, A., & Rovelli, F. (2017). The psychoneuroendocrine-immunotherapy of cancer: Historical evolution and clinical results. *Journal of Research in Medical Sciences: The Official Journal of Isfahan University of Medical Sciences*, *22*, 45. https://doi.org/10.4103/jrms.JRMS_255_16

Chapter 9: Influences on the Endocannabinoid System

1. Reviewed in Laurikainen, H., Tuominen, L., Tikka, M., Merisaari, H., Armio, R. L., Sormunen, E., ... & Solin, O. (2019). Sex difference in brain CB1 receptor availability in man. *Neuroimage*, 184, 834–842.

2. Reviewed in Craft, R. M., Marusich, J. A., & Wiley, J. L. (2013). Sex differences in cannabinoid pharmacology: A reflection of differences in the endocannabinoid system? *Life Sciences*, *92*(8–9), 476–481.

3. Wiley, J. L., O'Connell, M. M., Tokarz, M. E., & Wright, M. J. (2007). Pharmacological effects of acute and repeated administration of Δ^9-tetrahydrocannabinol in adolescent and adult rats. *Journal of Pharmacology and Experimental Therapeutics*, 320(3), 1097–1105.

4. Riebe, C. J., Hill, M. N., Lee, T. T., Hillard, C. J., & Gorzalka, B. B. (2010). Estrogenic regulation of limbic cannabinoid receptor binding. *Psychoneuroendocrinology*, 35(8), 1265–1269.

5. Scorticati, C., Fernández-Solari, J., De Laurentiis, A., Mohn, C., Prestifilippo, J. P., Lasaga, M., ... & Rettori, V. (2004). The inhibitory effect of anandamide on luteinizing hormone-releasing hormone secretion is reversed by estrogen. *Proceedings of the National Academy of Sciences*, 101(32), 11891–11896.

6. Reviewed in Laurikainen, H., Tuominen, L., Tikka, M., Merisaari, H., Armio, R. L., Sormunen, E., ... & Solin, O. (2019). Sex difference in brain CB1 receptor availability in man. *Neuroimage*, 184, 834–842.

7. Reviewed in McPartland, J. M., Guy, G. W., & Di Marzo, V. (2014). Care and feeding of the endocannabinoid system: A systematic review of potential clinical interventions that upregulate the endocannabinoid system. *PLOS ONE*, *9*(3), Article e89566.

8. Perez-Reyes, M., Burstein, S. H., White, W. R., McDonald, S. A., & Hicks, R. E. (1991). Antagonism of marihuana effects by indomethacin in humans. *Life sciences*, 48(6), 507–515.

9. Reviewed in McPartland, J. M., Guy, G. W., & Di Marzo, V. (2014). Care and feeding of the endocannabinoid system: A systematic review of potential clinical interventions that upregulate the endocannabinoid system. *PLOS ONE*, *9*(3), Article e89566.

10. Ghanem, C. I., Pérez, M. J., Manautou, J. E., & Mottino, A. D. (2016). Acetaminophen from liver to brain: new insights into drug pharmacological action and toxicity. *Pharmacological research*, 109, 119–131.

11. Reviewed in McPartland, J. M., Guy, G. W., & Di Marzo, V. (2014). Care and feeding of the endocannabinoid system: A systematic review of potential clinical interventions that upregulate the endocannabinoid system. *PLOS ONE*, *9*(3), Article e89566.

12. Reviewed in McPartland, J. M., Guy, G. W., & Di Marzo, V. (2014). Care and feeding of the endocannabinoid system: A systematic review of potential clinical interventions that upregulate the endocannabinoid system. *PLOS ONE*, *9*(3), Article e89566.

13. Nielsen, S., Sabioni, P., Trigo, J. M., Ware, M. A., Betz-Stablein, B. D., Murnion, B., Lintzeris, N., Khor, K. E., Farrell, M., Smith, A., & Le Foll, B. (2017). Opioid-sparing effect of cannabinoids: A systematic review and meta-analysis. *Neuropsychopharmacology*, *42*(9), 1752–1765.

14. Reviewed in McPartland, J. M., Guy, G. W., & Di Marzo, V. (2014). Care and feeding of the endocannabinoid system: A systematic review of potential clinical interventions that upregulate the endocannabinoid system. *PLOS ONE, 9*(3), Article e89566.

15. Reviewed in McPartland, J. M., Guy, G. W., & Di Marzo, V. (2014). Care and feeding of the endocannabinoid system: A systematic review of potential clinical interventions that upregulate the endocannabinoid system. *PLOS ONE, 9*(3), Article e89566.

16. Oppong-Damoah, A., Wood, B. J., Blough, B., & Murnane, K. S. (2019). Caryophyllene oxide is more potent than beta caryophyllene in attenuating the abuse-related effects of ethanol. *The FASEB Journal, 33*(1, supplement), 499.6.

17. Russo, E. B. (2016). Beyond cannabis: Plants and the endocannabinoid system. *Trends in Pharmacological Sciences, 37*(7), 594–605.

18. Zhang, Z., Guo, Y., Zhang, S., Zhang, Y., Wang, Y., Ni, W., ... & Zheng, S. (2013). Curcumin modulates cannabinoid receptors in liver fibrosis in vivo and inhibits extracellular matrix expression in hepatic stellate cells by suppressing cannabinoid receptor type-1 in vitro. *European journal of pharmacology, 721*(1-3), 133–140.

19. Reviewed in McPartland, J. M., Guy, G. W., & Di Marzo, V. (2014). Care and feeding of the endocannabinoid system: A systematic review of potential clinical interventions that upregulate the endocannabinoid system. *PLOS ONE, 9*(3), Article e89566.

20. Raichlen, D. A., Foster, A. D., Gerdeman, G. L., Seillier, A., & Giuffrida, A. (2012). Wired to run: exercise-induced endocannabinoid signaling in humans and cursorial mammals with implications for the 'runner's high'. *Journal of Experimental Biology, 215*(8), 1331–1336.

21. Stone, N. L., Millar, S. A., Herrod, P. J. J., Barrett, D. A., Ortori, C. A., Mellon, V. A., & O'Sullivan, S. E. (2018). An analysis of endocannabinoid concentrations and mood following singing and exercise in healthy volunteers. *Frontiers in Behavioral Neuroscience, 12*. https://doi.org/10.3389/fnbeh.2018.00269

22. Bazinet, R. P., & Layé, S. (2014). Polyunsaturated fatty acids and their metabolites in brain function and disease. *Nature Reviews Neuroscience, 15*(12), 771–785.

23. Ramsden, C. E., Zamora, D., Makriyannis, A., Wood, J. T., Mann, J. D., Faurot, K. R., ... & Davis, J. M. (2015). Diet-induced changes in n-3- and n-6-derived endocannabinoids and reductions in headache pain and psychological distress. *The Journal of Pain, 16*(8), 707–716.

24. Bosch-Bouju, C., & Layé, S. (2016). Dietary omega-6/omega-3 and endocannabinoids: Implications for brain health and diseases. In Meccariello, R. (Ed.), *Cannabinoids in health and disease* (pp. 111–142). IntechOpen.

25. Reviewed in McPartland, J. M., Guy, G. W., & Di Marzo, V. (2014). Care and feeding of the endocannabinoid system: A systematic review of potential clinical interventions that upregulate the endocannabinoid system. *PLOS ONE, 9*(3), Article e89566.

26. Kolettis, T. M., & Kolettis, M. T. (2003). Winter swimming: healthy or hazardous? Evidence and hypotheses. *Medical Hypotheses, 61*(5–6), 654–656.

27. Gibas-Dorna, M., Chęcińska, Z., Korek, E., Kupsz, J., Sowińska, A., & Krauss, H. (2016). Cold water swimming beneficially modulates insulin sensitivity in middle-aged individuals. *Journal of aging and physical activity, 24*(4), 547–554.

28. Pan, Y., Xiong, W., Yang, M., & Yan, D. (2015). Effect of winter swimming on blood lipid, Cr and UA of middle women." *Chongqing Medicine, 25*, 3529–3530.

29. Muzik, O., Reilly, K. T., & Diwadkar, V. A. (2018). "Brain over body"—A study on the willful regulation of autonomic function during cold exposure. *NeuroImage, 172*, 632–641.

30. van Eenige, R., van der Stelt, M., Rensen, P. C., & Kooijman, S. (2018). Regulation of adipose tissue metabolism by the endocannabinoid system. *Trends in Endocrinology & Metabolism, 29*(5), 326–337.

31. Gordon, K., Blondin, D. P., Friesen, B. J., Tingelstad, H. C., Kenny, G. P., & Haman, F. (2019). Seven days of cold acclimation substantially reduces shivering intensity and increases nonshivering thermogenesis in adult humans. *Journal of Applied Physiology, 126*(6), 1598–1606.

32. Buijze, G. A., De Jong, H. M. Y., Kox, M., van de Sande, M. G., Van Schaardenburg, D., Van Vugt, R. M., ... & Baeten, D. L. P. (2019). An add-on training program involving breathing exercises, cold exposure, and meditation attenuates inflammation and disease activity in axial spondyloarthritis–A proof of concept trial. *Plos one, 14*(12), e0225749.

33. Kox, M., van Eijk, L. T., Zwaag, J., van den Wildenberg, J., Sweep, F. C., van der Hoeven, J. G., & Pickkers, P. (2014). Voluntary activation of the sympathetic nervous system and attenuation of the innate immune response in humans. *Proceedings of the National Academy of Sciences, 111*(20), 7379–7384.

34. Grajower, M. M., & Horne, B. D. (2019). Clinical management of intermittent fasting in patients with diabetes mellitus. *Nutrients, 11*(4), 873.

35. Reviewed in Hillard, C. J. (2018). Circulating endocannabinoids: From whence do they come and where are they going? *Neuropsychopharmacology, 43*(1), 155.

36. Reviewed in McPartland, J. M., Guy, G. W., & Di Marzo, V. (2014). Care and feeding of the endocannabinoid system: A systematic review of potential clinical interventions that upregulate the endocannabinoid system. *PLOS ONE, 9*(3), Article e89566.

37. Onifer, S. M., Sozio, R. S., & Long, C. R. (2019). Role for endocannabinoids in spinal manipulative therapy analgesia? *Evidence-Based Complementary and Alternative Medicine*, *2019*, Article 2878352. https://doi.org/10.1155/2019/2878352

38. Chen, L., Zhang, J., Li, F., Qiu, Y., Wang, L., Li, Y. H., ... & Li, M. (2009). Endogenous anandamide and cannabinoid receptor-2 contribute to electroacupuncture analgesia in rats. *The Journal of Pain*, *10*(7), 732–739.

39. Xue, F., Xue, S. S., Liu, L., Sang, H. F., Ma, Q. R., Tan, Q. R., ... & Peng, Z. W. (2019). Early intervention with electroacupuncture prevents PTSD-like behaviors in rats through enhancing hippocampal endocannabinoid signaling. *Progress in Neuro-Psychopharmacology and Biological Psychiatry*, *93*, 171–181.

40. May, L. M., Kosek, P., Zeidan, F., & Berkman, E. T. (2018). Enhancement of meditation analgesia by opioid antagonist in experienced meditators. *Psychosomatic medicine*, *80*(9), 807.

Chapter 10: Endocannabinoid System Dysfunction

1. Reviewed in Russo, E. B. (2016). Clinical endocannabinoid deficiency reconsidered: current research supports the theory in migraine, fibromyalgia, irritable bowel, and other treatment-resistant syndromes. *Cannabis and Cannabinoid Research*, *1*(1), 154–165.

2. Bouaziz, J., Bar On, A., Seidman, D. S., & Soriano, D. (2017). The clinical significance of endocannabinoids in endometriosis pain management. *Cannabis and Cannabinoid Research*, *2*(1), 72–80.

3. Aran, A., Eylon, M., Harel, M., Polianski, L., Nemirovski, A., Tepper, S., ... & Tam, J. (2019). Lower circulating endocannabinoid levels in children with autism spectrum disorder. *Molecular autism*, *10*(1), 1–11.

4. Ambrose, T., & Simmons, A. (2019). Cannabis, cannabinoids, and the endocannabinoid system—is there therapeutic potential for inflammatory bowel disease? *Journal of Crohn's and Colitis*, *13*(4), 525–535.

5. Storr, M. A., Yüce, B., Andrews, C. N., & Sharkey, K. A. (2008). The role of the endocannabinoid system in the pathophysiology and treatment of irritable bowel syndrome. *Neurogastroenterology & Motility*, *20*(8), 857–868.

6. Reviewed in Russo, E. B. (2016). Clinical endocannabinoid deficiency reconsidered: current research supports the theory in migraine, fibromyalgia, irritable bowel, and other treatment-resistant syndromes. *Cannabis and Cannabinoid Research*, *1*(1), 154–165.

7. Hill, M. N., & Lee, F. S. (2016). Endocannabinoids and stress resilience: Is deficiency sufficient to promote vulnerability? *Biological Psychiatry*, *79*(10), 792.

8. Elliott, M. B., Ward, S. J., Abood, M. E., Tuma, R. F., & Jallo, J. I. (2017). Understanding the endocannabinoid system as a modulator of the trigeminal pain response to concussion. *Concussion*, *2*(4), CNC49.

9. Ujike, H., Takaki, M., Nakata, K., Tanaka, Y., Takeda, T., Kodama, M., ... & Kuroda, S. (2002). CNR1, central cannabinoid receptor gene, associated with susceptibility to hebephrenic schizophrenia. *Molecular psychiatry*, *7*(5), 515–518.

10. Schmidt, L. G., Samochowiec, J., Finckh, U., Fiszer-Piosik, E., Horodnicki, J., Wendel, B., ... & Hoehe, M. R. (2002). Association of a CB1 cannabinoid receptor gene (CNR1) polymorphism with severe alcohol dependence. *Drug and alcohol dependence*, *65*(3), 221–224.

11. Gazzerro, P., Caruso, M. G., Notarnicola, M., Misciagna, G., Guerra, V., Laezza, C., & Bifulco, M. (2007). Association between cannabinoid type-1 receptor polymorphism and body mass index in a southern Italian population. *International journal of obesity*, *31*(6), 908–912.

12. Jaeger, J. P., Mattevi, V. S., Callegari-Jacques, S. M., & Hutz, M. H. (2008). Cannabinoid type-1 receptor gene polymorphisms are associated with central obesity in a Southern Brazilian population. *Disease markers*, *25*(1), 67–74.

13. Lu, A. T., Ogdie, M. N., Järvelin, M. R., Moilanen, I. K., Loo, S. K., McCracken, J. T., ... & Cantor, R. M. (2008). Association of the cannabinoid receptor gene (CNR1) with ADHD and post-traumatic stress disorder. *American Journal of Medical Genetics Part B: Neuropsychiatric Genetics*, *147*(8), 1488–1494.

14. Matsunaga, M., Isowa, T., Yamakawa, K., Fukuyama, S., Shinoda, J., Yamada, J., & Ohira, H. (2014). Genetic variations in the human cannabinoid receptor gene are associated with happiness. *PloS one*, *9*(4), e93771.

15. De Luis, D. A., Ballesteros, M., Lopez Guzman, A., Ruiz, E., Muñoz, C., Penacho, M. A., ... & Delgado, M. (2016). Polymorphism G1359A of the cannabinoid receptor gene (CNR 1): allelic frequencies and influence on cardiovascular risk factors in a multicentre study of Castilla-Leon. *Journal of Human Nutrition and Dietetics*, *29*(1), 112–117.

16. Wasilewski, A., Lewandowska, U., Mosinska, P., Watala, C., Storr, M., Fichna, J., & Venkatesan, T. (2017). Cannabinoid receptor type 1 and mu-opioid receptor polymorphisms are associated with cyclic vomiting syndrome. *American Journal of Gastroenterology*, *112*(6), 933–939.

17. Habib, A. M., Okorokov, A. L., Hill, M. N., Bras, J. T., Lee, M.-C., Li, S., Gossage, S. J., van Drimmelen, M., Morena, M., Houlden, H., Ramirez, J. D., Bennett, D. L. H., Srivastava, D. & Cox, J. J. (2019). Microdeletion in a *FAAH* pseudogene identified in a patient with high anandamide concentrations and pain insensitivity. *British Journal of Anaesthesia*, *123*(2), e249–e253. https://doi.org/10.1016/j.bja.2019.02.019

18. Richards, J. R. (2017). Cannabinoid hyperemesis syndrome: a disorder of the HPA axis and sympathetic nervous system? *Medical Hypotheses*, *103*, 90–95.

19. Hodges, E. L., & Ashpole, N. M. (2019). Aging circadian rhythms and cannabinoids. *Neurobiology of Aging*, *79*, 110–118. https://doi.org/10.1016/j.neurobiolaging.2019.03.008

Chapter 11: Osteopathic Perspectives on the Endocannabinoid System

1. Still, A. T. (1897). *Autobiography of Andrew T. Still*. A. T. Still.
2. McPartland, J. M., Giuffrida, A., King, J., Skinner, E., Scotter, J., & Musty, R. E. (2005). Cannabimimetic effects of osteopathic manipulative treatment. *Journal of the American Osteopathic Association*, *105*(6), 283.
3. Jealous, J. Personal Communication. Cited by McPartland, J. M., & Skinner, E. (2005). The biodynamic model of osteopathy in the cranial field. *Explore (NY)*, *1*, 21–32.
4. McPartland, J. M. (2008). The endocannabinoid system: an osteopathic perspective. *The Journal of the American Osteopathic Association*, *108*(10), 586–600.
5. Still, A. T. (1899). *Philosophy of osteopathy*. Academy of Applied Osteopathy.
6. Still, A. T. (1897). *Autobiography of Andrew T. Still*. A. T. Still.
7. Hohmann, A. G., & Herkenham, M. (1999). Cannabinoid receptors undergo axonal flow in sensory nerves. *Neuroscience*, *92*(4), 1171–1175.
8. McPartland, J. M. (2008). The endocannabinoid system: an osteopathic perspective. *The Journal of the American Osteopathic Association*, *108*(10), 586–600.

Chapter 12: Clinically Relevant Botany

1. McPartland, J. M., Hegman, W., & Long, T. (2019). Cannabis in Asia: Its center of origin and early cultivation, based on a synthesis of subfossil pollen and archaeobotanical studies. *Vegetation History and Archaeobotany*, *28*, 691–702.
2. Bonini, S. A., Premoli, M., Tambaro, S., Kumar, A., Maccarinelli, G., Memo, M., & Mastinu, A. (2018). Cannabis sativa: A comprehensive ethnopharmacological review of a medicinal plant with a long history. *Journal of ethnopharmacology*, *227*, 300–315.
3. Russo, E. B., & Marcu, J. (2017). Cannabis pharmacology: The usual suspects and a few promising leads. *Advances in Pharmacology*, *80*, 67–134.
4. Lewis, M. A., Russo, E. B., & Smith, K. M. (2018). Pharmacological foundations of cannabis chemovars. *Planta Medica*, *84*(4), 225–233.
5. Winston, M. E., Hampton-Marcell, J., Zarraonaindia, I., Owens, S. M., Moreau, C. S., Gilbert, J. A., ... & Gibbons, S. M. (2014). Understanding cultivar-specificity and soil determinants of the cannabis microbiome. *PLoS one*, *9*(6), e99641.
6. McKernan, K., Spangler, J., Zhang, L., Tadigotla, V., Helbert, Y., Foss, T., & Smith, D. (2015). Cannabis microbiome sequencing reveals several mycotoxic fungi native to dispensary grade cannabis flowers. *F1000Research*, *4*, 1422. https://doi.org/10.12688/f1000research.7507.2
7. Ruchlemer, R., Amit-Kohn, M., Raveh, D., & Hanuš, L. (2015). Inhaled medicinal cannabis and the immunocompromised patient. *Supportive Care in Cancer*, *23*(3), 819–822.
8. Ryz, N. R., Remillard, D. J., & Russo, E. B. (2017). Cannabis roots: A traditional therapy with future potential for treating inflammation and pain. *Cannabis and Cannabinoid Research*, *2*(1), 210–216.
9. McPartland, J. M. (2018). Cannabis systematics at the levels of family, genus, and species. *Cannabis and Cannabinoid Research*, *3*(1), 203–212.
10. Russo, E. B. (2018). The case for the entourage effect and conventional breeding of clinical cannabis: No "strain," no gain. *Frontiers in Plant Science*, *9*, 1969.

Chapter 13: Phytocannabinoid Pharmacology

1. Hanuš, L. O., Meyer, S. M., Muñoz, E., Taglialatela-Scafati, O., & Appendino, G. (2016). Phytocannabinoids: a unified critical inventory. *Natural product reports*, 33(12), 1357–1392.
2. Baram, L., Peled, E., Berman, P., Yellin, B., Besser, E., Benami, M., ... & Meiri, D. (2019). The heterogeneity and complexity of Cannabis extracts as antitumor agents. *Oncotarget*, 10(41), 4091.
3. Pertwee, R. G. (2014). Part 2: Pharmacology, Pharmacokinetics, Metabolism, and Forensics. In *Handbook of Cannabis* (pp. 111–316). Oxford Scholarship Online. https://doi.org/10.1093/acprof:oso/9780199662685.011.0002
4. Russo, E. B., & Marcu, J. (2017). Cannabis pharmacology: the usual suspects and a few promising leads. *Advances in Pharmacology*, *80*, 67–134.
5. Hanuš, L. O., Meyer, S. M., Muñoz, E., Taglialatela-Scafati, O., & Appendino, G. (2016). Phytocannabinoids: a unified critical inventory. *Natural product reports*, 33(12), 1357–1392.
6. McPartland, J. M., MacDonald, C., Young, M., Grant, P. S., Furkert, D. P., & Glass, M. (2017). Affinity and efficacy stud-

ies of tetrahydrocannabinolic acid A at cannabinoid receptor types one and two. *Cannabis and cannabinoid research*, *2*(1), 87–95.

7. Grunfeld, Y., & Edery, H. (1969). Psychopharmacological activity of the active constituents of hashish and some related cannabinoids. *Psychopharmacologia*, *14*, 200–210.

8. Moreno-Sanz, G. (2016). Can you pass the acid test? Critical review and novel therapeutic perspectives of Δ⁹-tetrahydrocannabinolic acid A. *Cannabis and Cannabinoid Research*, *1*(1), 124–130.

9. Nallathambi, R., Mazuz, M., Ion, A., Selvaraj, G., Weininger, S., Fridlender, M., ... & Mendelovitz, M. (2017). Anti-inflammatory activity in colon models is derived from Δ⁹-tetrahydrocannabinolic acid that interacts with additional compounds in cannabis extracts. *Cannabis and cannabinoid research*, *2*(1), 167–182.

10. Rock, E. M., Kopstick, R. L., Limebeer, C. L., & Parker, L. A. (2013). Tetrahydrocannabinolic acid reduces nausea-induced conditioned gaping in rats and vomiting in S uncus murinus. *British journal of pharmacology*, *170*(3), 641–648.

11. Anderson, L. L., Low, I. K., Banister, S. D., McGregor, I. S., & Arnold, J. C. (2019). Pharmacokinetics of phytocannabinoid acids and anticonvulsant effect of cannabidiolic acid in a mouse model of Dravet syndrome. *Journal of Natural Products*, *82*(11), 3047–3055. https://doi.org/10.1021/acs.jnatprod.9b00600

12. Sulak, D., Saneto, R., & Goldstein, B. (2017). The current status of artisanal cannabis for the treatment of epilepsy in the United States. *Epilepsy & Behavior*, *70*, 328–333.

13. Hanael, E., Veksler, R., Friedman, A., Bar-Klein, G., Senatorov Jr, V. V., Kaufer, D., ... & Shamir, M. H. (2019). Blood-brain barrier dysfunction in canine epileptic seizures detected by dynamic contrast-enhanced magnetic resonance imaging. *Epilepsia*, *60*(5), 1005–1016.

14. Karler, R., & Turkanis, S. A. (1979). Cannabis and epilepsy. In G. G. Nahas and W. D. M. Paton (Eds.), *Marihuana biological effects: Analysis, metabolism, cellular responses, reproduction and brain* (pp. 619–641). Pergamon Press.

15. McPartland, J. M., MacDonald, C., Young, M., Grant, P. S., Furkert, D. P., & Glass, M. (2017). Affinity and efficacy studies of tetrahydrocannabinolic acid A at cannabinoid receptor types one and two. *Cannabis and cannabinoid research*, *2*(1), 87–95.

16. Hazekamp, A., Bastola, K., Rashidi, H., Bender, J., & Verpoorte, R. (2007). Cannabis tea revisited: A systematic evaluation of the cannabinoid composition of cannabis tea. *Journal of Ethnopharmacology*, *113*(1), 85–90.

17. Pellesi, L., Licata, M., Verri, P., Vandelli, D., Palazzoli, F., Marchesi, F., ... & Guerzoni, S. (2018). Pharmacokinetics and tolerability of oral cannabis preparations in patients with medication overuse headache (MOH)—a pilot study. *European Journal of Clinical Pharmacology*, *74*(11), 1427–1436.

18. Bih, C. I., Chen, T., Nunn, A. V., Bazelot, M., Dallas, M., & Whalley, B. J. (2015). Molecular targets of cannabidiol in neurological disorders. *Neurotherapeutics*, *12*(4), 699–730.

19. Laprairie, R. B., Bagher, A. M., Kelly, M. E. M., & Denovan-Wright, E. M. (2015). Cannabidiol is a negative allosteric modulator of the cannabinoid CB1 receptor. *British journal of pharmacology*, *172*(20), 4790–4805.

20. Morales, P., Goya, P., Jagerovic, N., & Hernandez-Folgado, L. (2016). Allosteric modulators of the CB1 cannabinoid receptor: a structural update review. *Cannabis and Cannabinoid Research*, *1*(1), 22–30.

21. Martínez-Pinilla, E., Varani, K., Reyes-Resina, I., Angelats, E., Vincenzi, F., Ferreiro-Vera, C., ... & Navarro, G. (2017). Binding and signaling studies disclose a potential allosteric site for cannabidiol in cannabinoid CB2 receptors. *Frontiers in pharmacology*, *8*, 744.

22. Navarro, G., Reyes-Resina, I., Rivas-Santisteban, R., de Medina, V. S., Morales, P., Casano, S., ... & Nadal, X. (2018). Cannabidiol skews biased agonism at cannabinoid CB1 and CB2 receptors with smaller effect in CB1-CB2 heteroreceptor complexes. *Biochemical Pharmacology*, *157*, 148–158.

23. Bih, C. I., Chen, T., Nunn, A. V., Bazelot, M., Dallas, M., & Whalley, B. J. (2015). Molecular targets of cannabidiol in neurological disorders. *Neurotherapeutics*, *12*(4), 699–730.

24. Raymundi, A. M., da Silva, T. R., Zampronio, A. R., Guimarães, F. S., Bertoglio, L. J., & Stern, C. A. J. (2020). A time-dependent contribution of hippocampal CB1, CB2, and PPARγ receptors to cannabidiol-induced disruption of fear memory consolidation. *British Journal of Pharmacology*, *177*(4), 945–957. https://doi.org/10.1111/bph.14895

25. Bi, G.-H., Galaj, E., He, Y., & Xi, Z.-X. (2020). Cannabidiol inhibits sucrose self-administration by CB1 and CB2 receptor mechanisms in rodents. *Addiction Biology*, *25*(4), Article e12783. https://doi.org/10.1111/adb.12783

26. Russo, E. B., Burnett, A., Hall, B., & Parker, K. K. (2005). Agonistic properties of cannabidiol at 5-HT1a receptors. *Neurochemical research*, *30*(8), 1037–1043.

27. Resstel, L. B., Tavares, R. F., Lisboa, S. F., Joca, S. R., Corrêa, F. M., & Guimarães, F. S. (2009). 5-HT1A receptors are involved in the cannabidiol-induced attenuation of behavioural and cardiovascular responses to acute restraint stress in rats. *British journal of pharmacology*, *156*(1), 181–188.

28. de Paula Soares, V., Campos, A. C., de Bortoli, V. C., Zangrossi Jr, H., Guimarães, F. S., & Zuardi, A. W. (2010). Intra-dorsal periaqueductal gray administration of cannabidiol blocks panic-like response by activating 5-HT1A receptors. *Behavioural brain research*, *213*(2), 225–229.

29. Mishima, K., Hayakawa, K., Abe, K., Ikeda, T., Egashira, N., Iwasaki, K., & Fujiwara, M. (2005). Cannabidiol prevents

cerebral infarction via a serotonergic 5-hydroxytryptamine1A receptor–dependent mechanism. *Stroke, 36*(5), 1071–1076.

30. Limebeer, C. L., Litt, D. E., & Parker, L. A. (2009). Effect of 5-HT3 antagonists and a 5-HT1A agonist on fluoxetine-induced conditioned gaping reactions in rats. *Psychopharmacology, 203*(4), 763.

31. Magen, I. (2009). *The Effects of Cannabidiol (CBD) on Brain Dysfunction Induced by Bile Duct Ligation in Mice.* Hebrew University.

32. Gonca, E., & Darıcı, F. (2015). The effect of cannabidiol on ischemia/reperfusion-induced ventricular arrhythmias: The role of adenosine A1 receptors. *Journal of Cardiovascular Pharmacology and Therapeutics, 20,* 76–83.

33. Mecha, M., Feliú, A., Iñigo, P. M., Mestre, L., Carrillo-Salinas, F. J., & Guaza, C. (2013). Cannabidiol provides long-lasting protection against the deleterious effects of inflammation in a viral model of multiple sclerosis: A role for A2A receptors. *Neurobiology of Disease, 59,* 141–150.

34. Castillo, A., Tolón, M. R., Fernández-Ruiz, J., Romero, J., & Martinez-Orgado, J. (2010). The neuroprotective effect of cannabidiol in an in vitro model of newborn hypoxic-ischemic brain damage in mice is mediated by CB(2) and adenosine receptors. *Neurobiology of Disease, 37,* 434–440.

35. Xiong, W., Cui, T., Cheng, K., Yang, F., Chen, S. R., Willenbring, D., ... & Zhang, L. (2012). Cannabinoids suppress inflammatory and neuropathic pain by targeting α3 glycine receptors. *Journal of Experimental Medicine, 209*(6), 1121–1134.

36. Lu, J., Fan, S., Zou, G., Hou, Y., Pan, T., Guo, W., ... & Zhang, L. (2018). Involvement of glycine receptor α1 subunits in cannabinoid-induced analgesia. *Neuropharmacology, 133,* 224–232.

37. Becker, C. M., Hermans-Borgmeyer, I., Schmitt, B., & Betz, H. (1986). The glycine receptor deficiency of the mutant mouse spastic: evidence for normal glycine receptor structure and localization. *Journal of Neuroscience, 6*(5), 1358–1364.

38. Seeman, P. (2016). Cannabidiol is a partial agonist at dopamine D2High receptors, predicting its antipsychotic clinical dose. *Translational Psychiatry, 6*(10), e920.

39. Chiurchiù, V., Lanuti, M., De Bardi, M., Battistini, L., & Maccarrone, M. (2015). The differential characterization of GPR55 receptor in human peripheral blood reveals a distinctive expression in monocytes and NK cells and a proinflammatory role in these innate cells. *International immunology, 27*(3), 153–160.

40. McHugh, D., Tanner, C., Mechoulam, R., Pertwee, R. G., & Ross, R. A. (2008). Inhibition of human neutrophil chemotaxis by endogenous cannabinoids and phytocannabinoids: evidence for a site distinct from CB1 and CB2. *Molecular pharmacology, 73*(2), 441–450.

41. Gray, R. A., & Whalley, B. J. (2020). The proposed mechanisms of action of CBD in epilepsy. *Epileptic Disorders, 22,* S10-S15.

42. Chahl, L. A. (2007). TRP's: links to schizophrenia? *Biochimica et Biophysica Acta (BBA)—Molecular Basis of Disease, 1772*(8), 968–977.

43. Campos, A. C., Moreira, F. A., Gomes, F. V., Del Bel, E. A., & Guimaraes, F. S. (2012). Multiple mechanisms involved in the large-spectrum therapeutic potential of cannabidiol in psychiatric disorders. Philosophical Transactions of the Royal Society B: Biological Sciences, 367(1607), 3364–3378.

44. Rimmerman, N., Ben-Hail, D., Porat, Z., Juknat, A., Kozela, E., Daniels, M. P., ... & Vogel, Z. (2013). Direct modulation of the outer mitochondrial membrane channel, voltage-dependent anion channel 1 (VDAC1) by cannabidiol: a novel mechanism for cannabinoid-induced cell death. Cell death & disease, 4(12), e949-e949.

45. Olivas-Aguirre, M., Torres-López, L., Valle-Reyes, J. S., Hernández-Cruz, A., Pottosin, I., & Dobrovinskaya, O. (2019). Cannabidiol directly targets mitochondria and disturbs calcium homeostasis in acute lymphoblastic leukemia. Cell death & disease, 10(10), 1–19.

46. Takeda, S., Misawa, K., Yamamoto, I., & Watanabe, K. (2008). Cannabidiolic acid as a selective cyclooxygenase-2 inhibitory component in cannabis. Drug metabolism and disposition, 36(9), 1917–1921.

47. Rock, E. M., & Parker, L. A. (2013). Effect of low doses of cannabidiolic acid and ondansetron on LiCl-induced conditioned gaping (a model of nausea-induced behaviour) in rats. British Journal of Pharmacology, 169(3), 685–692.

48. Rock, E. M., Limebeer, C. L., & Parker, L. A. (2018). Effect of cannabidiolic acid and Δ⁹-tetrahydrocannabinol on carrageenan-induced hyperalgesia and edema in a rodent model of inflammatory pain. Psychopharmacology, 235(11), 3259–3271.

49. Anderson, L. L., Low, I. K., Banister, S. D., McGregor, I. S., & Arnold, J. C. (2019). Pharmacokinetics of phytocannabinoid acids and anticonvulsant effect of cannabidiolic acid in a mouse model of Dravet syndrome. Journal of Natural Products, 82(11), 3047–3055. https://doi.org/10.1021/acs.jnatprod.9b00600

50. Bolognini, D., et al. (2013). Cannabidiolic acid prevents vomiting in Suncus murinus and nausea-induced behaviour in rats by enhancing 5-HT1A receptor activation. British Journal of Pharmacology, 168(6), 1456–1470.

51. Rock, E. M., Limebeer, C. L., Petrie, G. N., Williams, L. A., Mechoulam, R., & Parker, L. A. (2017). Effect of prior foot shock stress and Δ 9-tetrahydrocannabinol, cannabidiolic acid, and cannabidiol on anxiety-like responding in the light-dark emergence test in rats. Psychopharmacology, 234(14), 2207–2217.

52. Ligresti, A., Moriello, A. S., Starowicz, K., Matias, I., Pisanti, S., De Petrocellis, L., ... & Di Marzo, V. (2006). Antitumor

activity of plant cannabinoids with emphasis on the effect of cannabidiol on human breast carcinoma. Journal of Pharmacology and Experimental Therapeutics, 318(3), 1375–1387.

53. Rock, E. M., Limebeer, C. L., & Parker, L. A. (2018). Effect of cannabidiolic acid and Δ^9-tetrahydrocannabinol on carrageenan-induced hyperalgesia and edema in a rodent model of inflammatory pain. Psychopharmacology, 235(11), 3259–3271.

54. De Petrocellis, L., Vellani, V., Schiano-Moriello, A., Marini, P., Magherini, P. C., Orlando, P., & Di Marzo, V. (2008). Plant-derived cannabinoids modulate the activity of transient receptor potential channels of ankyrin type-1 and melastatin type-8. Journal of Pharmacology and Experimental Therapeutics, 325(3), 1007–1015.

55. Guimaraes, M. Z. P., & Jordt, S.-E. (2006). 11TRPA1: A Sensory Channel of Many Talents. In W. B. Liedtke & S. Heller (Eds.), TRP Ion Channel Function in Sensory Transduction and Cellular Signaling Cascades, (pp. 151–162). CRC Press/Taylor & Francis.

56. Kunkler, P. E., Ballard, C. J., Oxford, G. S., & Hurley, J. H. (2011). TRPA1 receptors mediate environmental irritant-induced meningeal vasodilatation. PAIN®, 152(1), 38–44.

57. De Petrocellis, L., Vellani, V., Schiano-Moriello, A., Marini, P., Magherini, P. C., Orlando, P., & Di Marzo, V. (2008). Plant-derived cannabinoids modulate the activity of transient receptor potential channels of ankyrin type-1 and melastatin type-8. Journal of Pharmacology and Experimental Therapeutics, 325(3), 1007–1015.

58. Wang, J., et al. (2019). Transient receptor potential melastatin 8 (TRPM8)-based mechanisms underlie both the cold temperature-induced inflammatory reactions and the synergistic effect of cigarette smoke in human bronchial epithelial (16HBE) cells. Frontiers in Physiology, 10, 285.

59. Iqbal, M., Mustafa, N. R., Henrie, A. A. J., Korthout, Y. H. C., & Verpoorte, R. (2013). Evaluation of anti-TNF-α activity of eight major cannabinoids isolated from Cannabis sativa. In M. Iqbal, NMR-based Metabolomics to Identify Bioactive Compounds in Herbs and Fruits (Chapter 4, pp. 97–112) [Doctoral thesis, Leiden University]. Leiden University Repository. http://hdl.handle.net/1887/20902

60. Takeda, S., Misawa, K., Yamamoto, I., & Watanabe, K. (2008). Cannabidiolic acid as a selective cyclooxygenase-2 inhibitory component in cannabis. Drug metabolism and disposition, 36(9), 1917–1921.

61. Ruhaak, L. R., Felth, J., Karlsson, P. C., Rafter, J. J., Verpoorte, R., & Bohlin, L. (2011). Evaluation of the cyclooxygenase inhibiting effects of six major cannabinoids isolated from Cannabis sativa. Biological and Pharmaceutical Bulletin, 34(5), 774–778.

62. Takeda, S., Himeno, T., Kakizoe, K., Okazaki, H., Okada, T., Watanabe, K., & Aramaki, H. (2017). Cannabidiolic acid-mediated selective down-regulation of c-fos in highly aggressive breast cancer MDA-MB-231 cells: Possible involvement of its down-regulation in the abrogation of aggressiveness. Journal of Natural Medicines, 71(1), 286–291.

63. Takeda, S., Okazaki, H., Kohro-Ikeda, E., Yoshida, K., Tokuyasu, M., Takemoto, Y., ... & Aramaki, H. (2015). DNA microarray analysis of genes in highly metastatic 4T1E/M3 murine breast cancer cells following exposure to cannabidiolic acid. Fundamental Toxicological Sciences, 2(2), 89–94.

64. Takeda, S., Okajima, S., Miyoshi, H., Yoshida, K., Okamoto, Y., Okada, T., ... & Aramaki, H. (2012). Cannabidiolic acid, a major cannabinoid in fiber-type cannabis, is an inhibitor of MDA-MB-231 breast cancer cell migration. Toxicology letters, 214(3), 314–319.

65. Takeda, S., Himeno, T., Kakizoe, K., Okazaki, H., Okada, T., Watanabe, K., & Aramaki, H. (2017). Cannabidiolic acid-mediated selective down-regulation of c-fos in highly aggressive breast cancer MDA-MB-231 cells: Possible involvement of its down-regulation in the abrogation of aggressiveness. Journal of Natural Medicines, 71(1), 286–291.

66. van de Donk, T., et al. (2019). An experimental randomized study on the analgesic effects of pharmaceutical-grade cannabis in chronic pain patients with fibromyalgia. PAIN, 160(4), 860.

67. Rock, E. M., Limebeer, C. L., & Parker, L. A. (2018). Effect of cannabidiolic acid and Δ^9-tetrahydrocannabinol on carrageenan-induced hyperalgesia and edema in a rodent model of inflammatory pain. Psychopharmacology, 235(11), 3259–3271.

68. Pellesi, L., Licata, M., Verri, P., Vandelli, D., Palazzoli, F., Marchesi, F., ... & Guerzoni, S. (2018). Pharmacokinetics and tolerability of oral cannabis preparations in patients with medication overuse headache (MOH)—a pilot study. European Journal of Clinical Pharmacology, 74(11), 1427–1436.

69. Ross, S. A., & ElSohly, M. A. (1997). CBN and Δ^9-THC concentration ratio as an indicator of the age of stored marijuana samples. Bulletin on Narcotics, 49(50), 139.

70. D'Aniello, E., Fellous, T., Iannotti, F. A., Gentile, A., Allarà, M., Balestrieri, F., ... & Di Marzo, V. (2019). Identification and characterization of phytocannabinoids as novel dual PPARα/γ agonists by a computational and in vitro experimental approach. Biochimica et Biophysica Acta (BBA)-General Subjects, 1863(3), 586–597.

71. Jadoon, K. A., Ratcliffe, S. H., Barrett, D. A., Thomas, E. L., Stott, C., Bell, J. D., ... & Tan, G. D. (2016). Efficacy and safety of cannabidiol and tetrahydrocannabivarin on glycemic and lipid parameters in patients with type 2 diabetes: a randomized, double-blind, placebo-controlled, parallel group pilot study. Diabetes Care, 39(10), 1777–1786.

72. Englund, A., Atakan, Z., Kralj, A., Tunstall, N., Murray, R., & Morrison, P. (2016). The effect of five day dosing with

THCV on THC-induced cognitive, psychological and physiological effects in healthy male human volunteers: a placebo-controlled, double-blind, crossover pilot trial. Journal of Psychopharmacology, 30(2), 140–151.

73. Pertwee, R. G. (2014). Part 2: Pharmacology, Pharmacokinetics, Metabolism, and Forensics. In Handbook of Cannabis (pp. 111–316). Oxford Scholarship Online. https://doi.org/10.1093/acprof:oso/9780199662685.011.0002

74. Lucas, C. J., Galettis, P., & Schneider, J. (2018). The pharmacokinetics and the pharmacodynamics of cannabinoids. British Journal of Clinical Pharmacology, 84(11), 2477–2482.

75. Oh, D. A., Parikh, N. Khurana, V., Smith, C. C., & Vetticaden, S. (2017). Effect of food on the pharmacokinetics of dronabinol oral solution versus dronabinol capsules in healthy volunteers. Clinical Pharmacology: Advances and Applications, 9, 9–17. https://doi.org/10.2147/CPAA.S119676

76. Karschner, E. L., Darwin, W. D., Goodwin, R. S., Wright, S., & Huestis, M. A. (2011). Plasma cannabinoid pharmacokinetics following controlled oral Δ^9-tetrahydrocannabinol and oromucosal cannabis extract administration. Clinical chemistry, 57(1), 66–75.

77. Oh, D. A., Parikh, N. Khurana, V., Smith, C. C., & Vetticaden, S. (2017). Effect of food on the pharmacokinetics of dronabinol oral solution versus dronabinol capsules in healthy volunteers. Clinical Pharmacology: Advances and Applications, 9, 9–17. https://doi.org/10.2147/CPAA.S119676

78. Taylor, L., Gidal, B., Blakey, G., Tayo, B., & Morrison, G. (2018). A phase I, randomized, double-blind, placebo-controlled, single ascending dose, multiple dose, and food effect trial of the safety, tolerability and pharmacokinetics of highly purified cannabidiol in healthy subjects. CNS drugs, 32(11), 1053–1067.

79. ElSohly, M. A., Gul, W., & Walker, L. A. (2018). Pharmacokinetics and tolerability of Δ^9-THC-hemisuccinate in a suppository formulation as an alternative to capsules for the systemic delivery of Δ^9-THC. Medical Cannabis and Cannabinoids, 1(1), 44–53.

80. Jiang, Q., Wu, Y., Zhang, H., Liu, P., Yao, J., Yao, P., ... & Duan, J. (2017). Development of essential oils as skin permeation enhancers: penetration enhancement effect and mechanism of action. Pharmaceutical Biology, 55(1), 1592–1600.

81. Stinchcomb, A. L., Valiveti, S., Hammell, D. C., & Ramsey, D. R. (2004). Human skin permeation of Δ^8-tetrahydrocannabinol, cannabidiol and cannabinol. Journal of pharmacy and pharmacology, 56(3), 291–297.

82. Anderson, L. L., Low, I. K., Banister, S. D., McGregor, I. S., & Arnold, J. C. (2019). Pharmacokinetics of phytocannabinoid acids and anticonvulsant effect of cannabidiolic acid in a mouse model of Dravet syndrome. Journal of Natural Products, 82(11), 3047–3055. https://doi.org/10.1021/acs.jnatprod.9b00600

83. Baker, T., Datta, P., Rewers-Felkins, K., Thompson, H., Kallem, R. R., & Hale, T. W. (2018). Transfer of inhaled cannabis into human breast milk. Obstetrics & Gynecology, 131(5), 783–788.

84. Ujváry, I., & Lopata, A. (2019). Towards understanding the phenytoin-like antiepileptic effect of cannabidiol and related phytocannabinoid metabolites: Insights from molecular modeling. ChemRxiv. Preprint. https://doi.org/10.26434/chemrxiv.7454252.v2

Chapter 14: Other Phytoconstituents in the Cannabis Entourage

1. Russo, E. B., & Marcu, J. (2017). Cannabis pharmacology: The usual suspects and a few promising leads. Advances in Pharmacology, 80, 67–134.

2. Gilbert, A. N., & DiVerdi, J. A. (2018). Consumer perceptions of strain differences in Cannabis aroma. PLOS ONE, 13(2), Article e0192247.

3. Agrawal, A. K., Kumar, P., Gulati, A., & Seth, P. K. (1989). Cannabis-induced neurotoxicity in mice-effect on cholinergic (muscarinic) receptors and blood-brain barrier permeability. Research Communications in Substances of Abuse, 10(3), 155–168.

4. Nóbrega de Almeida, R., Agra, M. D. F., Negromonte Souto Maior, F., & De Sousa, D. P. (2011). Essential oils and their constituents: anticonvulsant activity. Molecules, 16(3), 2726–2742.

5. Komori, T., Fujiwara, R., Tanida, M., Nomura, J., & Yokoyama, M. M. (1995). Effects of citrus fragrance on immune function and depressive states. Neuroimmunomodulation, 2(3), 174–180.

6. Pereira, I., Severino, P., Santos, A. C., Silva, A. M., & Souto, E. B. (2018). Linalool bioactive properties and potential applicability in drug delivery systems. Colloids and Surfaces B: Biointerfaces, 171, 566–578.

7. Pereira, I., Severino, P., Santos, A. C., Silva, A. M., & Souto, E. B. (2018). Linalool bioactive properties and potential applicability in drug delivery systems. Colloids and Surfaces B: Biointerfaces, 171, 566–578.

8. Pereira, I., Severino, P., Santos, A. C., Silva, A. M., & Souto, E. B. (2018). Linalool bioactive properties and potential applicability in drug delivery systems. Colloids and Surfaces B: Biointerfaces, 171, 566–578.

9. Pereira, I., Severino, P., Santos, A. C., Silva, A. M., & Souto, E. B. (2018). Linalool bioactive properties and potential applicability in drug delivery systems. Colloids and Surfaces B: Biointerfaces, 171, 566–578.

10. Ames-Sibin, A. P., Barizão, C. L., Castro-Ghizoni, C. V., Silva, F. M., Sá-Nakanishi, A. B., Bracht, L., ... & Comar, J. F. (2018). β-Caryophyllene, the major constituent of copaiba oil, reduces systemic inflammation and oxidative stress in arthritic rats. Journal of Cellular Biochemistry, 119(12), 10262-10277.

11. Ferro, M., Masso, S., de Souza, R. R., Moreno, M., & Moreira, E. (2018). Meta-analysis on copaiba oil: its functions in metabolism and its properties as an anti-inflammatory agent. *Journal of Morphological Sciences*, 35(03), 161–166.

12. Reviewed in Francomano, F., Caruso, A., Barbarossa, A., Fazio, A., La Torre, C., Ceramella, J., ... & Sinicropi, M. S. (2019). β-Caryophyllene: A Sesquiterpene with Countless Biological Properties. *Applied Sciences*, 9(24), 5420.

13. Varga, Z. V., Matyas, C., Erdelyi, K., Cinar, R., Nieri, D., Chicca, A., ... & Hasko, G. (2018). β-Caryophyllene protects against alcoholic steatohepatitis by attenuating inflammation and metabolic dysregulation in mice. *British journal of pharmacology*, 175(2), 320–334.

14. Meeran, M. N., Al Taee, H., Azimullah, S., Tariq, S., Adeghate, E., & Ojha, S. (2019). β-Caryophyllene, a natural bicyclic sesquiterpene attenuates doxorubicin-induced chronic cardiotoxicity via activation of myocardial cannabinoid type-2 (CB2) receptors in rats. *Chemico-biological interactions*, 304, 158–167.

15. Al Mansouri, S., Ojha, S., Al Maamari, E., Al Ameri, M., Nurulain, S. M., & Bahi, A. (2014). The cannabinoid receptor 2 agonist, β-caryophyllene, reduced voluntary alcohol intake and attenuated ethanol-induced place preference and sensitivity in mice. *Pharmacology Biochemistry and Behavior*, 124, 260–268.

16. Shim, H. I., Song, D. J., Shin, C. M., Yoon, H., Park, Y. S., Kim, N., & Lee, D. H. (2019). Inhibitory Effects of β-caryophyllene on Helicobacter pylori Infection: A Randomized Double-blind, Placebo-controlled Study. *The Korean Journal of Gastroenterology*, 74(4), 199–204.

17. Reviewed in Francomano, F., Caruso, A., Barbarossa, A., Fazio, A., La Torre, C., Ceramella, J., ... & Sinicropi, M. S. (2019). β-Caryophyllene: A Sesquiterpene with Countless Biological Properties. *Applied Sciences*, 9(24), 5420.

18. Russo, E. B. (2011). Taming THC: Potential cannabis synergy and phytocannabinoid–terpenoid entourage effects. *British Journal of Pharmacology*, 163(7), 1344–1364.

19. Oppong-Damoah, A., Blough, B. E., Makriyannis, A., & Murnane, K. S. (2019). The sesquiterpene beta-caryophyllene oxide attenuates ethanol drinking and place conditioning in mice. *Heliyon*, 5(6), e01915.

20. Legault, J., & Pichette, A. (2007). Potentiating effect of β-caryophyllene on anticancer activity of α-humulene, isocaryophyllene and paclitaxel. *Journal of Pharmacy and Pharmacology*, 59(12), 1643–1647.

21. Ambrož, M., Šmatová, M., Šadibolová, M., Pospíšilová, E., Hadravská, P., Kašparová, M., ... & Skálová, L. (2019). Sesquiterpenes α-humulene and β-caryophyllene oxide enhance the efficacy of 5-fluorouracil and oxaliplatin in colon cancer cells. *Acta Pharmaceutica*, 69(1), 121–128.

22. Chen, H., Yuan, J., Hao, J., Wen, Y., Lv, Y., Chen, L., & Yang, X. (2019). α-Humulene inhibits hepatocellular carcinoma cell proliferation and induces apoptosis through the inhibition of Akt signaling. *Food and Chemical Toxicology*, 134, 110830.

23. Loizzo, M. R., Saab, A. M., Tundis, R., Statti, G. A., Menichini, F., Lampronti, I., ... & Doerr, H. W. (2008). Phytochemical analysis and in vitro antiviral activities of the essential oils of seven Lebanon species. *Chemistry & biodiversity*, 5(3), 461–470.

24. McPartland, J. M., & Russo, E. B. (2014). Non-phytocannabinoid constituents of cannabis and herbal synergy. In R. Pertwee (Ed.), *Handbook of cannabis* (pp. 280–295). Oxford University Press.

25. Werz, O., Seegers, J., Schaible, A. M., Weinigel, C., Barz, D., Koeberle, A., Allegrone, G., Pollastro, F. Zampieri, L., Grassi, G., & Appendino, G. (2014). Cannflavins from hemp sprouts, a novel cannabinoid-free hemp food product, target microsomal prostaglandin E2 synthase-1 and 5-lipoxygenase. *PharmaNutrition* 2(3), 53–60.

26. Reviewed in Russo, E. B., & Marcu, J. (2017). Cannabis pharmacology: The usual suspects and a few promising leads. *Advances in Pharmacology*, 80, 67–134.

27. Eggers, C., Fujitani, M., Kato, R., & Smid, S. (2019). Novel cannabis flavonoid, cannflavin A displays both a hormetic and neuroprotective profile against amyloid β-mediated neurotoxicity in PC12 cells: Comparison with geranylated flavonoids, mimulone and diplacone. *Biochemical Pharmacology*, 169, 113609.

28. Moreau, M., Ibeh, U., Decosmo, K., Bih, N., Yasmin-Karim, S., Toyand, N., Lowe, H., & Ngwa, W. (2019). Flavonoid derivative of cannabis demonstrates therapeutic potential in preclinical models of metastatic pancreatic cancer. *Frontiers in Oncology*, 9, 660.

29. Callaway, J. C. (2004). Hempseed as a nutritional resource: An overview. *Euphytica*, 140(1–2), 65–72.

Chapter 15: Synthetic Cannabinoids and Endocannabinoid System Modulators

1. Haney, M., Cooper, Z. D., Bedi, G., Vosburg, S. K., Comer, S. D., & Foltin, R. W. (2013). Nabilone decreases marijuana withdrawal and a laboratory measure of marijuana relapse. *Neuropsychopharmacology*, 38(8), 1557–1565.

2. Castaneto, M. S., Gorelick, D. A., Desrosiers, N. A., Hartman, R. L., Pirard, S., & Huestis, M. A. (2014). Synthetic cannabinoids: epidemiology, pharmacodynamics, and clinical implications. *Drug and alcohol dependence*, 144, 12–41.

3. Castaneto, M. S., Gorelick, D. A., Desrosiers, N. A., Hartman, R. L., Pirard, S., & Huestis, M. A. (2014). Synthetic cannabinoids: epidemiology, pharmacodynamics, and clinical implications. *Drug and alcohol dependence*, 144, 12–41.

4. Kelkar, A. H., Smith, N. A., Martial, A., Moole, H., Tarantino, M. D., & Roberts, J. C. (2018). An outbreak of synthetic cannabinoid–associated coagulopathy in Illinois. *New England journal of medicine*, 379(13), 1216–1223.

5. Faroqui, R., Mena, P., Wolfe, A. R., Bibawy, J., Visvikis, G. A., & Mantello, M. T. (2018). Acute carotid thrombosis and ischemic stroke following overdose of the synthetic cannabinoid K2 in a previously healthy young adult male. *Radiology Case Reports*, *13*(3), 747–752.

6. Akram, H., Mokrysz, C., & Curran, H. V. (2019). What are the psychological effects of using synthetic cannabinoids? A systematic review. *Journal of Psychopharmacology*, *33*(3), 271–283.

7. Rodgers, R. J., Tschöp, M. H., & Wilding, J. P. H. (2012). Anti-obesity drugs: Past, present and future. *Disease Models & Mechanisms*, *5*(5), 621–626.

Chapter 16: Cannabis Preparation and Delivery Methods

1. Ind, P. W. (2019). Cannabis, cigarette smoking and lung function—Not all downhill? *Journal of Aerosol Medicine and Pulmonary Drug Delivery*, *32*(2). https://doi.org/10.1089/jamp.2019.ab01.abstracts

2. Gieringer, D. (1996). Marijuana water pipe and vaporizer study. *Newsletter of the Multidisciplinary Association for Psychedelic Studies*, *6*, 5–9.

3. Hazekamp, A., Ruhaak, R., Zuurman, L., van Gerven, J., & Verpoorte, R. (2006). Evaluation of a vaporizing device (Volcano®) for the pulmonary administration of tetrahydrocannabinol. *Journal of pharmaceutical sciences*, *95*(6), 1308–1317.

4. Gieringer, D., St. Laurent, J., & Goodrich, S. (2004). Cannabis vaporizer combines efficient delivery of THC with effective suppression of pyrolytic compounds. *Journal of Cannabis Therapeutics*, *4*(1), 7–27.

5. Earleywine, M., & Barnwell, S. S. (2007). Decreased respiratory symptoms in cannabis users who vaporize. *Harm Reduction Journal*, *4*(1), 11.

6. McPartland, J. M., & Russo, E. B. (2014). Non-phytocannabinoid constituents of cannabis and herbal synergy. In *Handbook of cannabis* (pp. 280–295). Oxford University Press.

7. Dreher, M. C. (1982). *Working men and ganja: Marihuana use in rural Jamaica*. Institute for the Study of Human Issues.

8. Merzouki, A., & Mesa, J. M. (1999). La chanvre (*Cannabis sativa* L.) dans la pharmacopée traditionnelle du rif (nord du Maroc). *Ars Pharmaceutica*, *40*(4), 233–240.

9. Hazekamp, A., Bastola, K., Rashidi, H., Bender, J., & Verpoorte, R. (2007). Cannabis tea revisited: A systematic evaluation of the cannabinoid composition of cannabis tea. *Journal of Ethnopharmacology*, *113*(1), 85–90.

10. Pellesi, L., Licata, M., Verri, P., Vandelli, D., Palazzoli, F., Marchesi, F., ... & Guerzoni, S. (2018). Pharmacokinetics and tolerability of oral cannabis preparations in patients with medication overuse headache (MOH)—a pilot study. *European Journal of Clinical Pharmacology*, *74*(11), 1427–1436.

11. Poli, P., Crestani, F., Salvadori, C., Valenti, I., & Sannino, C. (2018). Medical cannabis in patients with chronic pain: effect on pain relief, pain disability, and psychological aspects. A prospective non randomized single arm clinical trial. *La Clinica Terapeutica*, *169*(3), e102-e107.

12. Parikh, N., Kramer, W. G., Khurana, V., Smith, C. C., & Vetticaden, S. (2016). Bioavailability study of dronabinol oral solution versus dronabinol capsules in healthy volunteers. *Clinical pharmacology: advances and applications*, *8*, 155.

13. Oh, D. A., Parikh, N., Khurana, V., Smith, C. C., & Vetticaden, S. (2017). Effect of food on the pharmacokinetics of dronabinol oral solution versus dronabinol capsules in healthy volunteers. *Clinical Pharmacology: Advances and Applications*, *9*, 9.

14. Taylor, L., Gidal, B., Blakey, G., Tayo, B., & Morrison, G. (2018). A phase I, randomized, double-blind, placebo-controlled, single ascending dose, multiple dose, and food effect trial of the safety, tolerability and pharmacokinetics of highly purified cannabidiol in healthy subjects. *CNS drugs*, *32*(11), 1053–1067.

15. Sexton, M., Shelton, K., Haley, P., & West, M. (2018). Erratum: Evaluation of Cannabinoid and Terpenoid Content: Cannabis Flower Compared to Supercritical CO2 Concentrate. *Planta medica*, *84*(04), E3-E3.

16. Raber, J. C., Elzinga, S., & Kaplan, C. (2015). Understanding dabs: Contamination concerns of cannabis concentrates and cannabinoid transfer during the act of dabbing. *The Journal of Toxicological Sciences*, *40*(6), 797–803.

17. Meehan-Atrash, J., Luo, W., & Strongin, R. M. (2017). Toxicant formation in dabbing: The terpene story. *ACS Omega*, *2*(9), 6112–6117.

18. Richman, L. S., Whitaker, J., & Kinnard, W. V. (2018). A case of acute hypersensitivity pneumonitis due to cannabis dabbing. American Thoracic Society International Conference Abstracts, D35. Drug induced lung disease: Case reports, Abstract A6636.

19. Albrektson, K., Masroujeh, R., & Young, B. P. (2019). The dangers of dabbing: A case of ARDS following inhalation of vaporized butane-extracted cannabis product. American Thoracic Society International Conference Abstracts, A49. Case reports in lung disease associated with inhalational exposures, Abstract A1811. https://doi.org/10.1164/ajrccm-conference.2019.199.1_MeetingAbstracts.A1811

20. Troutt, W. D., & DiDonato, M. D. (2017). Carbonyl compounds produced by vaporizing cannabis oil thinning agents. *The Journal of Alternative and Complementary Medicine*, *23*(11), 879–884.

21. Boyar, K. (2019). Heavy Metal Contaminants from Cannabis Vaporizer Cartridges: Valid Concern or Blowing Smoke." CannMed 2019, Pasadena Convention Center, Pasadena, CA. 23 Sept 2019.

22. Elliott, D. R. F., Shah, R., Hess, C. A., Elicker, B., Henry, T. S., Rule, A. M., Chen, R., Golozar, M., & Jones, K. D. (2019). Giant cell interstitial pneumonia secondary to cobalt exposure from e-cigarette use. *European Respiratory Journal*, *54*(6), Article 1901922. https://doi.org/ 10.1183/13993003.01922-2019

23. Centers for Disease Control and Prevention. (2020, February 25). *Outbreak of lung injury associated with the use of e-cigarette, or vaping, products.* cdc.gov/tobacco/basic_information/e-cigarettes/severe-lung-disease. html#latest-information

24. Dogrul, A., Gul, H., Akar, A., Yildiz, O., Bilgin, F., & Guzeldemir, E. (2003). Topical cannabinoid antinociception: synergy with spinal sites. *Pain*, *105*(1-2), 11–16.

25. Yesilyurt, O., Dogrul, A., Gul, H., Seyrek, M., Kusmez, O., Ozkan, Y., & Yildiz, O. (2003). Topical cannabinoid enhances topical morphine antinociception. *Pain*, *105*(1-2), 303–308.

26. Gaffal, E., Cron, M., Glodde, N., & Tüting, T. (2013). Anti-inflammatory activity of topical THC in DNFB-mediated mouse allergic contact dermatitis independent of CB 1 and CB 2 receptors. *Allergy*, *68*(8), 994–1000.

27. Touitou, E., & Fabin, B. (1988). Altered skin permeation of a highly lipophilic molecule: tetrahydrocannabinol. *International journal of pharmaceutics*, *43*(1-2), 17–22.

28. Chelliah, M. P., Zinn, Z., Khuu, P., & Teng, J. M. (2018). Self-initiated use of topical cannabidiol oil for epidermolysis bullosa. *Pediatric Dermatology*, *35*(4), e224-e227.

29. Palmieri, B., Laurino, C., & Vadalà, M. (2019). A therapeutic effect of CBD-enriched ointment in inflammatory skin diseases and cutaneous scars. *La Clinica Terapeutica*, *170*(2), e93-e99.

30. Maida, V., & Corban, J. (2017). Topical medical cannabis: A new treatment for wound pain—Three cases of pyoderma gangrenosum. *Journal of Pain and Symptom Management*, *54*(5), 732–736.

31. Nitecka-Buchta, A., Nowak-Wachol, A., Wachol, K., Walczyńska-Dragon, K., Olczyk, P., Batoryna, O., ... & Baron, S. (2019). Myorelaxant Effect of Transdermal Cannabidiol Application in Patients with TMD: A Randomized, Double-Blind Trial. *Journal of clinical medicine*, *8*(11), 1886.

32. Phan, N. Q., Siepmann, D., Gralow, I., & Ständer, S. (2010). Adjuvant topical therapy with a cannabinoid receptor agonist in facial postherpetic neuralgia. *JDDG: Journal der Deutschen Dermatologischen Gesellschaft*, *8*(2), 88–91.

33. Hammell, D. C., Zhang, L. P., Ma, F., Abshire, S. M., McIlwrath, S. L., Stinchcomb, A. L., & Westlund, K. N. (2016). Transdermal cannabidiol reduces inflammation and pain-related behaviours in a rat model of arthritis. *European Journal of Pain*, *20*(6), 936–948.

34. Heussler, H., Cohen, J., Silove, N., Tich, N., Bonn-Miller, M. O., Du, W., ... & Sebree, T. (2019). A phase 1/2, open-label assessment of the safety, tolerability, and efficacy of transdermal cannabidiol (ZYN002) for the treatment of pediatric fragile X syndrome. *Journal of neurodevelopmental disorders*, *11*(1), 16.

35. Ryz, N. R., Remillard, D. J., & Russo, E. B. (2017). Cannabis roots: A traditional therapy with future potential for treating inflammation and pain. *Cannabis and Cannabinoid Research 2*(1), 210–216.

36. Nakajima, J., Nakae, D., & Yasukawa, K. (2013). Structure-dependent inhibitory effects of synthetic cannabinoids against 12-O-tetradecanoylphorbol-13-acetate-induced inflammation and skin tumour promotion in mice. *Journal of Pharmacy and Pharmacology*, *65*(8), 1223–1230.

37. Kander, J. (2020). *Cannabis for the Treatment of Cancer: The Anticancer Activity of Phytocannabinoids and Endocannabinoids.* http://freecannabiscancerbook.com/

38. Hess, C., Krämer, M., & Madea, B. (2017). Topical application of THC containing products is not able to cause positive cannabinoid finding in blood or urine. *Forensic Science International*, *272*, 68–71.

39. Boehnke, K. F., Scott, J. R., Litinas, E., Sisley, S., Clauw, D. J., Goesling, J., & Williams, D. A. (2019). Cannabis use preferences and decision making among a cross-sectional cohort of medical cannabis patients with chronic pain. *The Journal of Pain*, *20*(11), 1362–1372.

40. Marquez, E., and Buckley, N. (2017). "Delta-9-tetrahydrocannabinol and its effect of the Severity of Candida albicans induced Vulvovaginal Candidiasis."

Chapter 17: Cannabis Dosing

1. Kuhlen, M., Hoell, J. I., Gagnon, G., Balzer, S., Oommen, P. T., Borkhardt, A., & Janßen, G. (2016). Effective treatment of spasticity using dronabinol in pediatric palliative care. *European Journal of Paediatric Neurology*, *20*(6), 898–903.

2. Rosenberg, E. C., Louik, J., Conway, E., Devinsky, O., & Friedman, D. (2017). Quality of life in childhood epilepsy in pediatric patients enrolled in a prospective, open-label clinical study with cannabidiol. *Epilepsia*, *58*(8), e96-e100.

3. Thompson, G. R., Rosenkrantz, H., Schaeppi, U. H., & Braude, M. C. (1973). Comparison of acute oral toxicity of cannabinoids in rats, dogs and monkeys. *Toxicology and applied pharmacology*, *25*(3), 363–372.

4. Thompson, G. R., Fleischman, R. W., Rosenkrantz, H., & Braude, M. C. (1974). Oral and intravenous toxicity of Δ⁹-tetrahydrocannabinol in rhesus monkeys. *Toxicology and applied pharmacology*, *27*(3), 648–665.

5. Sañudo-Peña, M. C., Romero, J., Seale, G. E., Fernandez-Ruiz, J. J., & Walker, J. M. (2000). Activational role of cannabinoids on movement. *European Journal of Pharmacology*, *391*(3), 269–274.

6. Margulies, J. E., & Hammer, R. P., Jr. (1991). Δ⁹-Tetrahydrocannabinol alters cerebral metabolism in a biphasic, dose-dependent mannier in rat brain. *European Journal of Pharmacology, 202*(3), 373–378.

7. Reviewed in Patel, S., Hill, M. N., & Hillard, C. J. (2014). Effects of phytocannabinoids on anxiety, mood, and the endocrine system. In *Handbook of cannabis* (pp. 189–207). Oxford University Press.

8. Childs, E., Lutz, J. A., & de Wit, H. (2017). Dose-related effects of delta-9-THC on emotional responses to acute psychosocial stress. *Drug and Alcohol Dependence, 177*, 136–144.

9. Linares, I. M., Zuardi, A. W., Pereira, L. C., Queiroz, R. H., Mechoulam, R., Guimaraes, F. S., & Crippa, J. A. (2019). Cannabidiol presents an inverted U-shaped dose-response curve in a simulated public speaking test. *Brazilian Journal of Psychiatry, 41*(1), 9–14.

10. Zuardi, A. W., Rodrigues, N. P., Silva, A. L., Bernardo, S. A., Hallak, J. E., Guimarães, F. S., & Crippa, J. A. (2017). Inverted U-shaped dose-response curve of the anxiolytic effect of cannabidiol during public speaking in real life. *Frontiers in pharmacology, 8*, 259.

11. Zanelati, T. V., Biojone, C., Moreira, F. A., Guimaraes, F. S., & Joca, S. R. (2010). Antidepressant-like effects of cannabidiol in mice: possible involvement of 5-HT1A receptors. *British journal of pharmacology, 159*(1), 122–128.

12. Schiavon, A. P., Bonato, J. M., Milani, H., Guimarães, F. S., & de Oliveira, R. M. W. (2016). Influence of single and repeated cannabidiol administration on emotional behavior and markers of cell proliferation and neurogenesis in non-stressed mice. *Progress in Neuro-Psychopharmacology and Biological Psychiatry, 64*, 27–34.

13. Casarotto, P. C., Gomes, F. V., Resstel, L. B., & Guimarães, F. S. (2010). Cannabidiol inhibitory effect on marble-burying behaviour: involvement of CB1 receptors. *Behavioural pharmacology, 21*(4), 353–358.

14. Genaro, K., Fabris, D., Arantes, A. L., Zuardi, A. W., Crippa, J. A., & Prado, W. A. (2017). Cannabidiol is a potential therapeutic for the affective-motivational dimension of incision pain in rats. *Frontiers in Pharmacology, 8*, 391.

15. Portenoy, R. K., Ganae-Motan, E. D., Allende, S., Yanagihara, R., Shaiova, L., Weinstein, S., McQuade, R., Wright, S., & Fallon, M. T. (2012). Nabiximols for opioid-treated cancer patients with poorly-controlled chronic pain: A randomized, placebo-controlled, graded-dose trial. *The Journal of Pain, 13*(5), 438–449.

16. Wallace, M., Schulteis, G., Atkinson, J. H., Wolfson, T., Lazzaretto, D., Bentley, H., ... & Abramson, I. (2007). Dose-dependent effects of smoked cannabis on capsaicin-induced pain and hyperalgesia in healthy volunteers. *Anesthesiology: The Journal of the American Society of Anesthesiologists, 107*(5), 785–796.

17. Kraft, B., Frickey, N. A., Kaufmann, R. M., Reif, M., Frey, R., Gustorff, B., & Kress, H. G. (2008). Lack of analgesia by oral standardized cannabis extract on acute inflammatory pain and hyperalgesia in volunteers. *The Journal of the American Society of Anesthesiologists, 109*(1), 101–110.

18. Abel, E. L. (1971). Changes in anxiety feelings following marihuana smoking: The alternation in feelings of anxiety resulting from the smoking of marihuana (*Cannabis sativa* L.). *British Journal of Addiction to Alcohol & Other Drugs, 66*(3), 185–187.

19. Fishbein, M., Gov, S., Assaf, F., Gafni, M., Keren, O., & Sarne, Y. (2012). Long-term behavioral and biochemical effects of an ultra-low dose of Δ 9-tetrahydrocannabinol (THC): neuroprotection and ERK signaling. *Experimental brain research, 221*(4), 437–448.

20. Amal, H., Fridman-Rozevich, L., Senn, R., Strelnikov, A., Gafni, M., Keren, O., & Sarne, Y. (2010). Long-term consequences of a single treatment of mice with an ultra-low dose of Δ⁹-tetrahydrocannabinol (THC). *Behavioural brain research, 206*(2), 245–253.

21. Sarne, Y., Toledano, R., Rachmany, L., Sasson, E., & Doron, R. (2018). Reversal of age-related cognitive impairments in mice by an extremely low dose of tetrahydrocannabinol. *Neurobiology of Aging, 61*, 177–186.

22. Waldman, M., Hochhauser, E., Fishbein, M., Aravot, D., Shainberg, A., & Sarne, Y. (2013). An ultra-low dose of tetrahydrocannabinol provides cardioprotection. *Biochemical pharmacology, 85*(11), 1626–1633.

23. Hochhauser, E., Lahat, E., Sultan, M., Pappo, O., Waldman, M., Sarne, Y., ... & Ari, Z. B. (2015). Ultra low dose delta 9-tetrahydrocannabinol protects mouse liver from ischemia reperfusion injury. *Cellular Physiology and Biochemistry, 36*(5), 1971–1981.

24. Rock, E. M., Kopstick, R. L., Limebeer, C. L., & Parker, L. A. (2013). Tetrahydrocannabinolic acid reduces nausea-induced conditioned gaping in rats and vomiting in S uncus murinus. *British journal of pharmacology, 170*(3), 641–648.

25. Rock, E. M., & Parker, L. A. (2013). Effect of low doses of cannabidiolic acid and ondansetron on LiCl-induced conditioned gaping (a model of nausea-induced behaviour) in rats. *British Journal of Pharmacology, 169*(3), 685–692.

26. Kwiatkowska, M., Parker, L. A., Burton, P., & Mechoulam, R. (2004). A comparative analysis of the potential of cannabinoids and ondansetron to suppress cisplatin-induced emesis in the Suncus murinus (house musk shrew). *Psychopharmacology, 174*(2), 254–259.

27. Rock, E. M., Limebeer, C. L., & Parker, L. A. (2018). Effect of cannabidiolic acid and Δ9-tetrahydrocannabinol on carrageenan-induced hyperalgesia and edema in a rodent model of inflammatory pain. *Psychopharmacology, 235*(11), 3259–3271.

28. Calabrese, E. J., & Rubio-Casillas, A. (2018). Biphasic effects of THC in memory and cognition. *European Journal of Clinical Investigation, 48*(5), Article e12920.

29. D'souza, D. C., Ranganathan, M., Braley, G., Gueorguieva, R., Zimolo, Z., Cooper, T., ... & Krystal, J. (2008). Blunted psychotomimetic and amnestic effects of Δ-9-tetrahydrocannabinol in frequent users of cannabis. *Neuropsychopharmacology, 33*(10), 2505–2516.

30. Breivogel, C. S., Scates, S. M., Beletskaya, I. O., Lowery, O. B., Aceto, M. D., & Martin, B. R. (2003). The effects of Δ^9-tetrahydrocannabinol physical dependence on brain cannabinoid receptors. *European journal of pharmacology, 459*(2-3), 139–150.

31. De Vry, J., Jentzsch, K. R., Kuhl, E., & Eckel, G. (2004). Behavioral effects of cannabinoids show differential sensitivity to cannabinoid receptor blockade and tolerance development. *Behavioural pharmacology, 15*(1), 1–12.

32. Russo, E., & Guy, G. W. (2006). A tale of two cannabinoids: The therapeutic rationale for combining tetrahydrocannabinol and cannabidiol. *Medical Hypotheses, 66*(2), 234–246.

33. Johnson, J. R., Burnell-Nugent, M., Lossignol, D., Ganae-Motan, E. D., Potts, R., & Fallon, M. T. (2010). Multicenter, double-blind, randomized, placebo-controlled, parallel-group study of the efficacy, safety, and tolerability of THC: CBD extract and THC extract in patients with intractable cancer-related pain. *Journal of pain and symptom management, 39*(2), 167–179.

34. Haney, M., Malcolm, R. J., Babalonis, S., Nuzzo, P. A., Cooper, Z. D., Bedi, G., ... & Walsh, S. L. (2016). Oral cannabidiol does not alter the subjective, reinforcing or cardiovascular effects of smoked cannabis. *Neuropsychopharmacology, 41*(8), 1974–1982.

35. Karniol, I. G., Shirakawa, I., Kasinski, N., Pfeferman, A., & Carlini, E. A. (1974). Cannabidiol interferes with the effects of Δ^9-tetrahydrocannabinol in man. *European journal of pharmacology, 28*(1), 172–177.

36. van de Donk, T., Niesters, M., Kowal, M. A., Olofsen, E., Dahan, A., & van Velzen, M. (2019). An experimental randomized study on the analgesic effects of pharmaceutical-grade cannabis in chronic pain patients with fibromyalgia. *Pain, 160*(4), 860.

37. Whiting, P. F., Wolff, R. F., Deshpande, S., Di Nisio, M., Duffy, S., Hernandez, A. V., ... & Schmidlkofer, S. (2015). Cannabinoids for medical use: a systematic review and meta-analysis. *Jama, 313*(24), 2456–2473.

38. The American Heritage Dictionary of the English Language, 5th Edition. https://www.ahdictionary.com/word/search. html?q=euphoria. Accessed January 12, 2020.

39. Lavie-Ajayi, M., & Shvartzman, P. (2019). Restored self: A phenomenological study of pain relief by cannabis. *Pain Medicine 20*(11), 2086–2093. https://doi.org/10.1093/pm/pny176

40. Sativex Oromucosal Spray: Summary of Product Characteristics. https://www.medicines.org.uk/emc/product/602/ smpc Accessed January 12, 2020.

41. MacCallum, C. A., & Russo, E. B. (2018). Practical considerations in medical cannabis administration and dosing. *European Journal of Internal Medicine, 49*, 12–19.

42. D'Souza, D. C., Cortes-Briones, J. A., Ranganathan, M., Thurnauer, H., Creatura, G., Surti, T., ... & Kapinos, M. (2016). Rapid changes in cannabinoid 1 receptor availability in cannabis-dependent male subjects after abstinence from cannabis. *Biological psychiatry: cognitive neuroscience and neuroimaging, 1*(1), 60–67.

43. Burstein, S. H., & Hunter, S. A. (1995). Stimulation of anandamide biosynthesis in N-18TG2 neuroblastoma cells by Δ^9-tetrahydrocannabinol (THC). *Biochemical Pharmacology, 49*(6), 855–858.

44. Cichewicz, D. L., Haller, V. L., & Welch, S. P. (2001). Changes in opioid and cannabinoid receptor protein following short-term combination treatment with Δ^9-tetrahydrocannabinol and morphine. *Journal of Pharmacology and Experimental Therapeutics, 297*(1), 121–127.

45. Oviedo, A., Glowa, J., & Herkenham, M. (1993). Chronic cannabinoid administration alters cannabinoid receptor binding in rat brain: A quantitative autoradiographic study. *Brain Research, 616*(1–2), 293–302.

Chapter 18: Adverse Effects and Cautions

1. National Toxicology Program. (1996). *Toxicology and Carcinogenesis Studies of 1-Trans-Delta9-Tetrahydrocannabinol (CAS No. 1972-08-3) in F344 Rats and B6C3F1 Mice (Gavage Studies)* (National Toxicology Program Technical Report Series 446). https://ntp.niehs.nih.gov/ntp/htdocs/lt_rpts/tr446.pdf

2. Thompson, G. R., Rosenkrantz, H., Schaeppi, U. H., & Braude, M. C. (1973). Comparison of acute oral toxicity of cannabinoids in rats, dogs and monkeys. *Toxicology and applied pharmacology, 25*(3), 363–372.

3. Thompson, G. R., Fleischman, R. W., Rosenkrantz, H., & Braude, M. C. (1974). Oral and intravenous toxicity of Δ^9-tetrahydrocannabinol in rhesus monkeys. *Toxicology and applied pharmacology, 27*(3), 648–665.

4. Brutlag, A., & Hommerding, H. (2018). Toxicology of marijuana, synthetic cannabinoids, and cannabidiol in dogs and cats. *Veterinary Clinics: Small Animal Practice, 48*(6), 1087–1102.

5. Drummer, O. H., Gerostamoulos, D., & Woodford, N. W. (2019). Cannabis as a cause of death: A review. *Forensic Science International, 298*, 298–306. https://doi.org/10.1016/j.forsciint.2019.03.007

6. Cooper, Z. D., & Williams, A. R. (2019). Cannabis and cannabinoid intoxication and toxicity. In *Cannabis use disorders* (pp. 103–111). Springer.

7. Adapted from Cooper, Z. D., & Williams, A. R. (2019). Cannabis and cannabinoid intoxication and toxicity. In *Cannabis use disorders* (pp. 103–111). Springer.

8. Rosenkrantz, H., Fleischman, R. W., & Grant, R. J. (1981). Toxicity of short-term administration of cannabinoids to rhesus monkeys. *Toxicology and Applied Pharmacology, 58*(1), 118–131.

9. McGuire, P., Robson, P., Cubala, W. J., Vasile, D., Morrison, P. D., Barron, R., ... & Wright, S. (2018). Cannabidiol (CBD) as an adjunctive therapy in schizophrenia: a multicenter randomized controlled trial. *American Journal of Psychiatry, 175*(3), 225–231.

10. Devinsky, O., Marsh, E., Friedman, D., Thiele, E., Laux, L., Sullivan, J., ... & Wong, M. (2016). Cannabidiol in patients with treatment-resistant epilepsy: an open-label interventional trial. *The Lancet Neurology, 15*(3), 270–278.

11. Russo, E. B. (2015). Synthetic and natural cannabinoids: The cardiovascular risk." *British Journal of Cardiology, 22,* 7–9.

12. Pacher, P., Steffens, S., Haskó, G., Schindler, T. H., & Kunos, G. (2018). Cardiovascular effects of marijuana and synthetic cannabinoids: the good, the bad, and the ugly. *Nature Reviews Cardiology, 15*(3), 151.

13. Aronow, W. S., & Cassidy, J. (1974). Effect of marihuana and placebo-marihuana smoking on angina pectoris. *New England Journal of Medicine, 291*(2), 65–67.

14. Russo, E. B. (2015). Synthetic and natural cannabinoids: The cardiovascular risk." *British Journal of Cardiology, 22,* 7–9.

15. Sellers, E. M., Schoedel, K., Bartlett, C., Romach, M., Russo, E. B., Stott, C. G., ... & Chen, C. F. (2013). A Multiple-Dose, Randomized, Double-Blind, Placebo-Controlled, Parallel-Group QT/QTc Study to Evaluate the Electrophysiologic Effects of THC/CBD Spray. *Clinical Pharmacology in Drug Development, 2*(3), 285–294.

16. Shayesteh, M. R., Haghi-Aminjan, H., Mousavi, M. J., Momtaz, S., & Abdollahi, M. (2019). The Protective Mechanism of Cannabidiol in Cardiac Injury: A Systematic Review of Non-Clinical Studies. *Current pharmaceutical design, 25*(22), 2499–2507.

17. Reviewed in Ind, P. W. "Cannabis, cigarette smoking and lung function—Not all downhill? *Journal of Aerosol Medicine and Pulmonary Drug Delivery, 32*(2), 140

18. Reviewed in Tashkin, D. P. (2013). Effects of marijuana smoking on the lung. *Annals of the American Thoracic Society, 10*(3), 239–247.

19. Hashibe, M., Morgenstern, H., Cui, Y., Tashkin, D. P., Zhang, Z. F., Cozen, W., ... & Greenland, S. (2006). Marijuana use and the risk of lung and upper aerodigestive tract cancers: results of a population-based case-control study. *Cancer Epidemiology and Prevention Biomarkers, 15*(10), 1829–1834.

20. McPartland, J. M. (1994). Microbiological contaminants of marijuana. *Journal of the International Hemp Association, 1,* 41–44.

21. Ruchlemer, R., Amit-Kohn, M., Raveh, D., & Hanuš, L. (2015). Inhaled medicinal cannabis and the immunocompromised patient. *Supportive Care in Cancer, 23*(3), 819–822.

22. Levitz, S. M., & Diamond, R. D. (1991). Aspergillosis and marijuana. *Annals of Internal Medicine, 115*(7), 578–579.

23. Evans, M. E., Twentyman, E., Click, E. S., Goodman, A. B., Weissman, D. N., Kiernan, E., Hocevar, S. A., Mikosz, C. A., Danielson, M., Anderson, K. N., Ellington, S., Lozier, M. J., Pollack, L. A., Rose, D. A., Krishnasamy, V., Jones, C. M., Briss, P., King, B. A., Wiltz, J. L., Lung Injury Response Clinical Task Force, & Lung Injury Response Clinical Working Group. (2020). Update: Interim guidance for health care professionals evaluating and caring for patients with suspected e-cigarette, or vaping, product use–associated lung injury and for reducing the risk for rehospitalization and death following hospital discharge — United States, December 2019. *Morbidity and Mortality Weekly Report, 68*(5152), 1189–1194. https://doi.org/10.15585/mmwr.mm685152e2

24. Hazekamp, A., Ruhaak, R., Zuurman, L., van Gerven, J., & Verpoorte, R. (2006). Evaluation of a vaporizing device (Volcano®) for the pulmonary administration of tetrahydrocannabinol. *Journal of pharmaceutical sciences, 95*(6), 1308–1317.

25. Gieringer, D., St. Laurent, J., & Goodrich, S. (2004). Cannabis vaporizer combines efficient delivery of THC with effective suppression of pyrolytic compounds. *Journal of Cannabis Therapeutics, 4*(1), 7–27.

26. Earleywine, M., & Barnwell, S. S. (2007). Decreased respiratory symptoms in cannabis users who vaporize. *Harm Reduction Journal, 4*(1), 11.

27. Whiting, P. F., Wolff, R. F., Deshpande, S., Di Nisio, M., Duffy, S., Hernandez, A. V., ... & Schmidlkofer, S. (2015). Cannabinoids for medical use: a systematic review and meta-analysis. *Jama, 313*(24), 2456–2473.

28. Etges, T., Karolia, K., Grint, T., Taylor, A., Lauder, H., Daka, B., & Wright, S. (2016). An observational postmarketing safety registry of patients in the UK, Germany, and Switzerland who have been prescribed Sativex®(THC: CBD, nabiximols) oromucosal spray. *Therapeutics and Clinical Risk Management, 12,* 1667.

29. Reviewed in Joshi, S., & Ashley, M. (2016). Cannabis: A joint problem for patients and the dental profession. *British Dental Journal, 220*(11), 597.

30. Reviewed in Le, A., & Palamar, J. J. (2019). Oral health implications of increased cannabis use among older adults: Another public health concern? *Journal of Substance Use, 24*(1), 61–65.

31. Prestifilippo, J. P., Fernandez-Solari, J., Cal, C. D. L., Iribarne, M., Suburo, A. M., Rettori, V., ... & Elverdin, J. C. (2006).

Inhibition of salivary secretion by activation of cannabinoid receptors. *Experimental Biology and Medicine*, *231*(8), 1421–1429.

32. Darling, M. R., & Arendorf, T. M. (1993). Effects of cannabis smoking on oral soft tissues. *Community Dentistry and Oral Epidemiology*, *21*(2), 78–81.

33. Schulz-Katterbach, M., Imfeld, T., & Carola Imfeld, C. (2009). Cannabis and caries–Does regular cannabis use increase the risk of caries in cigarette smokers. *Schweizer Monatsschrift für Zahnmedizin*, *119*(6), 576–583.

34. Stout, S. M., & Cimino, N. M. (2014). Exogenous cannabinoids as substrates, inhibitors, and inducers of human drug metabolizing enzymes: A systematic review. *Drug Metabolism Reviews*, *46*(1), 86–95.

35. Jusko, W. J., Schentag, J. J., Clark, J. H., Gardner, M., & Yurchak, A. M. (1978). Enhanced biotransformation of theophylline in marihuana and tobacco smokers. *Clinical Pharmacology & Therapeutics*, *24*(4), 406–410.

36. Alsherbiny, M. A., & Li, C. G. (2019). Medicinal cannabis—Potential drug interactions. *Medicines*, *6*(1), 3.

37. Reviewed in Cox, E. J., Maharao, N., Patilea-Vrana, G., Unadkat, J. D., Rettie, A. E., McCune, J. S., & Paine, M. F. (2019). A marijuana–drug interaction primer: Precipitants, pharmacology, and pharmacokinetics. *Pharmacology & Therapeutics*, *201*, 25–38. https://doi.org/10.1016/j.pharmthera.2019.05.001

38. Reviewed in Cox, E. J., Maharao, N., Patilea-Vrana, G., Unadkat, J. D., Rettie, A. E., McCune, J. S., & Paine, M. F. (2019). A marijuana–drug interaction primer: Precipitants, pharmacology, and pharmacokinetics. *Pharmacology & Therapeutics*, *201*, 25–38. https://doi.org/10.1016/j.pharmthera.2019.05.001

39. Stott, C., White, L., Wright, S., Wilbraham, D., & Guy, G. (2013). A phase I, open-label, randomized, crossover study in three parallel groups to evaluate the effect of rifampicin, ketoconazole, and omeprazole on the pharmacokinetics of THC/CBD oromucosal spray in healthy volunteers. *Springerplus*, *2*(1), 236. https://doi.org/10.1186/2193-1801-2-236

40. Damkier, P., Lassen, D., Christensen, M. M. H., Madsen, K. G., Hellfritzsch, M., & Pottegård, A. (2019). Interaction between warfarin and cannabis. *Basic & clinical pharmacology & toxicology*, *124*(1), 28–31.

41. Gaston, T. E., Bebin, E. M., Cutter, G. R., Liu, Y., Szaflarski, J. P., & UAB CBD Program. (2017). Interactions between cannabidiol and commonly used antiepileptic drugs. *Epilepsia*, *58*(9), 1586–1592.

42. Paoletti, R., Corsini, A., & Bellosta, S. (2002). Pharmacological interactions of statins. *Atherosclerosis. Supplements*, *3*(1), 35–40.

43. Qu, H., Guo, M., Chai, H., Wang, W. T., Gao, Z. Y., & Shi, D. Z. (2018). Effects of coenzyme Q10 on statin-induced myopathy: an updated meta-analysis of randomized controlled trials. *Journal of the American Heart Association*, *7*(19), e009835.

44. Perez-Reyes, M., Burstein, S. H., White, W. R., McDonald, S. A., & Hicks, R. E. (1991). Antagonism of marihuana effects by indomethacin in humans. *Life sciences*, *48*(6), 507–515.

45. Green, K., Kearse, E. C., & McIntyre, O. L. (2001). Interaction between delta-9-tetrahydrocannabinol and indomethacin. *Ophthalmic Research*, *33*(4), 217–220.

46. Opdivo for Health Care Professionals. (n.d.). *Management of adverse reactions*. Bristol Myers Squibb. Retrieved January 26, 2020, from https://www.opdivohcp.com/safety/adverse-reactions-management.

47. Connell, C. M., Raby, S., Beh, I., Flint, T. R., Williams, E. H., Fearon, D. T., … & Janowitz, T. (2017). Cancer immunotherapy trial registrations increase exponentially but chronic immunosuppressive glucocorticoid therapy may compromise outcomes. *Annals of Oncology*, *28*(7), 1678–1679.

48. Taha, T., Meiri, D., Talhamy, S., Wollner, M., Peer, A., & Bar-Sela, G. (2019). Cannabis impacts tumor response rate to nivolumab in patients with advanced malignancies. *The oncologist*, *24*(4), 549.

49. Center for Behavioral Health Statistics and Quality. (2017). *Results from the 2016 National Survey on Drug Use and Health: Detailed tables*. Substance Abuse and Mental Health Services Administration. https://www.samhsa.gov/data/sites/default/files/NSDUH-DetTabs-2016/NSDUH-DetTabs-2016.pdf

50. Lopez-Quintero, C., de los Cobos, J. P., Hasin, D. S., Okuda, M., Wang, S., Grant, B. F., & Blanco, C. (2011). Probability and predictors of transition from first use to dependence on nicotine, alcohol, cannabis, and cocaine: Results of the National Epidemiologic Survey on Alcohol and Related Conditions (NESARC). *Drug and Alcohol Dependence*, *115*(1–2), 120–130. https://doi.org/10.1016/j.drugalcdep.2010.11.004

51. National Academies of Sciences, Engineering, and Medicine. (2017). *The health effects of cannabis and cannabinoids: The current state of evidence and recommendations for research*. National Academies Press.

52. Etges, T., Karolia, K., Grint, T., Taylor, A., Lauder, H., Daka, B., & Wright, S. (2016). An observational postmarketing safety registry of patients in the UK, Germany, and Switzerland who have been prescribed Sativex®(THC: CBD, nabiximols) oromucosal spray. *Therapeutics and Clinical Risk Management*, *12*, 1667.

53. Calhoun, S. R., Galloway, G. P., & Smith, D. E. (1998). Abuse potential of dronabinol (Marinol). *Journal of Psychoactive Drugs*, *30*(2), 187–196.

54. Schoedel, K. A., Chen, N., Hilliard, A., White, L., Stott, C., Russo, E., … & Sellers, E. M. (2011). A randomized, double-blind, placebo-controlled, crossover study to evaluate the subjective abuse potential and cognitive effects of nabiximols oromucosal spray in subjects with a history of recreational cannabis use. *Human Psychopharmacology: Clinical and Experimental*, *26*(3), 224–236.

55. Schlienz, N. J., & Vandrey, R. (2018). Cannabis Withdrawal. In *Cannabis use disorders* (Chapter 11). Springer. https://doi.org/10.1007/978-3-319-90365-1_11

56. Schlienz, N. J., Budney, A. J., Lee, D. C., & Vandrey, R. (2017). Cannabis withdrawal: A review of neurobiological mechanisms and sex differences." *Current Addiction Reports, 4*(2), 75–81.

57. Levin, K. H., Copersino, M. L., Heishman, S. J., Liu, F., Kelly, D. L., Boggs, D. L., & Gorelick, D. A. (2010). Cannabis withdrawal symptoms in non-treatment-seeking adult cannabis smokers. *Drug and alcohol dependence, 111*(1-2), 120–127.

58. Schlienz, N. J., & Vandrey, R. (2018). Cannabis Withdrawal. In *Cannabis use disorders* (Chapter 11). Springer. https://doi.org/10.1007/978-3-319-90365-1_11

59. Perron, B. E., Holt, K. R., Yeagley, E., & Ilgen, M. (2019). Mental health functioning and severity of cannabis withdrawal among medical cannabis users with chronic pain. *Drug and Alcohol Dependence, 194*, 401–409.

60. D'Souza, D. C., Cortes-Briones, J. A., Ranganathan, M., Thurnauer, H., Creatura, G., Surti, T., ... & Kapinos, M. (2016). Rapid changes in cannabinoid 1 receptor availability in cannabis-dependent male subjects after abstinence from cannabis. *Biological psychiatry: cognitive neuroscience and neuroimaging, 1*(1), 60–67.

61. Werneck, M. A., Kortas, G. T., de Andrade, A. G., & Castaldelli-Maia, J. M. (2018). A systematic review of the efficacy of cannabinoid agonist replacement therapy for cannabis withdrawal symptoms. *CNS drugs, 32*(12), 1113–1129.

62. Hostiuc, S., Moldoveanu, A., Negoi, I., & Drima, E. (2018). The association of unfavorable traffic events and cannabis usage: a meta-analysis. *Frontiers in pharmacology, 9*, 99.

63. Hostiuc, S., Moldoveanu, A., Negoi, I., & Drima, E. (2018). The association of unfavorable traffic events and cannabis usage: a meta-analysis. *Frontiers in pharmacology, 9*, 99.

64. Owens, J. M., Dingus, T. A., Guo, F., Fang, Y., Perez, M., & McClafferty, J. (2018). Crash risk of cell phone use while driving: A case-crossover analysis of naturalistic driving data. AAA Foundation for Traffic Safety. https://aaafoundation.org/wp-content/uploads/2018/01/CellPhoneCrashRisk_FINAL.pdf

65. Huisingh, C., Owsley, C., Levitan, E. B., Irvin, M. R., MacLennan, P., & McGwin, G. (2019). Distracted driving and risk of crash or near-crash involvement among older drivers using naturalistic driving data with a case-crossover study design. *The Journals of Gerontology: Series A, 74*(4), 550–555.

66. Sexton, B. F., Tunbridge, R. J., Brook-Carter, N., Jackson, P. G., Wright, K., Stark, M. M., & Englehart, K. (2000). The influence of cannabis on driving. *TRL report, 477*, 106.

67. Brands, B., Mann, R. E., Wickens, C. M., Sproule, B., Stoduto, G., Sayer, G. S., ... & George, T. P. (2019). Acute and residual effects of smoked cannabis: Impact on driving speed and lateral control, heart rate, and self-reported drug effects. *Drug and alcohol dependence, 205*, 107641.

68. Hartman, R. L., Richman, J. E., Hayes, C. E., & Huestis, M. A. (2016). Drug Recognition Expert (DRE) examination characteristics of cannabis impairment. *Accident Analysis & Prevention, 92*, 219–229.

69. Celius, E. G., & Vila, C. (2018). The influence of THC:CBD oromucosal spray on driving ability in patients with multiple sclerosis-related spasticity. *Brain and Behavior, 8*(5), Article e00962.

70. MacCallum, C. A., & Russo, E. B. (2018). Practical considerations in medical cannabis administration and dosing. *European Journal of Internal Medicine, 49*, 12–19.

71. Bonar, E. E., Cranford, J. A., Arterberry, B. J., Walton, M. A., Bohnert, K. M., & Ilgen, M. A. (2019). Driving under the influence of cannabis among medical cannabis patients with chronic pain. *Drug and alcohol dependence, 195*, 193–197.

72. Arkell, T. R., Lintzeris, N., Kevin, R. C., Ramaekers, J. G., Vandrey, R., Irwin, C., ... & McGregor, I. S. (2019). Cannabidiol (CBD) content in vaporized cannabis does not prevent tetrahydrocannabinol (THC)-induced impairment of driving and cognition. *Psychopharmacology, 236*(9), 2713–2724.

73. Walsh, Z., Gonzalez, R., Crosby, K., Thiessen, M. S., Carroll, C., & Bonn-Miller, M. O. (2017). Medical cannabis and mental health: a guided systematic review. *Clinical psychology review, 51*, 15–29.

74. Watson, C. W. M., Paolillo, E. W., Morgan, E. E., Umlauf, A., Sundermann, E. E., Ellis, R. J., ... & Grant, I. (2020). Cannabis exposure is associated with a lower likelihood of neurocognitive impairment in people living with HIV. *JAIDS Journal of Acquired Immune Deficiency Syndromes, 83*(1), 56–64.

75. Thames, A. D., Mahmood, Z., Burggren, A. C., Karimian, A., & Kuhn, T. P. (2016). Combined effects of HIV and marijuana use on neurocognitive functioning and immune status. *AIDS care, 28*(5), 628–632.

76. Cristiani, S. A., Pukay-Martin, N. D., & Bornstein, R. A. (2004). Marijuana use and cognitive function in HIV-infected people. *The Journal of Neuropsychiatry and Clinical Neurosciences, 16*(3), 330–335.

77. Gruber, S. A., Sagar, K. A., Dahlgren, M. K., Gonenc, A., Smith, R. T., Lambros, A. M., ... & Lukas, S. E. (2018). The grass might be greener: medical marijuana patients exhibit altered brain activity and improved executive function after 3 months of treatment. *Frontiers in pharmacology, 8*, 983.

78. Morrison, P. D., Zois, V., McKeown, D. A., Lee, T. D., Holt, D. W., Powell, J. F., ... & Murray, R. M. (2009). The acute effects of synthetic intravenous [Delta] 9-tetrahydrocannabinol on psychosis, mood and cognitive functioning. *Psychological medicine, 39*(10), 1607.

79. Morrison, P. D., & Stone, J. M. (2011). Synthetic delta-9-tetrahydrocannabinol elicits schizophrenia-like negative symptoms which are distinct from sedation. *Human Psychopharmacology: Clinical and Experimental, 26*(1), 77–80.

80. Compton, M. T., Kelley, M. E., Ramsay, C. E., Pringle, M., Goulding, S. M., Esterberg, M. L., ... & Walker, E. F. (2009). Association of pre-onset cannabis, alcohol, and tobacco use with age at onset of prodrome and age at onset of psychosis in first-episode patients. *American Journal of Psychiatry, 166*(11), 1251–1257.

81. Galvez-Buccollini, J. A., Proal, A. C., Tomaselli, V., Trachtenberg, M., Coconcea, C., Chun, J., ... & Delisi, L. E. (2012). Association between age at onset of psychosis and age at onset of cannabis use in non-affective psychosis. *Schizophrenia research, 139*(1-3), 157–160.

82. Zammit, S., Allebeck, P., Andreasson, S., Lundberg, I., & Lewis, G. (2002). Self reported cannabis use as a risk factor for schizophrenia in Swedish conscripts of 1969: historical cohort study. *Bmj, 325*(7374), 1199.

83. Di Forti, M., Quattrone, D., Freeman, T. P., Tripoli, G., Gayer-Anderson, C., Quigley, H., ... & La Barbera, D. (2019). The contribution of cannabis use to variation in the incidence of psychotic disorder across Europe (EU-GEI): a multi-centre case-control study. *The Lancet Psychiatry, 6*(5), 427–436.

84. Frisher, M., Crome, I., Martino, O., & Croft, P. (2009). Assessing the impact of cannabis use on trends in diagnosed schizophrenia in the United Kingdom from 1996 to 2005. *Schizophrenia Research, 113*(2-3), 123–128.

85. Proal, A. C., Fleming, J., Galvez-Buccollini, J. A., & DeLisi, L. E. (2014). A controlled family study of cannabis users with and without psychosis. *Schizophrenia research, 152*(1), 283–288.

86. Ksir, C., & Hart, C. L. (2016). Cannabis and psychosis: A critical overview of the relationship. *Current Psychiatry Reports, 18*(2), 12.

87. Reviewed in Radhakrishnan, R., Wilkinson, S. T., & D'Souza, D. C. (2014). Gone to pot—A review of the association between cannabis and psychosis. *Frontiers in Psychiatry, 5*, 54.

88. Peralta, V., & Cuesta, M. J. (1992). Influence of cannabis abuse on schizophrenic psychopathology. *Acta Psychiatrica Scandinavica, 85*(2), 127–130.

89. Bersani, G., Orlandi, V., Kotzalidis, G. D., & Pancheri, P. (2002). Cannabis and schizophrenia: impact on onset, course, psychopathology and outcomes. *European Archives of Psychiatry and Clinical Neuroscience, 252*(2), 86–92.

90. Compton, M. T., Furman, A. C, & Kaslow, N. J. (2004). Lower negative symptom scores among cannabis-dependent patients with schizophrenia-spectrum disorders: Preliminary evidence from an African American first-episode sample. *Schizophrenia Research, 71*(1), 61–64.

91. Hickman, M., Vickerman, P., Macleod, J., Lewis, G., Zammit, S., Kirkbride, J., & Jones, P. (2009). If cannabis caused schizophrenia—how many cannabis users may need to be prevented in order to prevent one case of schizophrenia? England and Wales calculations. *Addiction, 104*(11), 1856–1861.

92. Reviewed in Brents, L. K. (2016). Focus: Sex and gender health: Marijuana, the endocannabinoid system and the female reproductive system. *The Yale Journal of Biology and Medicine, 89*(2), 175.

93. Reviewed in Du Plessis, S. S., Agarwal, A., & Syriac, A. (2015). Marijuana, phytocannabinoids, the endocannabinoid system, and male fertility. *Journal of Assisted Reproduction and Genetics, 32*(11), 1575–1588.

94. Reviewed in Payne, K. S., Mazur, D. J., Hotaling, J. M., & Pastuszak, A. W. (2019). Cannabis and male fertility: A systematic review. *The Journal of urology, 202*(4), 674–681.

95. Rodriguez, C. E., Sheeder, J., Allshouse, A. A., Scott, S., Wymore, E., Hopfer, C., ... & Metz, T. D. (2019). Marijuana use in young mothers and adverse pregnancy outcomes: a retrospective cohort study. *BJOG: An International Journal of Obstetrics & Gynaecology, 126*(12), 1491–1497.

96. National Academies of Sciences, Engineering, and Medicine. (2017). *The health effects of cannabis and cannabinoids: The current state of evidence and recommendations for research*. The National Academies Press. https://doi.org/10.17226/24625

97. Gunn, J. K. L., Rosales, C. B., Center, K. E., Nuñez, A., Gibson, S. J., Christ, C., & Ehiri, J. E. (2016). Prenatal exposure to cannabis and maternal and child health outcomes: a systematic review and meta-analysis. *BMJ open, 6*(4).

98. Ko, J. Y., Tong, V. T., Bombard, J. M., Hayes, D. K., Davy, J., & Perham-Hester, K. A. (2018). Marijuana use during and after pregnancy and association of prenatal use on birth outcomes: A population-based study. *Drug and alcohol dependence, 187*, 72–78.

99. Sturrock, S., Williams, E., Ambulkar, H., Dassios, T., & Greenough, A. (2020). Maternal smoking and cannabis use during pregnancy and infant outcomes. *Journal of Perinatal Medicine, 48*(2), 168–172.

100. Conner, S. N., Bedell, V., Lipsey, K., Macones, G. A., Cahill, A. G., & Tuuli, M. G. (2016). Maternal marijuana use and adverse neonatal outcomes. *Obstetrics & Gynecology, 128*(4), 713–723.

101. Rodriguez, C. E., Sheeder, J., Allshouse, A. A., Scott, S., Wymore, E., Hopfer, C., ... & Metz, T. D. (2019). Marijuana use in young mothers and adverse pregnancy outcomes: a retrospective cohort study. *BJOG: An International Journal of Obstetrics & Gynaecology, 126*(12), 1491–1497.

102. Corsi, D. J., Walsh, L., Weiss, D., Hsu, H., El-Chaar, D., Hawken, S., ... & Walker, M. (2019). Association between self-reported prenatal cannabis use and maternal, perinatal, and neonatal outcomes. *Jama, 322*(2), 145–152.

103. Grant, K. S., Petroff, R., Isoherranen, N., Stella, N., & Burbacher, T. M. (2018). Cannabis use during pregnancy: pharmacokinetics and effects on child development. *Pharmacology & therapeutics, 182*, 133–151.

104. Dreher, M. C., Nugent, K., & Hudgins, R. (1994). Prenatal marijuana exposure and neonatal outcomes in Jamaica: An ethnographic study. *Pediatrics*, *93*(2), 254–260.

105. Dalterio, S., Steger, R., Mayfield, D., & Bartke, A. (1984). Early cannabinoid exposure influences neuroendocrine and reproductive functions in male mice: I. Prenatal exposure. *Pharmacology Biochemistry and Behavior*, *20*(1), 107–113.

106. Brigante, T. A. V., Abe, F. R., Zuardi, A. W., Hallak, J. E. C., Crippa, J. A. S., & de Oliveira, D. P. (2018). Cannabidiol did not induce teratogenicity or neurotoxicity in exposed zebrafish embryos. *Chemico-biological Interactions*, *291*, 81–86.

107. Sarrafpour, Syena, et al. "Considerations and Implications of Cannabidiol Use During Pregnancy." *Current Pain and Headache Reports* 24.7 (2020): 1-10.

108. El Marroun, H., Bolhuis, K., Franken, I. H., Jaddoe, V. W., Hillegers, M. H., Lahey, B. B., & Tiemeier, H. (2019). Preconception and prenatal cannabis use and the risk of behavioural and emotional problems in the offspring; a multi-informant prospective longitudinal study. *International Journal of Epidemiology*, *48*(1), 287–296.

109. Fine, J. D., Moreau, A. L., Karcher, N. R., Agrawal, A., Rogers, C. E., Barch, D. M., & Bogdan, R. (2019). Association of prenatal cannabis exposure with psychosis proneness among children in the adolescent brain cognitive development (ABCD) Study. *JAMA psychiatry*, *76*(7), 762–764.

110. Chakraborty, A., Anstice, N. S., Jacobs, R. J., LaGasse, L. L., Lester, B. M., Wouldes, T. A., & Thompson, B. (2015). Prenatal exposure to recreational drugs affects global motion perception in preschool children. *Scientific reports*, *5*, 16921.

111. Torres, C. A., Medina-Kirchner, C., O'malley, K. Y., & Hart, C. L. (2020). Totality of the Evidence Suggests Prenatal Cannabis Exposure Does Not Lead to Cognitive Impairments: A Systematic and Critical Review. *Frontiers in Psychology*, *11*, 816.

112. Westfall, R. E., Janssen, P. A., Lucas, P., & Capler, R. (2006). Survey of medicinal cannabis use among childbearing women: patterns of its use in pregnancy and retroactive self-assessment of its efficacy against 'morning sickness'. *Complementary Therapies in Clinical Practice*, *12*(1), 27–33.

113. Koren, G., & Cohen, R. (2020). Medicinal use of cannabis in children and pregnant women. *Rambam Maimonides Medical Journal*, *11*(1), Article e0005.

114. Dole, N., Savitz, D. A., Hertz-Picciotto, I., Siega-Riz, A. M., McMahon, M. J., & Buekens, P. (2003). Maternal stress and preterm birth. *American journal of epidemiology*, *157*(1), 14–24.

115. Aizer, A., Stroud, L., & Buka, S. (2016). Maternal stress and child outcomes: Evidence from siblings. *Journal of Human Resources*, *51*(3), 523–555.

116. Van den Bergh, B. R. H., van den Heuvel, M. I., Lahti, M., Braeken, M., de Rooij, S. R., Entringer, S., Hoyer, D., Roseboom, T., Räikkönen, K., King, S., & Schwab, M. (2017). Prenatal developmental origins of behavior and mental health: The influence of maternal stress in pregnancy. *Neuroscience & Biobehavioral Reviews*. https://doi.org/10.1016/j.neubiorev.2017.07.003

117. Wexelblatt, S. L., McAllister, J. M., Nathan, A. T., & Hall, E. S. (2018). Opioid neonatal abstinence syndrome: an overview. *Clinical Pharmacology & Therapeutics*, *103*(6), 979–981.

118. Shyken, J. M., Babbar, S., Babbar, S., & Forinash, A. (2019). Benzodiazepines in pregnancy. *Clinical Obstetrics and Gynecology*, *62*(1), 156–167.

119. Kramer, E., Patnella, M., Bulko, R., Harrison, A., Lamb, H., & D'Souza, M. (2017). Neonatal Abstinence Syndrome from Selective Serotonin Reuptake Inhibitor Use During Pregnancy. *Pharmacy and Wellness Review*, *8*(1), 22–26.

120. Huizink, A. C. (2014). Prenatal cannabis exposure and infant outcomes: Overview of studies. *Progress in Neuro-Psychopharmacology and Biological Psychiatry*, *52*, 45–52.

121. Hoechstetter, S. S. (1930). Effects of alcohol and cannabis during labor. *Journal of the American Medical Association*, *94*(15), 1165.

122. Gaskin, I. M. (2010). *Spiritual midwifery*. Book Publishing Company.

123. Kerr, S. (2017, August 29). *Cannabis Use During Pregnancy: Is It Safe?* Project CBD: Medical Marijuana & Cannabinoid Science. www.projectcbd.org/medicine/cannabis-use-during-pregnancy-is-safe

124. Stanisiere, J., Mousset, P.-Y., & Lafay, S. (2018). How safe is ginger rhizome for decreasing nausea and vomiting in women during early pregnancy? *Foods*, *7*(4), 50.

125. Adlan, A.-S., Chooi, K. Y., & Adenan, N. A. M. (2017). Acupressure as adjuvant treatment for the inpatient management of nausea and vomiting in early pregnancy: A double-blind randomized controlled trial. *Journal of Obstetrics and Gynaecology Research*, *43*(4), 662–668.

126. Allais, G., Chiarle, G., Sinigaglia, S., Airola, G., Schiapparelli, P., Bergandi, F., & Benedetto, C. (2019). Acupuncture treatment of migraine, nausea, and vomiting in pregnancy. *Neurological Sciences*, *40*(1), 213–215.

127. Sahakian, V., Rouse, D., Sipes, S., Rose, N., & Niebyl, J. (1991). Vitamin B6 is effective therapy for nausea and vomiting of pregnancy: a randomized, double-blind placebo-controlled study. *Obstetrics and gynecology*, *78*(1), 33–36.

128. Danielsson, B., Wikner, B. N., & Källén, B. (2014). Use of ondansetron during pregnancy and congenital malformations in the infant. *Reproductive Toxicology*, *50*, 134–137.

129. Gaitán, A. V., Wood, J. T., Zhang, F., Makriyannis, A., & Lammi-Keefe, C. J. (2018). Endocannabinoid metabolome characterization of transitional and mature human milk. *Nutrients*, *10*(9), 1294.

130. Djulus, J., Moretti, M., & Koren, G. (2005). Marijuana use and breastfeeding. *Canadian Family Physician*, *51*(3), 349–350.

131. Baker, T., Datta, P., Rewers-Felkins, K., Thompson, H., Kallem, R. R., & Hale, T. W. (2018). Transfer of inhaled cannabis into human breast milk. *Obstetrics & Gynecology*, *131*(5), 783–788.

132. Bertrand, K. A., Hanan, N. J., Honerkamp-Smith, G., Best, B. M., & Chambers, C. D. (2018). Marijuana use by breastfeeding mothers and cannabinoid concentrations in breast milk. *Pediatrics*, *142*(3).

133. Gaitán, A. V., Wood, J. T., Zhang, F., Makriyannis, A., & Lammi-Keefe, C. J. (2018). Endocannabinoid metabolome characterization of transitional and mature human milk. *Nutrients*, *10*(9), 1294.

134. Astley, S. J., & Little, R. E. (1990). Maternal marijuana use during lactation and infant development at one year. *Neurotoxicology and Teratology*, *12*(2), 161–168.

135. Tennes, K., Avitable, N., Blackard, C., Boyles, C., Hassoun, B., Holmes, L., & Kreye, M. (1985). Marijuana: prenatal and postnatal exposure in the human. *NIDA Res Monogr*, *59*, 48–60.

136. Wang, G. S. (2017). Pediatric concerns due to expanded cannabis use: Unintended consequences of legalization. *Journal of Medical Toxicology*, *13*(1), 99–105.

137. Ryan, S. A., Ammerman, S. D., & O'Connor, M. E. (2018). Marijuana use during pregnancy and breastfeeding: Implications for neonatal and childhood outcomes. *Pediatrics*, *142*(3), Article e20181889.

138. Hill, M., & Reed, K. (2013). Pregnancy, breast-feeding, and marijuana: A review article. *Obstetrical & Gynecological Survey*, *68*(10), 710–718.

139. Ryan, S. A., Ammerman, S. D., & O'Connor, M. E. (2018). Marijuana use during pregnancy and breastfeeding: Implications for neonatal and childhood outcomes. *Pediatrics*, *142*(3), Article e20181889.

140. Sulak, D., Saneto, R., & Goldstein, B. (2017). The current status of artisanal cannabis for the treatment of epilepsy in the United States. *Epilepsy & Behavior*, *70*, 328–333.

141. Kwan, P., & Brodie, M. J. (2000). Early identification of refractory epilepsy. *New England Journal of Medicine*, *342*(5), 314–319.

142. Wong, S. S., & Wilens, T. E. (2017). Medical cannabinoids in children and adolescents: A systematic review. *Pediatrics*, *140*(5), Article e20171818.

143. Lorenz, R. (2004). On the application of cannabis in paediatrics and epileptology. *Neuroendocrinology Letters*, *25*(1/2), 40–44.

144. Gottschling, S. (2011). Gute Erfahrungen bei Schmerzen, Spastik und in der Onkologie. *Angewandte Schmerztherapie und Palliativmedizin*, *4*(1), 37–39.

145. Levine, A., Clemenza, K., Rynn, M., & Lieberman, J. (2017). Evidence for the risks and consequences of adolescent cannabis exposure. *Journal of the American Academy of Child & Adolescent Psychiatry*, *56*(3), 214–225.

146. Wong, S. S., & Wilens, T. E. (2017). Medical cannabinoids in children and adolescents: A systematic review. *Pediatrics*, *140*(5), Article e20171818.

147. Wang, T., Collet, J.-P., Shapiro, S., & Ware, M. A. (2008). Adverse effects of medical cannabinoids: A systematic review. *CMAJ*, *178*(13), 1669–1678.

148. Claudet, I., Le Breton, M., Bréhin, C., & Franchitto, N. (2017). A 10-year review of cannabis exposure in children under 3-years of age: do we need a more global approach?. *European journal of pediatrics*, *176*(4), 553–556.

149. Fride, E. (2004). The endocannabinoid-CB receptor system: Importance for development and in pediatric disease. *Neuroendocrinology Letters*, *25*(1/2), 24–30.

150. Russo, E. B. (2014). The pharmacological history of cannabis. In R. Pertwee (Ed.), *Handbook of cannabis* (pp. 23–43). Oxford University Press.

151. Abrahamov, A., Abrahamov, A., & Mechoulam, R. (1995). An efficient new cannabinoid antiemetic in pediatric oncology. *Life Sciences*, *56*(23–24), 2097–2102.

152. Decuyper, I. I., Rihs, H. P., Van Gasse, A. L., Elst, J., De Puysseleyr, L., Faber, M. A., ... & De Clerck, L. (2019). Cannabis allergy: what the clinician needs to know in 2019. *Expert Review of Clinical Immunology*, *15*(6), 599–606.

153. Stokes, J. R., Hartel, R., Ford, L. B., & Casale, T. B. (2000). Cannabis (hemp) positive skin tests and respiratory symptoms. *Annals of Allergy, Asthma & Immunology*, *85*(3), 238–240.

154. Decuyper, I. I., Van Gasse, A. L., Cop, N., Sabato, V., Faber, M. A., Mertens, C., ... & Ebo, D. G. (2017). Cannabis sativa allergy: looking through the fog. *Allergy*, *72*(2), 201–206.

155. Armentia, A., Herrero, M., Martín-Armentia, B., Rihs, H. P., Postigo, I., & Martínez-Quesada, J. (2014). Molecular diagnosis in cannabis allergy. *The Journal of Allergy and Clinical Immunology: In Practice*, *2*(3), 351–352.

156. De Larramendi, C. H., Carnés, J., García-Abujeta, J. L., García-Endrino, A., Muñoz-Palomino, E., Huertas, Á. J., ... & Ferrer, Á. (2008). Sensitization and allergy to Cannabis sativa leaves in a population of tomato (Lycopersicon esculentum)-sensitized patients. *International archives of allergy and immunology*, *146*(3), 195–202.

157. Ebo, D. G., Swerts, S., Sabato, V., Hagendorens, M. M., Bridts, C. H., Jorens, P. G., & De Clerck, L. S. (2013). New food allergies in a European non-Mediterranean region: is Cannabis sativa to blame?. *International archives of allergy and immunology*, *161*(3), 220–228.

158. Allen, J. H., De Moore, G. M., Heddle, R., & Twartz, J. (2004). Cannabinoid hyperemesis: cyclical hyperemesis in association with chronic cannabis abuse. *Gut*, *53*(11), 1566–1570.

159. Lu, M. L., & Agito, M. D. (2015). Cannabinoid hyperemesis syndrome: Marijuana is both antiemetic and proemetic. *Cleveland Clinic Journal of Medicine*, *82*(7), 429–434.

160. Bhandari, S., & Venkatesan, T. (2016). Novel treatments for cyclic vomiting syndrome: Beyond ondansetron and amitriptyline. *Current Treatment Options in Gastroenterology*, *14*(4), 495–506.

161. Stanghellini, V., Chan, F. K., Hasler, W. L., Malagelada, J. R., Suzuki, H., Tack, J., & Talley, N. J. (2016). Gastroduodenal disorders. *Gastroenterology*, *150*(6), 1380–1392.

162. Sorensen, C. J., DeSanto, K., Borgelt, L., Phillips, K. T., & Monte, A. A. (2017). Cannabinoid hyperemesis syndrome: diagnosis, pathophysiology, and treatment—a systematic review. *Journal of Medical Toxicology*, *13*(1), 71–87.

163. Sulak, D., & Theisen, E. (2019). Atypical presentation of cannabinoid hyperemesis syndrome: Two case reports. *American Journal of Endocannabinoid Medicine*, *1*(1), 31–36.

164. Richards, J. R. (2017). Cannabinoid hyperemesis syndrome: A disorder of the HPA axis and sympathetic nervous system? *Medical Hypotheses*, *103*, 90–95.

165. DeVuono, M. V., & Parker, L. A. (2020). Cannabinoid hyperemesis syndrome: A review of potential mechanisms. *Cannabis and Cannabinoid Research*, *5*(2). https://doi.org/10.1089/can.2019.0059

166. Bick, B. L., Szostek, J. H., & Mangan, T. F. (2014). Synthetic cannabinoid leading to cannabinoid hyperemesis syndrome." *Mayo Clinic Proceedings*, *89*(8), 1168–1169. https://doi.org/10.1016/j.mayocp.2014.06.013

167. Blumentrath, C. G., Dohrmann, B., & Ewald, N. (2017). Cannabinoid hyperemesis and the cyclic vomiting syndrome in adults: Recognition, diagnosis, acute and long-term treatment. *GMS German Medical Science*, *15*, Article 6. https://doi.org/10.3205/000247

168. Wagner, S., Hoppe, J., Zuckerman, M., Schwarz, K., & McLaughlin, J. (2019). Efficacy and safety of topical capsaicin for cannabinoid hyperemesis syndrome in the emergency department. *Clinical Toxicology*, *58*(6), 471–475. https://doi.org/10.1080/15563650.2019.1660783 1-5.

169. Perrotta, G., Miller, J., Stevens, T., Chauhan, A., Musunuru, H., Salciccioli, J., Cocchi, M., Donnino, M., & Walsh, M. (2012). Cannabinoid hyperemesis: Relevance to emergency medicine." *Academic Emergency Medicine*, *19*, S286–S287.

Chapter 19: Strategies for Improving Efficacy and Access

1. Grimaldi, A. E., De Giglio, L., Haggiag, S., Bianco, A., Cortese, A., Crisafulli, S. G., Monteleone, F., Marfia, G., Prosperini, L., Galgani, S., Mirabella, M., Centonze, D., Pozzilli, C., & Castelli, L. (2019). The influence of physiotherapy intervention on patients with multiple sclerosis–related spasticity treated with nabiximols (THC:CBD oromucosal spray). *PLOS ONE*, *14*(7), Article e0219670. https://doi.org/10.1371/journal.pone.0219670

2. Hammoud, M. Z., Peters, C., Hatfield, J. R. B., Gorka, S. M., Phan, K. L., Milad, M. R., & Rabinak, C. A. (2019). Influence of Δ⁹-tetrahydrocannabinol on long-term neural correlates of threat extinction memory retention in humans. *Neuropsychopharmacology*, *44*, 1769–1777. https://doi.org/10.1038/s41386-019-0416-6

3. Das, R. K., Kamboj, S. K., Ramadas, M., Yogan, K., Gupta, V., Redman, E., ... & Morgan, C. J. (2013). Cannabidiol enhances consolidation of explicit fear extinction in humans. *Psychopharmacology*, *226*(4), 781–792.

4. Ruglass, L. M., Shevorykin, A., Radoncic, V., Smith, K. M., Smith, P. H., Galatzer-Levy, I. R., ... & Hien, D. A. (2017). Impact of cannabis use on treatment outcomes among adults receiving cognitive-behavioral treatment for PTSD and substance use disorders. *Journal of Clinical Medicine*, *6*(2), 14.

5. Greeson, J. M., & Chin, G. R. (2019). Mindfulness and physical disease: A concise review. *Current Opinion in Psychology*, *28*, 204–210.

6. Aldrich, M. R. (1977). Tantric cannabis use in India. *Journal of Psychedelic Drugs*, *9*(3), 227–233.

7. Garland, E. L., Howard, M. O., Zubieta, J. K., & Froeliger, B. (2017). Restructuring hedonic dysregulation in chronic pain and prescription opioid misuse: effects of mindfulness-oriented recovery enhancement on responsiveness to drug cues and natural rewards. *Psychotherapy and psychosomatics*, *86*(2), 111.

8. Garland, E. L., Atchley, R. M., Hanley, A. W., Zubieta, J. K., & Froeliger, B. (2019). Mindfulness-Oriented Recovery Enhancement remediates hedonic dysregulation in opioid users: Neural and affective evidence of target engagement. *Science advances*, *5*(10), eaax1569.

9. Luba, R. R., Earleywine, M., Melse, B., & Gordis, E. B. (2019). Savoring moderates the link between marijuana use and marijuana problems. *Substance Use & Misuse*, *55*(2), 291–295. https://doi.org/10.1080/10826084.2019.1666145

10. Bossong, M. G., van Hell, H. H., Jager, G., Kahn, R. S., Ramsey, N. F., & Jansma, J. M. (2013). The endocannabinoid

system and emotional processing: A pharmacological fMRI study withΔ 9-tetrahydrocannabinol. *European Neuro-psychopharmacology*, *23*(12), 1687–1697.

11. Russo, E. (2005). Cannabis in India: Ancient lore and modern medicine. In *Cannabinoids as therapeutics* (pp. 1–22). Birkhäuser.

12. Jamshidi, N., & Cohen, M. M. (2017). The clinical efficacy and safety of Tulsi in humans: A systematic review of the literature. *Evidence-Based Complementary and Alternative Medicine*, *2017*, Article 9217567. https://doi.org/10.1155/2017/9217567

13. Yende, S., Harle, U., Rajgure, D., Tuse, T., & Vyawahare, N. (2008). Pharmacological profile of Acorus calamus: an overview. *Pharmacognosy Reviews*, *2*(4), 23.

14. Mukherjee, P. K., Kumar, V., Mal, M., & Houghton, P. J. (2007). In vitro acetylcholinesterase inhibitory activity of the essential oil from Acorus calamus and its main constituents. *Planta medica*, *73*(3), 283.

15. Rajput, S. B., Tonge, M. B., & Karuppayil, S. M. (2014). An overview on traditional uses and pharmacological profile of *Acorus calamus* Linn.(sweet flag) and other *Acorus* species. *Phytomedicine*, *21*(3), 268–276.

16. McPartland, J. M. (2008). Adulteration of cannabis with tobacco, calamus, and other cholinergic compounds. *Cannabinoids*, *3*, 16–20.

17. McPartland, J. M., Blanchon, D. J., & Musty, R. E. (2008). Cannabimimetic effects modulated by cholinergic compounds. *Addiction Biology*, *13*(3–4), 411–415. https://doi.org/10.1111/j.1369-1600.2008.00126.x

18. Frost, E. A. M. (2019). Kratom: A cure for chronic pain or a deadly herb? *Topics in Pain Management*, *35*(5), 1–6.

19. Coe, M. A., Pillitteri, J. L., Sembower, M. A., Gerlach, K. K., & Henningfield, J. E. (2019). Kratom as a substitute for opioids: results from an online survey. *Drug and alcohol dependence*, *202*, 24–32.

20. Caruso, I., Puttini, P. S., Cazzola, M., & Azzolini, V. (1990). Double-blind study of 5-hydroxytryptophan versus placebo in the treatment of primary fibromyalgia syndrome. *Journal of international medical research*, *18*(3), 201–209.

21. Soulairac, A., & Lambinet, H. (1988). Etudes cliniques de líaction du precurseur de la serotonine le l-5-hydroxy-tryptophane, sur les troubles du sommeil. *Schweizerische Rundschau für Medizin (PRAXIS)*, *77*(34A), 19–23.

22. Petrosino, S., & Di Marzo, V. (2017). The pharmacology of palmitoylethanolamide and first data on the therapeutic efficacy of some of its new formulations. *British Journal of Pharmacology*, *174*(11), 1349–1365.

23. Clemente, S. (2012). Amyotrophic lateral sclerosis treatment with ultramicronized palmitoylethanolamide: A case report." *CNS & Neurological Disorders-Drug Targets*, *11*(7), 933–936.

24. Palma, E., Reyes-Ruiz, J. M., Lopergolo, D., Roseti, C., Bertollini, C., Ruffolo, G., ... & Inghilleri, M. (2016). Acetylcholine receptors from human muscle as pharmacological targets for ALS therapy. *Proceedings of the National Academy of Sciences*, *113*(11), 3060–3065.

25. Brotini, S., Schievano, C., & Guidi, L. (2017). Ultra-micronized palmitoylethanolamide: An efficacious adjuvant therapy for Parkinson's disease. *CNS & Neurological Disorders-Drug Targets*, *16*(6), 705–713.

26. Caltagirone, C., Cisari, C., Schievano, C., Di Paola, R., Cordaro, M., Bruschetta, G., ... & Stroke Study Group. (2016). Co-ultramicronized palmitoylethanolamide/luteolin in the treatment of cerebral ischemia: from rodent to man. *Translational stroke research*, *7*(1), 54–69.

27. Khalaj, M., Saghazadeh, A., Shirazi, E., Shalbafan, M. R., Alavi, K., Shooshtari, M. H., ... & Akhondzadeh, S. (2018). Palmitoylethanolamide as adjunctive therapy for autism: Efficacy and safety results from a randomized controlled trial. *Journal of psychiatric research*, *103*, 104–111.

28. Reviewed in Davis, M. P., Behm, B., Mehta, Z., & Fernandez, C. (2019). The potential benefits of palmitoylethanolamide in palliation: a qualitative systematic review. *American Journal of Hospice and Palliative Medicine®*, *36*(12), 1134–1154.

29. Steels, E., Venkatesh, R., Steels, E., Vitetta, G., & Vitetta, L. (2019). A double-blind randomized placebo controlled study assessing safety, tolerability and efficacy of palmitoylethanolamide for symptoms of knee osteoarthritis. *Inflammopharmacology*, *27*(3), 475–485.

30. Ghazizadeh-Hashemi, M., Ghajar, A., Shalbafan, M. R., Ghazizadeh-Hashemi, F., Afarideh, M., Malekpour, F., ... & Akhondzadeh, S. (2018). Palmitoylethanolamide as adjunctive therapy in major depressive disorder: a double-blind, randomized and placebo-controlled trial. *Journal of Affective Disorders*, *232*, 127–133.

31. Cremon, C., Stanghellini, V., Barbaro, M. R., Cogliandro, R. F., Bellacosa, L., Santos, J., ... & Azpiroz, F. (2017). Randomised clinical trial: the analgesic properties of dietary supplementation with palmitoylethanolamide and polydatin in irritable bowel syndrome. *Alimentary Pharmacology & Therapeutics*, *45*(7), 909–922.

32. Palace, Z. J., & Reingold, D. A. (2019). Medical cannabis in the skilled nursing facility: A novel approach to improving symptom management and quality of life. *Journal of the American Medical Directors Association*, *20*(1), 94–98.

33. Haney, M., Cooper, Z. D., Bedi, G., Vosburg, S. K., Comer, S. D., & Foltin, R. W. (2013). Nabilone decreases marijuana withdrawal and a laboratory measure of marijuana relapse. *Neuropsychopharmacology*, *38*(8), 1557–1565.

34. Abu-Sawwa, R., & Stehling, C. (2020). Epidiolex (cannabidiol) primer: Frequently asked questions for patients and caregivers." *The Journal of Pediatric Pharmacology and Therapeutics*, *25*(1), 75–77.

Chapter 20: Chronic Pain and Spasticity

1. Sexton, M., Cuttler, C., Finnell, J. S., & Mischley, L. K. (2016). A cross-sectional survey of medical cannabis users: patterns of use and perceived efficacy. *Cannabis and cannabinoid research*, *1*(1), 131–138.

2. National Academies of Sciences, Engineering, and Medicine. (2017). *The health effects of cannabis and cannabinoids: The current state of evidence and recommendations for research*. National Academies Press.

3. Dahlhamer, J., Lucas, J., Zelaya, C., Nahin, R., Mackey, S., DeBar, L., ... & Helmick, C. (2018). Prevalence of chronic pain and high-impact chronic pain among adults—United States, 2016. *Morbidity and Mortality Weekly Report*, *67*(36), 1001.

4. Saxena, A. K., Jain, P. N., & Bhatnagar, S. (2018). The prevalence of chronic pain among adults in India. *Indian Journal of Palliative Care*, *24*(4), 472.

5. Fayaz, A., Croft, P., Langford, R. M., Donaldson, L. J., & Jones, G. T. (2016). Prevalence of chronic pain in the UK: A systematic review and meta-analysis of population studies. *BMJ Open*, *6*(6), Article e010364. https://doi.org/10.1136/bmjopen-2015-010364

6. Institute of Medicine. (2011). Relieving pain in America: A blueprint for transforming prevention, care, education, and research. National Academies Press.

7. Cohen, K. (2017, November 18). White House puts the cost of the opioid crisis at $504 billion in 2015. *Washington Examiner*. http://www.washingtonexaminer.com/white-house-puts-the-cost-of-the-opioid-crisis-at-504-billion-in-2015/article/2641206

8. Whiting, P. F., Wolff, R. F., Deshpande, S., Di Nisio, M., Duffy, S., Hernandez, A. V., ... & Schmidlkofer, S. (2015). Cannabinoids for medical use: a systematic review and meta-analysis. *Jama*, *313*(24), 2456–2473.

9. Koppel, B. S., Brust, J. C., Fife, T., Bronstein, J., Youssof, S., Gronseth, G., & Gloss, D. (2014). Systematic review: efficacy and safety of medical marijuana in selected neurologic disorders: report of the Guideline Development Subcommittee of the American Academy of Neurology. *Neurology*, *82*(17), 1556–1563.

10. Corey-Bloom, J., Wolfson, T., Gamst, A., Jin, S., Marcotte, T. D., Bentley, H., & Gouaux, B. (2012). Smoked cannabis for spasticity in multiple sclerosis: a randomized, placebo-controlled trial. *Cmaj*, *184*(10), 1143–1150.

11. Andreae, M. H., Carter, G. M., Shaparin, N., Suslov, K., Ellis, R. J., Ware, M. A., ... & Johnson, M. (2015). Inhaled cannabis for chronic neuropathic pain: a meta-analysis of individual patient data. *The Journal of Pain*, *16*(12), 1221–1232.

12. Vergara, D., Bidwell, L. C., Gaudino, R., Torres, A., Du, G., Ruthenburg, T. C., ... & Kane, N. C. (2017). Compromised external validity: federally produced cannabis does not reflect legal markets. *Scientific Reports*, *7*, 46528.

13. Schwabe, A. L., Hansen, C. J., Hyslop, R. M., & McGlaughlin, M. E. (2019). Research grade marijuana supplied by the National Institute on Drug Abuse is genetically divergent from commercially available cannabis. *bioRxiv*, Article 592725. https://doi.org/10.1101/592725

14. Boehnke, K. F., Scott, J. R., Litinas, E., Sisley, S., Clauw, D. J., Goesling, J., & Williams, D. A. (2019). Cannabis use preferences and decision making among a cross-sectional cohort of medical cannabis patients with chronic pain. *The Journal of Pain*, *20*(11), 1362–1372. https://doi.org/10.1016/j.jpain.2019.05.009

15. Reviewed in Karst, M., Wippermann, S., & Ahrens, J. (2010). Role of cannabinoids in the treatment of pain and (painful) spasticity. *Drugs*, *70*(18), 2409–2438.

16. Stockings, E., Campbell, G., Hall, W. D., Nielsen, S., Zagic, D., Rahman, R., ... & Degenhardt, L. (2018). Cannabis and cannabinoids for the treatment of people with chronic noncancer pain conditions: a systematic review and meta-analysis of controlled and observational studies. *Pain*, *159*(10), 1932–1954.

17. Reviewed in Karst, M., Wippermann, S., & Ahrens, J. (2010). Role of cannabinoids in the treatment of pain and (painful) spasticity. *Drugs*, *70*(18), 2409–2438.

18. Martin, B. R. (1986). Cellular effects of cannabinoids. *Pharmacological Reviews*, *38*(1), 45–74.

19. Walker, J. M., & Hohmann, A. G. (2005). Cannabinoid mechanisms of pain suppression. *Cannabinoids* (pp. 509–554). Springer.

20. Walker, J. M., & Hohmann, A. G. (2005). Cannabinoid mechanisms of pain suppression. *Cannabinoids* (pp. 509–554). Springer.

21. Garland, E. L. (2012). Pain processing in the human nervous system: A selective review of nociceptive and biobehavioral pathways. *Primary Care: Clinics in Office Practice*, *39*(3), 561–571.

22. Weizman, L., Dayan, L., Brill, S., Nahman-Averbuch, H., Hendler, T., Jacob, G., & Sharon, H. (2018). Cannabis analgesia in chronic neuropathic pain is associated with altered brain connectivity. *Neurology*, *91*(14), e1285-e1294.

23. Walker, J. M., & Hohmann, A. G. (2005). Cannabinoid mechanisms of pain suppression. *Cannabinoids* (pp. 509–554). Springer.

24. De Gregorio, D., McLaughlin, R. J., Posa, L., Ochoa-Sanchez, R., Enns, J., Lopez-Canul, M., ... & Gobbi, G. (2019). Cannabidiol modulates serotonergic transmission and reverses both allodynia and anxiety-like behavior in a model of neuropathic pain. *Pain*, *160*(1), 136.

25. Xiong, W., Cui, T., Cheng, K., Yang, F., Chen, S. R., Willenbring, D., ... & Zhang, L. (2012). Cannabinoids suppress

inflammatory and neuropathic pain by targeting α3 glycine receptors. *Journal of Experimental Medicine*, *209*(6), 1121–1134.

26. Lu, J., Fan, S., Zou, G., Hou, Y., Pan, T., Guo, W., ... & Zhang, L. (2018). Involvement of glycine receptor α1 subunits in cannabinoid-induced analgesia. *Neuropharmacology*, *133*, 224–232.

27. Rock, E. M., Limebeer, C. L., & Parker, L. A. (2018). Effect of cannabidiolic acid and Δ9-tetrahydrocannabinol on carrageenan-induced hyperalgesia and edema in a rodent model of inflammatory pain. *Psychopharmacology*, *235*(11), 3259–3271.

28. Russo, E. B. (2011). Taming THC: Potential cannabis synergy and phytocannabinoid-terpenoid entourage effects. *British Journal of Pharmacology*, *163*(7), 1344–1364.

29. Gallily, R., Yekhtin, Z., & Hanuš, L. O. (2018). The anti-inflammatory properties of terpenoids from cannabis. *Cannabis and Cannabinoid Research*, *3*(1), 282–290.

30. Pryce, G., & Baker, D. (2007). Control of spasticity in a multiple sclerosis model is mediated by CB1, not CB2, cannabinoid receptors. *British Journal of Pharmacology*, *150*(4), 519–525.

31. Reviewed in Russo, E. B. (2007). History of cannabis and its preparations in saga, science, and sobriquet. *Chemistry & Biodiversity*, *4*(8), 1614–1648.

32. Becker, C. M., Hermans-Borgmeyer, I., Schmitt, B., & Betz, H. (1986). The glycine receptor deficiency of the mutant mouse spastic: evidence for normal glycine receptor structure and localization. *Journal of Neuroscience*, *6*(5), 1358–1364.

33. Cichewicz, D. L. (2004). Synergistic interactions between cannabinoid and opioid analgesics. *Life Sciences*, *74*(11), 1317–1324.

34. Nielsen, S., Sabioni, P., Trigo, J. M., Ware, M. A., Betz-Stablein, B. D., Murnion, B., ... & Le Foll, B. (2017). Opioid-sparing effect of cannabinoids: a systematic review and meta-analysis. *Neuropsychopharmacology*, *42*(9), 1752–1765.

35. Cichewicz, D. L., & Welch, S. P. (2003). Modulation of oral morphine antinociceptive tolerance and naloxone-precipitated withdrawal signs by oral Δ⁹-tetrahydrocannabinol. *Journal of Pharmacology and Experimental Therapeutics*, *305*(3), 812–817.

36. Cichewicz, D. L., Haller, V. L., & Welch, S. P. (2001). Changes in opioid and cannabinoid receptor protein following short-term combination treatment with Δ⁹-tetrahydrocannabinol and morphine. *Journal of Pharmacology and Experimental Therapeutics*, *297*(1), 121–127.

37. Cichewicz, D. L., & McCarthy. E. A. (2003). Antinociceptive synergy between Δ⁹-tetrahydrocannabinol and opioids after oral administration. *Journal of Pharmacology and Experimental Therapeutics*, *304*(3), 1010–1015.

38. Scavone, J. L., Sterling, R. C., & Van Bockstaele, E. J. (2013). Cannabinoid and opioid interactions: Implications for opiate dependence and withdrawal. *Neuroscience, 248*, 637–654.

39. Cooper, Z. D., Bedi, G., Ramesh, D., Balter, R., Comer, S. D., & Haney, M. (2018). Impact of co-administration of oxycodone and smoked cannabis on analgesia and abuse liability. *Neuropsychopharmacology*, *43*(10), 2046–2055.

40. Abrams, D. I., Couey, P., Shade, S. B., Kelly, M. E., & Benowitz, N. L. (2011). Cannabinoid–opioid interaction in chronic pain. *Clinical Pharmacology & Therapeutics*, *90*(6), 844–851.

41. Narang, S., Gibson, D., Wasan, A. D., Ross, E. L., Michna, E., Nedeljkovic, S. S., & Jamison, R. N. (2008). Efficacy of dronabinol as an adjuvant treatment for chronic pain patients on opioid therapy. *The Journal of Pain*, *9*(3), 254–264.

42. Harris, H. M., Gul, W., ElSohly, M. A., & Sufka, K. J. (2018). Effects of Cannabidiol and a Novel Cannabidiol Analog against Tactile Allodynia in a Murine Model of Cisplatin-Induced Neuropathy: Enhanced Effects of Sub-Analgesic Doses of Morphine. *Medical Cannabis and Cannabinoids*, *1*(1), 54–59.

43. Capano, A., Weaver, R., & Burkman, E. (2020). Evaluation of the effects of CBD hemp extract on opioid use and quality of life indicators in chronic pain patients: A prospective cohort study. *Postgraduate Medicine*, *132*(1), 56–61.

44. Hurd, Y. L., Spriggs, S., Alishayev, J., Winkel, G., Gurgov, K., Kudrich, C., ... & Salsitz, E. (2019). Cannabidiol for the reduction of cue-induced craving and anxiety in drug-abstinent individuals with heroin use disorder: a double-blind randomized placebo-controlled trial. *American Journal of Psychiatry*, *176*(11), 911–922.

45. Roehrs, T., Hyde, M., Blaisdell, B., Greenwald, M., & Roth, T. (2006). Sleep loss and REM sleep loss are hyperalgesic. *Sleep*, *29*(2), 145–151.

Chapter 21: Anxiety and Trauma-Related Disorders

1. Bandelow, B., & Michaelis, S. (2015). Epidemiology of anxiety disorders in the 21st century. *Dialogues in Clinical Neuroscience*, *17*(3), 327.

2. Kosiba, J. D., Maisto, S. A., & Ditre, J. W. (2019). Patient-reported use of medical cannabis for pain, anxiety, and depression symptoms: Systematic review and meta-analysis. *Social Science & Medicine*, *233*, 181–192. https://doi.org/10.1016/j.socscimed.2019.06.005.

3. American Psychiatric Association. (2013). *Diagnostic and statistical manual of mental disorders (5th ed.)*. American Psychiatric Association.

4. Tambs, K., Czajkowsky, N., Neale, M. C., Reichborn-Kjennerud, T., Aggen, S. H., Harris, J. R., & Kendler, K. S. (2009).

Structure of genetic and environmental risk factors for dimensional representations of DSM–IV anxiety disorders. *The British Journal of Psychiatry, 195*(4), 301–307.

5. Lu, A. T., Ogdie, M. N., Järvelin, M. R., Moilanen, I. K., Loo, S. K., McCracken, J. T., … & Cantor, R. M. (2008). Association of the cannabinoid receptor gene (CNR1) with ADHD and post-traumatic stress disorder. *American Journal of Medical Genetics Part B: Neuropsychiatric Genetics, 147*(8), 1488–1494.

6. Rauch, S. L., Shin, L. M., & Wright, C. I. (2003). Neuroimaging studies of amygdala function in anxiety disorders. *Annals of the New York Academy of Sciences, 985*(1), 389–410.

7. Thayer, J. F., Friedman, B. H., & Borkovec, T. D. (1996). Autonomic characteristics of generalized anxiety disorder and worry. *Biological Psychiatry, 39*(4), 255–266.

8. Roth, W. T., Doberenz, S., Dietel, A., Conrad, A., Mueller, A., Wollburg, E., … & Kim, S. (2008). Sympathetic activation in broadly defined generalized anxiety disorder. *Journal of psychiatric research, 42*(3), 205–212.

9. Katona, I., Rancz, E. A., Acsády, L., Ledent, C., Mackie, K., Hájos, N., & Freund, T. F. (2001). Distribution of CB1 cannabinoid receptors in the amygdala and their role in the control of GABAergic transmission. *Journal of Neuroscience, 21*(23), 9506–9518.

10. Pertwee, R. G. (2008). The therapeutic potential of drugs that target cannabinoid receptors or modulate the tissue levels or actions of endocannabinoids. In *Drug Addiction* (pp. 637–686). Springer.

11. Barna, I., Zelena, D., Arszovszki, A. C., & Ledent, C. (2004). The role of endogenous cannabinoids in the hypothalamo-pituitary-adrenal axis regulation: in vivo and in vitro studies in CB1 receptor knockout mice. *Life sciences, 75*(24), 2959–2970.

12. Allen, J., Holder, M. D., & Walsh, Z. (2017). Cannabis use and well-being. In *The handbook of cannabis and related pathologies* (pp. 308–316). Elsevier.

13. Kedzior, K. K., & Laeber, L. T. (2014). A positive association between anxiety disorders and cannabis use or cannabis use disorders in the general population—A meta-analysis of 31 studies. *BMC Psychiatry, 14*(1), 136.

14. Blanco, C., Hasin, D. S., Wall, M. M., Flórez-Salamanca, L., Hoertel, N., Wang, S., … & Olfson, M. (2016). Cannabis use and risk of psychiatric disorders: prospective evidence from a US national longitudinal study. *JAMA psychiatry, 73*(4), 388–395.

15. Cougle, J. R., Hakes, J. K., Macatee, R. J., Chavarria, J., & Zvolensky, M. J. (2015). Quality of life and risk of psychiatric disorders among regular users of alcohol, nicotine, and cannabis: An analysis of the National Epidemiological Survey on Alcohol and Related Conditions (NESARC). *Journal of psychiatric research, 66*, 135–141.

16. Gage, S. H., Hickman, M., Heron, J., Munafò, M. R., Lewis, G., Macleod, J., & Zammit, S. (2015). Associations of cannabis and cigarette use with depression and anxiety at age 18: findings from the Avon Longitudinal Study of Parents and Children. *PloS one, 10*(4), e0122896.

17. Linares, I. M., Zuardi, A. W., Pereira, L. C., Queiroz, R. H., Mechoulam, R., Guimaraes, F. S., & Crippa, J. A. (2019). Cannabidiol presents an inverted U-shaped dose-response curve in a simulated public speaking test. *Brazilian Journal of Psychiatry, 41*(1), 9–14.

18. Zuardi, A. W., Rodrigues, N. P., Silva, A. L., Bernardo, S. A., Hallak, J. E., Guimarães, F. S., & Crippa, J. A. (2017). Inverted U-shaped dose-response curve of the anxiolytic effect of cannabidiol during public speaking in real life. *Frontiers in pharmacology, 8*, 259.

19. Orsolini, L., Chiappini, S., Volpe, U., De Berardis, D., Latini, R., Papanti, G. D., & Corkery, J. M. (2019). Use of medicinal cannabis and synthetic cannabinoids in post-traumatic stress disorder (PTSD): A Systematic Review. *Medicina, 55*(9), 525.

20. Hill, M. N., Bierer, L. M., Makotkine, I., Golier, J. A., Galea, S., McEwen, B. S., … & Yehuda, R. (2013). Reductions in circulating endocannabinoid levels in individuals with post-traumatic stress disorder following exposure to the World Trade Center attacks. *Psychoneuroendocrinology, 38*(12), 2952–2961.

21. Berardi, A., Schelling, G., & Campolongo, P. (2016). The endocannabinoid system and post traumatic stress disorder (PTSD): From preclinical findings to innovative therapeutic approaches in clinical settings. *Pharmacological Research, 111*, 668–678.

22. Fabre, L. F., McLendon, D. M., & Stark, P. (1978). Nabilone, a cannabinoid, in the treatment of anxiety: An open-label and double-blind study. *Current Therapeutic Research, 24*(2), 161–169.

23. Fabre, L. F., & McLendon, D. (1981). The efficacy and safety of nabilone (a synthetic cannabinoid) in the treatment of anxiety. *The Journal of Clinical Pharmacology, 21*(S1), 377S–382S.

24. Lee, M. (2009). Anxiolytic effect of an oral cannabinoid in patients with anxiety. *European Journal of Pain, 13*, S200, Article 695. https://doi.org/10.1016/S1090-3801(09)60698-4

25. Cameron, C., Watson, D., & Robinson, J. (2014). Use of a synthetic cannabinoid in a correctional population for post-traumatic stress disorder–related insomnia and nightmares, chronic pain, harm reduction, and other indications: A retrospective evaluation. *Journal of Clinical Psychopharmacology, 34*(5), 559.

26. Roitman, P., Mechoulam, R., Cooper-Kazaz, R., & Shalev, A. (2014). Preliminary, open-label, pilot study of add-on oral Δ 9-tetrahydrocannabinol in chronic post-traumatic stress disorder. *Clinical drug investigation, 34*(8), 587–591.

27. Jetly, R., Heber, A., Fraser, G., & Boisvert, D. (2015). The efficacy of nabilone, a synthetic cannabinoid, in the treat-

ment of PTSD-associated nightmares: a preliminary randomized, double-blind, placebo-controlled cross-over design study. *Psychoneuroendocrinology, 51*, 585–588.

28. Clinical Trial NCT02517424. Placebo-controlled, triple-blind, crossover study of the safety and efficacy of three different potencies of vaporized cannabis in 42 participants with chronic, treatment-resistant posttraumatic stress disorder (PTSD). https://clinicaltrials.gov/ct2/show/NCT02517424

29. Clinical Trial NCT02759185. Placebo-controlled, triple-blind, randomized crossover pilot study of the safety and efficacy of four different potencies of smoked marijuana in 76 veterans with posttraumatic stress disorder (PTSD). https://clinicaltrials.gov/ct2/show/NCT02759185

30. Walsh, Z., Gonzalez, R., Crosby, K., Thiessen, M. S., Carroll, C., & Bonn-Miller, M. O. (2017). Medical cannabis and mental health: a guided systematic review. *Clinical psychology review, 51*, 15–29.

31. Bergamaschi, M. M., Queiroz, R. H. C., Chagas, M. H. N., De Oliveira, D. C. G., De Martinis, B. S., Kapczinski, F., ... & Martín-Santos, R. (2011). Cannabidiol reduces the anxiety induced by simulated public speaking in treatment-naive social phobia patients. *Neuropsychopharmacology, 36*(6), 1219–1226.

32. Shannon, S., Lewis, N., Lee, H., & Hughes, S. (2019). Cannabidiol in Anxiety and Sleep: A Large Case Series. *The Permanente journal, 23*, 18–041.

33. Elms, L., Shannon, S., Hughes, S., & Lewis, N. (2019). Cannabidiol in the treatment of post-traumatic stress disorder: a case series. *The Journal of Alternative and Complementary Medicine, 25*(4), 392–397.

34. Lucas, P., & Walsh, Z. (2017). Medical cannabis access, use, and substitution for prescription opioids and other substances: A survey of authorized medical cannabis patients. *International Journal of Drug Policy, 42*, 30–35.

35. Corroon, J. M., Jr., Mischley, L. K., & Sexton, M. (2017). Cannabis as a substitute for prescription drugs—A cross-sectional study. *Journal of Pain Research, 10*, 989.

36. Piper, B. J., DeKeuster, R. M., Beals, M. L., Cobb, C. M., Burchman, C. A., Perkinson, L., ... & Abess, A. T. (2017). Substitution of medical cannabis for pharmaceutical agents for pain, anxiety, and sleep. *Journal of Psychopharmacology, 31*(5), 569–575.

37. Greer, G. R., Grob, C. S., & Halberstadt, A. L. (2014). PTSD symptom reports of patients evaluated for the New Mexico Medical Cannabis Program. *Journal of Psychoactive Drugs, 46*(1), 73–77.

38. Lake, S., Kerr, T., Buxton, J., Walsh, Z., Marshall, B. D., Wood, E., & Milloy, M. J. (2020). Does cannabis use modify the effect of post-traumatic stress disorder on severe depression and suicidal ideation? Evidence from a population-based cross-sectional study of Canadians. *Journal of psychopharmacology, 34*(2), 181–188.

39. Johnson, M. J., Pierce, J. D., Mavandadi, S., Klaus, J., Defelice, D., Ingram, E., & Oslin, D. W. (2016). Mental health symptom severity in cannabis using and non-using Veterans with probable PTSD. *Journal of affective disorders, 190*, 439–442.

40. Kamal, B. S., Kamal, F., & Lantela, D. E. (2018). Cannabis and the anxiety of fragmentation—A systems approach for finding an anxiolytic cannabis chemotype. *Frontiers in Neuroscience, 12*, Article 730. https://doi.org/10.3389/fnins.2018.00730

41. Reviewed in Saito, V. M., Wotjak, C. T., & Moreira, F. A. (2010). Pharmacological exploitation of the endocannabinoid system: New perspectives for the treatment of depression and anxiety disorders? *Revista Brasileira de Psiquiatria, 32*, 57–514.

42. Reviewed in Ruehle, S., Rey, A. A., Remmers, F., & Lutz, B. (2012). The endocannabinoid system in anxiety, fear memory and habituation. *Journal of Psychopharmacology, 26*(1), 23–39.

43. Rey, A. A., Purrio, M., Viveros, M. P., & Lutz, B. (2012). Biphasic effects of cannabinoids in anxiety responses: CB1 and GABA B receptors in the balance of GABAergic and glutamatergic neurotransmission. *Neuropsychopharmacology, 37*(12), 2624–2634.

44. Hill, M. N., & Gorzalka, B. B. (2006). Increased sensitivity to restraint stress and novelty-induced emotionality following long-term, high dose cannabinoid exposure. *Psychoneuroendocrinology, 31*(4), 526–536.

45. Reviewed in Van Ameringen, M., Zhang, J., Patterson, B., & Turna, J. (2020). The role of cannabis in treating anxiety: an update. *Current Opinion in Psychiatry, 33*(1), 1–7.

46. Berardi, A., Schelling, G., & Campolongo, P. (2016). The endocannabinoid system and post traumatic stress disorder (PTSD): From preclinical findings to innovative therapeutic approaches in clinical settings. *Pharmacological Research, 111*, 668–678.

47. Pertwee, R. G., Greentree, S. G., & Swift, P. A. (1988). Drugs which stimulate or facilitate central GABAergic transmission interact synergistically with delta-9-tetrahydrocannabinol to produce marked catalepsy in mice. *Neuropharmacology, 27*(12), 1265–1270.

48. Pertwee, R. G., & Greentree, S. G. (1988). Synergistic interactions between delta-9-THC and flurazepam: Further studies. In *Marijuana: An International Research Report*. Proceedings of the Melbourne Symposium on Cannabis, September 2–4, 1987. Australian Government Publishing Service.

Chapter 22: Sleep Disorders

1. Liu, Y., Wheaton, A. G., Chapman, D. P., Cunningham, T. J., Lu, H., & Croft, J. B. (2016). Prevalence of healthy sleep duration among adults—United States, 2014. *Morbidity and Mortality Weekly Report*, *65*(6), 137–141.

2. Liu, Y., Croft, J. B., Wheaton, A. G., Perry, G. S., Chapman, D. P., Strine, T. W., ... & Presley-Cantrell, L. (2013). Association between perceived insufficient sleep, frequent mental distress, obesity and chronic diseases among US adults, 2009 behavioral risk factor surveillance system. *BMC public health*, *13*(1), 84.

3. Gomes, A. A., Tavares, J., & de Azevedo, M. H. P. (2011). Sleep and academic performance in undergraduates: A multi-measure, multi-predictor approach. *Chronobiology International*, *28*(9), 786–801.

4. Thorne, D. R., Thomas, M. L., Russo, M. B., Sing, H. C., Balkin, T. J., Wesensten, N. J., ... & Cephus, R. (1999). Performance on a driving-simulator divided attention task during one week of restricted nightly sleep. *Sleep*, *22*(Suppl 1), 301.

5. Freeman, D., Sheaves, B., Goodwin, G. M., Yu, L. M., Nickless, A., Harrison, P. J., ... & Hinds, C. (2017). The effects of improving sleep on mental health (OASIS): a randomised controlled trial with mediation analysis. *The Lancet Psychiatry*, *4*(10), 749–758.

6. Reviewed in Haack, M., Simpson, N., Sethna, N., Kaur, S., & Mullington, J. (2020). Sleep deficiency and chronic pain: potential underlying mechanisms and clinical implications. *Neuropsychopharmacology*, *45*(1), 205–216.

7. Tang, N. K., Goodchild, C. E., Sanborn, A. N., Howard, J., & Salkovskis, P. M. (2012). Deciphering the temporal link between pain and sleep in a heterogeneous chronic pain patient sample: a multilevel daily process study. *Sleep*, *35*(5), 675–687.

8. Ho, K. K. N., Ferreira, P. H., Pinheiro, M. B., Silva, D. A., Miller, C. B., Grunstein, R., & Simic, M. (2019). Sleep interventions for osteoarthritis and spinal pain: a systematic review and meta-analysis of randomized controlled trials. *Osteoarthritis and cartilage*, *27*(2), 196–218.

9. Reviewed in Haack, M., Simpson, N., Sethna, N., Kaur, S., & Mullington, J. (2020). Sleep deficiency and chronic pain: potential underlying mechanisms and clinical implications. *Neuropsychopharmacology*, *45*(1), 205–216.

10. Van Gastel, A. (2018). Drug-induced insomnia and excessive sleepiness. *Sleep Medicine Clinics*, *13*(2), 147–159.

11. Kundermann, B., Krieg, J. C., Schreiber, W., & Lautenbacher, S. (2004). The effects of sleep deprivation on pain. *Pain Research and Management*, *9*.

12. Reviewed in Aguirre, C. C. (2016). Sleep deprivation: A mind-body approach. *Current Opinion in Pulmonary Medicine*, *22*(6), 583–588.

13. Reviewed in Aguirre, C. C. (2016). Sleep deprivation: A mind-body approach. *Current Opinion in Pulmonary Medicine*, *22*(6), 583–588.

14. Küry, P., Nath, A., Créange, A., Dolei, A., Marche, P., Gold, J., ... & Perron, H. (2018). Human endogenous retroviruses in neurological diseases. *Trends in molecular medicine*, *24*(4), 379–394.

15. Spiegel, K., Sheridan, J. F., & Van Cauter, E. (2002). Effect of sleep deprivation on response to immunization. *JAMA*, *288*(12), 1471–1472.

16. Reinoso-Suárez, F., de Andrés I., & Garzón, M. (2011). The sleep–wakefulness cycle. In *Functional anatomy of the sleep–wakefulness cycle: Wakefulness*. Advances in Anatomy, Embryology and Cell Biology, vol 208. Springer. https://doi.org/10.1007/978-3-642-14626-8_1

17. Reviewed in Ramful, A. (2005). Psychological disturbances caused by sleep deprivation in intensive care patients. *British Journal of Anaesthetic & Recovery Nursing*, *6*(4), 63–67.

18. Chokroverty, S. (1994). Physiologic changes in sleep. In *Sleep disorders medicine* (pp. 57–76). Butterworth-Heinemann.

19. Kashiwagi, M., & Hayashi, Y. (2016). The function of REM sleep: Implications from transgenic mouse models. *Shinkei Kenkyu no Shinpo [Brain and Nerve]*, *68*(10), 1205–1211.

20. Reviewed in Schierenbeck, T., Riemann, D., Berger, M., & Hornyak, M. (2008). Effect of illicit recreational drugs upon sleep: cocaine, ecstasy and marijuana. *Sleep medicine reviews*, *12*(5), 381–389.

21. Fronmüller, B. (1869). *Klinische Studien über die schlafmachende Wirkung der narkotischen Arzneimittel [Clinical studies on the sleep inducing effects of narcotic medicines]*. Enke.

22. Cousens, K., & DiMascio, A. (1973). (-)Δ⁹THC as an hypnotic: An experimental study of three dose levels. *Psychopharmacologia*, *33*(4), 355–364.

23. Carlini, E. A., & Cunha, J. M. (1981). Hypnotic and antiepileptic effects of cannabidiol. *The Journal of Clinical Pharmacology*, *21*(S1), 417S–427S.

24. Nicholson, A. N., Turner, C., Stone, B. M., & Robson, P. J. (2004). Effect of Δ-9-tetrahydrocannabinol and cannabidiol on nocturnal sleep and early-morning behavior in young adults. *Journal of clinical psychopharmacology*, *24*(3), 305–313.

25. Linares, I. M., Guimaraes, F. S., Eckeli, A., Crippa, A., Zuardi, A. W., Souza, J. D., ... & Crippa, J. A. (2018). No acute effects of cannabidiol on the sleep-wake cycle of healthy subjects: a randomized, double-blind, placebo-controlled, crossover study. *Frontiers in pharmacology*, *9*, 315.

26. Carley, D. W., Prasad, B., Reid, K. J., Malkani, R., Attarian, H., Abbott, S. M., ... & Zee, P. C. (2018). Pharmacotherapy

of apnea by cannabimimetic enhancement, the PACE clinical trial: effects of dronabinol in obstructive sleep apnea. *Sleep*, *41*(1).

27. Calik, M. W., & Carley, D. W. (2016). Intracerebroventricular injections of dronabinol, a cannabinoid receptor agonist, does not attenuate serotonin-induced apnea in Sprague-Dawley rats. *Journal of Negative Results in Biomedicine*, *15*(1), 8.

28. Toth, C., Mawani, S., Brady, S., Chan, C., Liu, C., Mehina, E., ... & Korngut, L. (2012). An enriched-enrolment, randomized withdrawal, flexible-dose, double-blind, placebo-controlled, parallel assignment efficacy study of nabilone as adjuvant in the treatment of diabetic peripheral neuropathic pain. *PAIN®*, *153*(10), 2073–2082.

29. Narang, S., Gibson, D., Wasan, A. D., Ross, E. L., Michna, E., Nedeljkovic, S. S., & Jamison, R. N. (2008). Efficacy of dronabinol as an adjuvant treatment for chronic pain patients on opioid therapy. *The Journal of Pain*, *9*(3), 254–264.

30. Ware, M. A., Wang, T., Shapiro, S., Robinson, A., Ducruet, T., Huynh, T., ... & Collet, J. P. (2010). Smoked cannabis for chronic neuropathic pain: a randomized controlled trial. *Cmaj*, *182*(14), E694-E701.

31. Ware, M. A., Fitzcharles, M. A., Joseph, L., & Shir, Y. (2010). The effects of nabilone on sleep in fibromyalgia: results of a randomized controlled trial. *Anesthesia & Analgesia*, *110*(2), 604–610.

32. Russo, E. B., Guy, G. W, & Robson, P. J. (2007). Cannabis, pain, and sleep: Lessons from therapeutic clinical trials of Sativex, a cannabis-based medicine. *Chemistry & Biodiversity*, *4*(8), 1729–1743.

33. Sznitman, S. R., Vulfsons, S., Meiri, D., & Weinstein, G. (2020). Medical cannabis and insomnia in older adults with chronic pain: A cross-sectional study. *BMJ Supportive & Palliative Care*. Online ahead of print. https://doi.org/10.1136/bmjspcare-2019-001938

34. Shannon, S., Lewis, N., Lee, H., & Hughes, S. (2019). Cannabidiol in anxiety and sleep: A large case series. *The Permanente Journal*, *23*, Article 18-041. https://doi.org/10.7812/TPP/18-041

35. Fraser, G. A. (2009). The use of a synthetic cannabinoid in the management of treatment-resistant nightmares in posttraumatic stress disorder (PTSD). *CNS Neuroscience & Therapeutics*, *15*(1), 84–88.

36. Roitman, P., Mechoulam, R., Cooper-Kazaz, R., & Shalev, A. (2014). Preliminary, open-label, pilot study of add-on oral Δ 9-tetrahydrocannabinol in chronic post-traumatic stress disorder. *Clinical drug investigation*, *34*(8), 587–591.

37. Woodward, M. R., Harper, D. G., Stolyar, A., Forester, B. P., & Ellison, J. M. (2014). Dronabinol for the treatment of agitation and aggressive behavior in acutely hospitalized severely demented patients with noncognitive behavioral symptoms. *The American Journal of Geriatric Psychiatry*, *22*(4), 415–419.

38. Walther, S., Mahlberg, R., Eichmann, U., & Kunz, D. (2006). Delta-9-tetrahydrocannabinol for nighttime agitation in severe dementia. *Psychopharmacology (Berlin)*, *185*(4), 524–528.

39. Neff, G. W., O'Brien, C. B., Reddy, K. R., Bergasa, N. V., Regev, A., Molina, E., ... & Schiff, E. (2002). Preliminary observation with dronabinol in patients with intractable pruritus secondary to cholestatic liver disease. *The American journal of gastroenterology*, *97*(8), 2117–2119.

40. Chagas, M. H., Eckeli, A. L., Zuardi, A. W., Pena-Pereira, M. A., Sobreira-Neto, M. A., Sobreira, E. T., ... & Tumas, V. (2014). Cannabidiol can improve complex sleep-related behaviours associated with rapid eye movement sleep behaviour disorder in Parkinson's disease patients: a case series. *Journal of clinical pharmacy and therapeutics*, *39*(5), 564–566.

41. Vigil, J. M., Stith, S. S., Diviant, J. P., Brockelman, F., Keeling, K., & Hall, B. (2018). Effectiveness of raw, natural medical Cannabis flower for treating insomnia under naturalistic conditions. *Medicines*, *5*(3), 75.

42. Bowles, N. P., Herzig, M. X., Bhide, M., & Shea, S. A. (2019). 0130 Cannabis Use, Sleep, and Sleepiness: An Online Survey. *Sleep*, *42*(Supplement_1), A53-A54.

43. Bachhuber, M., Arnsten, J. H., & Wurm, G. (2019). Use of cannabis to relieve pain and promote sleep by customers at an adult use dispensary. *Journal of Psychoactive Drugs*, *51*(5), 400–404.

44. Doremus, J. M., Stith, S. S., & Vigil, J. M. (2019). Using recreational cannabis to treat insomnia: Evidence from over-the-counter sleep aid sales in Colorado. *Complementary Therapies in Medicine*, *47*, Article 102207. https://doi.org/10.1016/j.ctim.2019.102207

45. Reviewed in Suraev, A. S., Marshall, N. S., Vandrey, R., McCartney, D. M., Benson, M. J., McGregor, I. S., Grunstein, R. R., & Hoyos, C. M. (2020). Cannabinoid therapies in the management of sleep disorders: A systematic review of preclinical and clinical studies. *Sleep Medicine Reviews*, *53*, Article 101339. https://doi.org/10.1016/j.smrv.2020.101339

Chapter 23: Cancer

1. Abrams, D. I. (2016). Integrating cannabis into clinical cancer care." *Current Oncology*, *23*(Suppl 2), S8.

2. Ladin, D. A., Soliman, E., Griffin, L., & Van Dross, R. (2016). Preclinical and clinical assessment of cannabinoids as anti-cancer agents. *Frontiers in pharmacology*, *7*, 361.

3. Abrams, D. I. (2016). Integrating cannabis into clinical cancer care." *Current Oncology*, *23*(Suppl 2), S8.

4. Mei, Z., Shi, L., Wang, B., Yang, J., Xiao, Z., Du, P., ... & Yang, W. (2017). Prognostic role of pretreatment blood neutro-

phil-to-lymphocyte ratio in advanced cancer survivors: a systematic review and meta-analysis of 66 cohort studies. *Cancer treatment reviews*, *58*, 1–13.

5. Petrie, H. T., Klassen, L. W., & Kay, H. D. (1985). Inhibition of human cytotoxic T lymphocyte activity in vitro by autologous peripheral blood granulocytes. *The Journal of Immunology*, *134*(1), 230–234.

6. Elliott, R. L., & Blobe, G. C. (2005). Role of transforming growth factor beta in human cancer. *Journal of Clinical Oncology*, *23*(9), 2078–2093.

7. Pedrazzani, C., Mantovani, G., Fernandes, E., Bagante, F., Salvagno, G. L., Surci, N., … & Guglielmi, A. (2017). Assessment of neutrophil-to-lymphocyte ratio, platelet-to-lymphocyte ratio and platelet count as predictors of long-term outcome after R0 resection for colorectal cancer. *Scientific reports*, *7*(1), 1–10.

8. Miao, P., Sheng, S., Sun, X., Liu, J., & Huang, G. (2013). Lactate dehydrogenase A in cancer: a promising target for diagnosis and therapy. *IUBMB life*, *65*(11), 904–910.

9. Holloway A. (2014, October 15). *Did ancient Siberian princess use cannabis to cope with breast cancer?* Ancient Origins. http://www.ancient-origins.net/news-history-archaeology/did-ancient-siberian-princess-use-cannabis-cope-breast-cancer-002207

10. National Academies of Sciences, Engineering, and Medicine. (2017). *The health effects of cannabis and cannabinoids: The current state of evidence and recommendations for research*. The National Academies Press. https://doi.org/10.17226/24625

11. Fallon, M. T., Albert Lux, E., McQuade, R., Rossetti, S., Sanchez, R., Sun, W., … & Kornyeyeva, E. (2017). Sativex oromucosal spray as adjunctive therapy in advanced cancer patients with chronic pain unalleviated by optimized opioid therapy: two double-blind, randomized, placebo-controlled phase 3 studies. *British journal of pain*, *11*(3), 119–133.

12. Fallon, M. T., Albert Lux, E., McQuade, R., Rossetti, S., Sanchez, R., Sun, W., … & Kornyeyeva, E. (2017). Sativex oromucosal spray as adjunctive therapy in advanced cancer patients with chronic pain unalleviated by optimized opioid therapy: two double-blind, randomized, placebo-controlled phase 3 studies. *British journal of pain*, *11*(3), 119–133.

13. Steele, G., Arneson, T., & Zylla, D. (2019). A comprehensive review of cannabis in patients with cancer: Availability in the USA, general efficacy, and safety. *Current Oncology Reports*, *21*(1), 10.

14. Rosewall, T., Feuz, C., & Bayley, A. (2020). Cannabis and radiation therapy: A scoping review of human clinical trials. *Journal of Medical Imaging and Radiation Sciences*, *51*(2), 342–349.

15. Côté, M., Trudel, M., Wang, C., & Fortin, A. (2016). Improving quality of life with nabilone during radiotherapy treatments for head and neck cancers: a randomized double-blind placebo-controlled trial. *Annals of Otology, Rhinology & Laryngology*, *125*(4), 317–324.

16. Elliott, D. A., Nabavizadeh, N., Romer, J. L., Chen, Y., & Holland, J. M. (2016). Medical marijuana use in head and neck squamous cell carcinoma patients treated with radiotherapy. *Supportive Care in Cancer*, *24*(8), 3517–3524.

17. Anderson, S. P., Zylla, D. M., McGriff, D. M., & Arneson, T. J. (2019). Impact of medical cannabis on patient-reported symptoms for patients with cancer enrolled in Minnesota's medical cannabis program. *Journal of oncology practice*, *15*(4), e338-e345.

18. Schleider, L. B.-L., Mechoulam, R., Lederman, V., Hilou, M., Lencovsky, O., Betzalel, O., Shbiro, L., & Novack, V. (2018). Prospective analysis of safety and efficacy of medical cannabis in large unselected population of patients with cancer. *European Journal of Internal Medicine*, *49*, 37–43.

19. Zylla, D. M., Eklund, J., Gilmore, G., Gavenda, A., Vazquez-Benitez, G., Pawloski, P. A., … & Dudek, A. Z. (2019). A randomized trial of medical cannabis (MC) in patients with advanced cancer (AC) to assess impact on opioid use and cancer-related symptoms. *Journal of Clinical Oncology*, *37*(31_suppl), Abstract 109.

20. Guzman, M., Duarte, M. J., Blazquez, C., Ravina, J., Rosa, M. C., Galve-Roperh, I., … & González-Feria, L. (2006). A pilot clinical study of Δ 9-tetrahydrocannabinol in patients with recurrent glioblastoma multiforme. *British journal of cancer*, *95*(2), 197–203.

21. Singh, Y., & Bali, C. (2013). Cannabis extract treatment for terminal acute lymphoblastic leukemia with a Philadelphia chromosome mutation. *Case Reports in Oncology*, *6*(3), 585–592.

22. Twelves, C., Short, S., & Wright, S. (2017). A two-part safety and exploratory efficacy randomized double-blind, placebo-controlled study of a 1 : 1 ratio of the cannabinoids cannabidiol and delta-9-tetrahydrocannabinol (CBD:THC) plus dose-intense temozolomide in patients with recurrent glioblastoma multiforme (GBM). *Journal of Clinical Oncology*, *35*(15_suppl), Abstract 2046. https://doi.org/10.1200/JCO.2017.35.15_suppl.2046

23. Dall'Stella, P. B., Docema, M. F., Maldaun, M. V., Feher, O., & Lancellotti, C. L. (2019). Case report: Clinical outcome and image response of two patients with secondary high-grade glioma treated with chemoradiation, PCV, and cannabidiol. *Frontiers in oncology*, *8*, 643.

24. Kenyon, J., Liu, W. A. I., & Dalgleish, A. (2018). Report of objective clinical responses of cancer patients to pharmaceutical-grade synthetic cannabidiol. *Anticancer Research*, *38*(10), 5831–5835.

25. Likar, R., Koestenberger, M., Stultschnig, M., & Nahler, G. (2019). Concomitant Treatment of Malignant Brain Tumours With CBD–A Case Series and Review of the Literature. *Anticancer Research*, *39*(10), 5797–5801.

26. Sulé-Suso, J., Watson, N. A., van Pittius, D. G., & Jegannathen, A. (2019). Striking lung cancer response to self-administration of cannabidiol: A case report and literature review. *SAGE Open Medical Case Reports, 7*, Article 2050313X19832160. https://doi.org/10.1177/2050313X19832160

27. Kander, J. (2020). *Cannabis for the treatment of cancer: The anticancer activity of phytocannabinoids and endocannabinoids* (6th ed.).

28. Ligresti, A., Bisogno, T., Matias, I., De Petrocellis, L., Cascio, M. G., Cosenza, V., ... & Di Marzo, V. (2003). Possible endocannabinoid control of colorectal cancer growth. *Gastroenterology, 125*(3), 677–687.

29. Cianchi, F., Papucci, L., Schiavone, N., Lulli, M., Magnelli, L., Vinci, M. C., ... & Donnini, M. (2008). Cannabinoid receptor activation induces apoptosis through tumor necrosis factor α–mediated ceramide de novo synthesis in colon cancer cells. *Clinical Cancer Research, 14*(23), 7691–7700.

30. Xu, X., Liu, Y., Huang, S., Liu, G., Xie, C., Zhou, J., ... & Miao, X. (2006). Overexpression of cannabinoid receptors CB1 and CB2 correlates with improved prognosis of patients with hepatocellular carcinoma. *Cancer genetics and cytogenetics, 171*(1), 31–38.

31. Reviewed in Kovalchuk, O., & Kovalchuk, I. (2020). Cannabinoids as anticancer therapeutic agents. *Cell Cycle 19*(9), 961–989. https://doi.org/10.1080/15384101.2020.1742952

32. Torres, S., Lorente, M., Rodríguez-Fornés, F., Hernández-Tiedra, S., Salazar, M., García-Taboada, E., ... & Velasco, G. (2011). A combined preclinical therapy of cannabinoids and temozolomide against glioma. *Molecular cancer therapeutics, 10*(1), 90–103.

33. Armstrong, J. L., Hill, D. S., McKee, C. S., Hernandez-Tiedra, S., Lorente, M., Lopez-Valero, I., ... & Velasco, G. (2015). Exploiting cannabinoid-induced cytotoxic autophagy to drive melanoma cell death. *Journal of Investigative Dermatology, 135*(6), 1629–1637.

34. Armstrong, J. L., Hill, D. S., McKee, C. S., Hernandez-Tiedra, S., Lorente, M., Lopez-Valero, I., ... & Velasco, G. (2015). Exploiting cannabinoid-induced cytotoxic autophagy to drive melanoma cell death. *Journal of Investigative Dermatology, 135*(6), 1629–1637.

35. De Petrocellis, L., Ligresti, A., Schiano Moriello, A., Iappelli, M., Verde, R., Stott, C. G., ... & Di Marzo, V. (2013). Non-THC cannabinoids inhibit prostate carcinoma growth in vitro and in vivo: pro-apoptotic effects and underlying mechanisms. *British journal of pharmacology, 168*(1), 79–102.

36. Nallathambi, R., Mazuz, M., Namdar, D., Shik, M., Namintzer, D., Vinayaka, A. C., ... & Konikoff, F. M. (2018). Identification of synergistic interaction between cannabis-derived compounds for cytotoxic activity in colorectal cancer cell lines and colon polyps that induces apoptosis-related cell death and distinct gene expression. *Cannabis and cannabinoid research, 3*(1), 120–135.

37. Kuttan, G., Pratheeshkumar, P., Manu, K. A., & Kuttan, R. (2011). Inhibition of tumor progression by naturally occurring terpenoids. *Pharmaceutical biology, 49*(10), 995–1007.

38. Holland, M. L., Allen, J. D., & Arnold, J. C. (2008). Interaction of plant cannabinoids with the multidrug transporter ABCC1 (MRP1). *European Journal of Pharmacology, 591*(1–3), 128–131.

39. Blasco-Benito, S., Seijo-Vila, M., Caro-Villalobos, M., Tundidor, I., Andradas, C., García-Taboada, E., ... & Gordon, M. (2018). Appraising the "entourage effect": antitumor action of a pure cannabinoid versus a botanical drug preparation in preclinical models of breast cancer. *Biochemical pharmacology, 157*, 285–293.

40. Baram, L., Peled, E., Berman, P., Yellin, B., Besser, E., Benami, M., ... & Meiri, D. (2019). The heterogeneity and complexity of Cannabis extracts as antitumor agents. *Oncotarget, 10*(41), 4091.

41. Baram, L., Peled, E., Berman, P., Yellin, B., Besser, E., Benami, M., ... & Meiri, D. (2019). The heterogeneity and complexity of Cannabis extracts as antitumor agents. *Oncotarget, 10*(41), 4091.

42. Donadelli, M., Dando, I., Zaniboni, T., Costanzo, C., Dalla Pozza, E., Scupoli, M. T., ... & Bifulco, M. (2011). Gemcitabine/cannabinoid combination triggers autophagy in pancreatic cancer cells through a ROS-mediated mechanism. *Cell death & disease, 2*(4), e152-e152.

43. Miyato, H., Kitayama, J., Yamashita, H., Souma, D., Asakage, M., Yamada, J., & Nagawa, H. (2009). Pharmacological synergism between cannabinoids and paclitaxel in gastric cancer cell lines. *Journal of Surgical Research, 155*(1), 40–47.

44. Preet, A., Qamri, Z., Nasser, M. W., Prasad, A., Shilo, K., Zou, X., ... & Ganju, R. K. (2011). Cannabinoid receptors, CB1 and CB2, as novel targets for inhibition of non–small cell lung cancer growth and metastasis. *Cancer prevention research, 4*(1), 65–75.

45. Blasco-Benito, S., Seijo-Vila, M., Caro-Villalobos, M., Tundidor, I., Andradas, C., García-Taboada, E., ... & Gordon, M. (2018). Appraising the "entourage effect": antitumor action of a pure cannabinoid versus a botanical drug preparation in preclinical models of breast cancer. *Biochemical pharmacology, 157*, 285–293.

46. Gustafsson, S. B., Lindgren, T., Jonsson, M., & Jacobsson, S. O. (2009). Cannabinoid receptor-independent cytotoxic effects of cannabinoids in human colorectal carcinoma cells: synergism with 5-fluorouracil. *Cancer chemotherapy and pharmacology, 63*(4), 691–701.

47. Reviewed in Velasco, G., Sánchez, C., & Guzmán, M. (2016). Anticancer mechanisms of cannabinoids. *Current Oncology, 23*(Suppl 2), S23.

48. Torres, S., Lorente, M., Rodríguez-Fornés, F., Hernández-Tiedra, S., Salazar, M., García-Taboada, E., ... & Velasco, G. (2011). A combined preclinical therapy of cannabinoids and temozolomide against glioma. *Molecular cancer therapeutics*, *10*(1), 90–103.

49. Scott, K. A., Dalgleish, A. G., & Liu, W. M. (2014). The combination of cannabidiol and Δ⁹-tetrahydrocannabinol enhances the anticancer effects of radiation in an orthotopic murine glioma model. *Molecular Cancer Therapeutics*, *13*(12), 2955–2967. https://doi.org/10.1158/1535-7163.MCT-14-0402

50. Reviewed in Blanton, H. L., Brelsfoard, J., DeTurk, N., Pruitt, K., Narasimhan, M., Morgan, D. J., & Guindon, J. (2019). Cannabinoids: Current and future options to treat chronic and chemotherapy-induced neuropathic pain. *Drugs*, *79*(9), 969–995. https://doi.org/10.1007/s40265-019-01132-x

51. Reviewed in Masocha, W. (2018). Targeting the endocannabinoid system for prevention or treatment of chemotherapy-induced neuropathic pain: Studies in animal models. *Pain Research and Management*, *2018*, Article 5234943. https://doi.org/10.1155/2018/5234943

52. Taha, T., Meiri, D., Talhamy, S., Wollner, M., Peer, A., & Bar-Sela, G. (2019). Cannabis impacts tumor response rate to nivolumab in patients with advanced malignancies. *The oncologist*, *24*(4), 549.

53. Liu, C., Sadat, S. H., Ebisumoto, K., Sakai, A., Panuganti, B. A., Ren, S., Goto, Y., Haft, S., Fukusumi, T., Ando, M., Saito, Y., Guo, T., Tayamo, P., Yeema, H., Kim, W., Hubbard, J., Sharabi, A. B, Gutkind, J. S., & Califano, J. A. (2020). Cannabinoids promote progression of HPV positive head and neck squamous cell carcinoma via p38 MAPK activation. *Clinical Cancer Research*, *26*(11), 2693–2703. https://doi.org/10.1158/1078-0432.CCR-18-3301

54. Zhang, H., Xie, M., Levin, M., Archibald, S. D., Jackson, B. S., Young, J. E. M., & Gupta, M. K. (2019). Survival outcomes of marijuana users in p16 positive oropharynx cancer patients. *Journal of Otolaryngology-Head & Neck Surgery*, *48*(1), 43.

Chapter 24: Alzheimer's Disease and Other Forms of Dementia

1. 2019 American Geriatrics Society Beers Criteria Update Expert Panel. (2019). American Geriatrics Society 2019 updated AGS Beers Criteria for potentially inappropriate medication use in older adults. *Journal of the American Geriatrics Society*, *67*(4), 674–694.

2. Jirón, M., Pate, V., Hanson, L. C., Lund, J. L., Jonsson Funk, M., & Stürmer, T. (2016). Trends in prevalence and determinants of potentially inappropriate prescribing in the United States: 2007 to 2012. *Journal of the American Geriatrics Society*, *64*(4), 788–797.

3. Alhawassi, T. M., Alatawi, W., & Alwhaibi, M. (2019). Prevalence of potentially inappropriate medications use among older adults and risk factors using the 2015 American Geriatrics Society Beers criteria. *BMC Geriatrics*, *19*(1), 154.

4. Chiapella, L. C., Menna, J. M., Marzi, M., & Mamprin, M. E. (2019). Prevalence of potentially inappropriate medications in older adults in Argentina using Beers criteria and the IFAsPIAM List. *International Journal of Clinical Pharmacy*, *41*(4), 913–919.

5. Anrys, P. M., Strauven, G. C., Foulon, V., Degryse, J. M., Henrard, S., & Spinewine, A. (2018). Potentially inappropriate prescribing in Belgian nursing homes: prevalence and associated factors. *Journal of the American Medical Directors Association*, *19*(10), 884–890.

6. Volicer, L., Stelly, M., Morris, J., McLaughlin, J., & Volicer, B. J. (1997). Effects of dronabinol on anorexia and disturbed behavior in patients with Alzheimer's disease. International journal of geriatric psychiatry, 12(9), 913–919.

7. Woodward, M. R., Harper, D. G., Stolyar, A., Forester, B. P., & Ellison, J. M. (2014). Dronabinol for the treatment of agitation and aggressive behavior in acutely hospitalized severely demented patients with noncognitive behavioral symptoms. *The American Journal of Geriatric Psychiatry*, *22*(4), 415–419.

8. Walther, S., Mahlberg, R., Eichmann, U., & Kunz, D. (2006). Delta-9-tetrahydrocannabinol for nighttime agitation in severe dementia. *Psychopharmacology (Berlin)*, *185*(4), 524–528.

9. van den Elsen, G. A., Ahmed, A. I., Verkes, R. J., Feuth, T., van der Marck, M. A., & Rikkert, M. G. O. (2015). Tetrahydrocannabinol in behavioral disturbances in dementia: a crossover randomized controlled trial. *The American Journal of Geriatric Psychiatry*, *23*(12), 1214–1224.

10. Shelef, A., Barak, Y., Berger, U., Paleacu, D., Tadger, S., Plopsky, I., & Baruch, Y. (2016). Safety and efficacy of medical cannabis oil for behavioral and psychological symptoms of dementia: an open label, add-on, pilot study. *Journal of Alzheimer's disease*, *51*(1), 15–19.

11. Broers, B., Pata, Z., Mina, A., Wampfler, J., De Saussure, C., & Pautex, S. (2019). Prescription of a THC/CBD-based medication to patients with dementia: a pilot study in Geneva. *Medical Cannabis and Cannabinoids*, *2*(1), 56–59.

12. Gómez, P. M. H., Ochoa-Orozco, S. A., & Toro, C. J. (in press). Cannabinoids for major neurocognitive disorder: Case report and literature review. *Revista Colombiana de Psiquiatría*. https://doi.org/10.1016/j.rcp.2019.07.002

13. Herrmann, N., Ruthirakuhan, M., Gallagher, D., Verhoeff, N. P. L., Kiss, A., Black, S. E., & Lanctôt, K. L. (2019). Randomized placebo-controlled trial of nabilone for agitation in Alzheimer's disease. *The American Journal of Geriatric Psychiatry*, *27*(11), 1161–1173.

14. Wang, L., Liu, J., Harvey-White, J., Zimmer, A., & Kunos, G. (2003). Endocannabinoid signaling via cannabinoid recep-

tor 1 is involved in ethanol preference and its age-dependent decline in mice. *Proceedings of the National Academy of Sciences of the United States of America*, *100*, 1393–1398.

15. Piyanova, A., Lomazzo, E., Bindila, L., Lerner, R., Albayram, O., Ruhl, T., Lutz, B., Zimmer, A., & Bilkei-Gorzo, A. (2015). Age-related changes in the endocannabinoid system in the mouse hippocampus. *Mechanisms of Ageing and Development*, *150*, 55–64.

16. Ferrer, I. (2014). Cannabinoids for treatment of Alzheimer's disease: Moving toward the clinic. *Frontiers in Pharmacology*, *5*, 37.

17. Bilkei-Gorzo, A., Albayram, O., Draffehn, A., Michel, K., Piyanova, A., Oppenheimer, H., ... & Bab, I. (2017). A chronic low dose of Δ 9-tetrahydrocannabinol (THC) restores cognitive function in old mice. *Nature Medicine*, *23*(6), 782.

18. Sarne, Y., Toledano, R., Rachmany, L., Sasson, E., & Doron, R. (2018). Reversal of age-related cognitive impairments in mice by an extremely low dose of tetrahydrocannabinol. *Neurobiology of Aging*, *61*, 177–186.

19. American Geriatrics Society 2015 Beers Criteria Update Expert Panel. (2015). American Geriatrics Society 2015 updated Beers Criteria for potentially inappropriate medication use in older adults. *Journal of the American Geriatrics Society*, *63*(11), 2227–2246.

20. Leweke, F. M., Piomelli, D., Pahlisch, F., Muhl, D., Gerth, C. W., Hoyer, C., ... & Koethe, D. (2012). Cannabidiol enhances anandamide signaling and alleviates psychotic symptoms of schizophrenia. *Translational psychiatry*, *2*(3), e94-e94.

21. Farrimond, J. A., Whalley, B. J., & Williams, C. M. (2012). Cannabinol and cannabidiol exert opposing effects on rat feeding patterns. *Psychopharmacology*, *223*(1), 117–129.

22. Patel, S., & Hillard, C. J. (2001). Cannabinoid CB(1) receptor agonists produce cerebellar dysfunction in mice. *The Journal of Pharmacology and Experimental Therapeutics*, *297*, 629–637.

23. Muir, S. W., Gopaul, K., & Odasso, M. M. M. (2012). The role of cognitive impairment in fall risk among older adults: A systematic review and meta-analysis. *Age and Ageing*, *41*(3), 299–308.

24. van den Elsen, G. A., Tobben, L., Ahmed, A. I., Verkes, R. J., Kramers, C., Marijnissen, R. M., ... & van der Marck, M. A. (2017). Effects of tetrahydrocannabinol on balance and gait in patients with dementia: a randomised controlled crossover trial. *Journal of psychopharmacology*, *31*(2), 184–191.

25. McPartland, J. M., Blanchon, D. J., & Musty, R. E. (2008). Cannabimimetic effects modulated by cholinergic compounds. *Addiction Biology*, *13*(3–4), 411–415.

Chapter 25: Seizure Disorders

1. St. Louis, E. K., & Cascino, G. D. (2016). Diagnosis of epilepsy and related episodic disorders. *CONTINUUM: Lifelong Learning in Neurology*, *22*(1), 15–37.

2. Kwan, P., Schachter, S. C., & Brodie, M. J. (2011). Drug-resistant epilepsy. *New England Journal of Medicine*, *365*(10), 919–926.

3. Kwan, P., Schachter, S. C., & Brodie, M. J. (2011). Drug-resistant epilepsy. *New England Journal of Medicine*, *365*(10), 919–926.

4. French, J. A. (2007). Refractory epilepsy: Clinical overview. *Epilepsia*, *48*, 3–7.

5. Reviewed in Russo, E. B. (2017). Cannabis and epilepsy: An ancient treatment returns to the fore. *Epilepsy & Behavior* *70*, 292–297.

6. Anderson, L. L., Low, I. K., Banister, S. D., McGregor, I. S., & Arnold, J. C. (2019). Pharmacokinetics of phytocannabinoid acids and anticonvulsant effect of cannabidiolic acid in a mouse model of Dravet syndrome. *Journal of Natural Products*, *82*(11), 3047–3055.

7. Oby, E., & Janigro, D. (2006). The blood–brain barrier and epilepsy. *Epilepsia*, *47*(11), 1761–1774.

8. Devinsky, O., Cross, J. H., Laux, L., Marsh, E., Miller, I., Nabbout, R., ... & Wright, S. (2017). Trial of cannabidiol for drug-resistant seizures in the Dravet syndrome. *New England Journal of Medicine*, *376*(21), 2011–2020.

9. Devinsky, O., Patel, A. D., Cross, J. H., Villanueva, V., Wirrell, E. C., Privitera, M., ... & Zuberi, S. M. (2018). Effect of cannabidiol on drop seizures in the Lennox–Gastaut syndrome. *New England Journal of Medicine*, *378*(20), 1888–1897.

10. Thiele, E. A., Marsh, E. D., French, J. A., Mazurkiewicz-Beldzinska, M., Benbadis, S. R., Joshi, C., ... & Gunning, B. (2018). Cannabidiol in patients with seizures associated with Lennox-Gastaut syndrome (GWPCARE4): a randomised, double-blind, placebo-controlled phase 3 trial. *The Lancet*, *391*(10125), 1085–1096.

11. Devinsky, O., Patel, A. D., Thiele, E. A., Wong, M. H., Appleton, R., Harden, C. L., ... & GWPCARE1 Part A Study Group. (2018). Randomized, dose-ranging safety trial of cannabidiol in Dravet syndrome. *Neurology*, *90*(14), e1204-e1211.

12. Lattanzi, S., Brigo, F., Trinka, E., Zaccara, G., Cagnetti, C., Del Giovane, C., & Silvestrini, M. (2018). Efficacy and safety of cannabidiol in epilepsy: a systematic review and meta-analysis. *Drugs*, *78*(17), 1791–1804.

13. Lattanzi, S., Brigo, F., Trinka, E., Zaccara, G., Cagnetti, C., Del Giovane, C., & Silvestrini, M. (2018). Efficacy and safety of cannabidiol in epilepsy: a systematic review and meta-analysis. *Drugs*, *78*(17), 1791–1804.

14. Sands, T. T., Rahdari, S., Oldham, M. S., Nunes, E. C., Tilton, N., & Cilio, M. R. (2019). Long-term safety, tolerability, and efficacy of cannabidiol in children with refractory epilepsy: results from an expanded access program in the US. *Cns Drugs*, *33*(1), 47–60.

15. Stockings, E., Zagic, D., Campbell, G., Weier, M., Hall, W. D., Nielsen, S., ... & Degenhardt, L. (2018). Evidence for cannabis and cannabinoids for epilepsy: a systematic review of controlled and observational evidence. *Journal of Neurology, Neurosurgery & Psychiatry*, *89*(7), 741–753.

16. Pamplona, F. A., Rolim da Silva, L., & Coan, A. C. (2018). Potential clinical benefits of CBD-rich *Cannabis* extracts over purified CBD in treatment-resistant epilepsy: Observational data meta-analysis." *Frontiers in Neurology*, *9*, 759.

17. Pamplona, F. A., Rolim da Silva, L., & Coan, A. C. (2019). Corrigendum: Potential clinical benefits of CBD-rich *Cannabis* extracts over purified CBD in treatment-resistant epilepsy: Observational data meta-analysis. *Frontiers in Neurology*, *9*, 1050.

18. Pamplona, F. A., Rolim da Silva, L., & Coan, A. C. (2018). Potential clinical benefits of CBD-rich *Cannabis* extracts over purified CBD in treatment-resistant epilepsy: Observational data meta-analysis." *Frontiers in Neurology*, *9*, 759.

19. Gaston, T. E., Szaflarski, M., Hansen, B., Bebin, E. M., & Szaflarski, J. P. (2019). Quality of life in adults enrolled in an open-label study of cannabidiol (CBD) for treatment-resistant epilepsy. *Epilepsy & Behavior*, *95*, 10–17.

20. Gaston, T. E., Bebin, E. M., Cutter, G. R., Liu, Y., Szaflarski, J. P., & UAB CBD Program. (2017). Interactions between cannabidiol and commonly used antiepileptic drugs. *Epilepsia*, *58*(9), 1586–1592.

21. Sulak, D., Saneto, R., & Goldstein, B. (2017). The current status of artisanal cannabis for the treatment of epilepsy in the United States. *Epilepsy & Behavior*, *70*, 328–333.

22. Chen, K. A., Farrar, M., Cardamone, M., Gill, D., Smith, R., Cowell, C. T., ... & Lawson, J. A. (2018). Cannabidiol for treating drug-resistant epilepsy in children: the New South Wales experience. *Medical Journal of Australia*, *209*(5), 217–221.

23. Massot-Tarrús, A., & McLachlan, R. S. (2016). Marijuana use in adults admitted to a Canadian epilepsy monitoring unit. *Epilepsy & Behavior*, *63*, 73–78.

24. Tzadok, M., Uliel-Siboni, S., Linder, I., Kramer, U., Epstein, O., Menascu, S., ... & Dor, M. (2016). CBD-enriched medical cannabis for intractable pediatric epilepsy: the current Israeli experience. *Seizure*, *35*, 41–44..

25. Sulak, D., Saneto, R., & Goldstein, B. (2017). The current status of artisanal cannabis for the treatment of epilepsy in the United States. *Epilepsy & Behavior*, *70*, 328–333.

26. Pane, C., & Saccà, F. (2020). The use of medical grade cannabis in Italy for drug-resistant epilepsy: A case series. *Neurological Sciences*, *41*(3), 695–698.

27. Massot-Tarrús, A., & McLachlan, R. S. (2016). Marijuana use in adults admitted to a Canadian epilepsy monitoring unit. *Epilepsy & Behavior*, *63*, 73–78.

28. Yap, M., Easterbrook, L., Connors, J., & Koopmans, L. (2015). Use of cannabis in severe childhood epilepsy and child protection considerations. *Journal of paediatrics and child health*, *51*(5), 491–496.

29. Perucca, P., Carter, J., Vahle, V., & Gilliam, F. G. (2009). Adverse antiepileptic drug effects: toward a clinically and neurobiologically relevant taxonomy. *Neurology*, *72*(14), 1223–1229.

30. Devinsky, O., Cilio, M. R., Cross, H., Fernandez-Ruiz, J., French, J., Hill, C., ... & Martinez-Orgado, J. (2014). Cannabidiol: pharmacology and potential therapeutic role in epilepsy and other neuropsychiatric disorders. *Epilepsia*, *55*(6), 791–802.

31. Karler, R., & Turkanis, S. A. (1979). Cannabis and epilepsy. In *Marihuana Biological Effects* (pp. 619–641). Pergamon. https://doi.org/10.1016/B978-0-08-023759-6.50052-4

32. Reviewed in Ben-Zeev, B. (2020). Medical cannabis for intractable epilepsy in childhood: A review. *Rambam Maimonides Medical Journal*, *11*(1), Article e0004. https://doi.org/10.5041/RMMJ.10387

33. Huizenga, M. N., Sepulveda-Rodriguez, A., & Forcelli, P. A. (2019). Preclinical safety and efficacy of cannabidivarin for early life seizures. *Neuropharmacology*, *148*, 189–198.

34. Anderson, L. L., Low, I. K., Banister, S. D., McGregor, I. S., & Arnold, J. C. (2019). Pharmacokinetics of phytocannabinoid acids and anticonvulsant effect of cannabidiolic acid in a mouse model of Dravet syndrome. *Journal of Natural Products*, *82*(11), 3047–3055.

35. Fisher, R. S., Cross, J. H., French, J. A., Higurashi, N., Hirsch, E., Jansen, F. E., ... & Scheffer, I. E. (2017). Operational classification of seizure types by the International League Against Epilepsy: Position Paper of the ILAE Commission for Classification and Terminology. *Epilepsia*, *58*(4), 522–530.

36. Hegde, M., Santos-Sanchez, C., Hess, C. P., Kabir, A. A., & Garcia, P. A. (2012). Seizure exacerbation in two patients with focal epilepsy following marijuana cessation. *Epilepsy & Behavior*, *25*(4), 563–566.

37. Christiansen, C., Rødbro, P., & Sjö, O. (1974). "Anticonvulsant action" of vitamin D in epileptic patients? A controlled pilot study. *British Medical Journal*, *2*(5913), 258–259.

38. DeGiorgio, C. M., Hertling, D., Curtis, A., Murray, D., & Markovic, D. (2019). Safety and tolerability of Vitamin D3 5000 IU/day in epilepsy. *Epilepsy & Behavior*, *94*, 195–197.

39. Mehrotra, P., Marwaha, R. K., Aneja, S., Seth, A., Singla, B. M., Ashraf, G., ... & Tandon, N. (2010). Hypovitaminosis d and hypocalcemic seizures in infancy. *Indian pediatrics*, *47*(7), 581–586.

40. Uwitonze, A. M., & Razzaque, M. S. (2018). Role of magnesium in vitamin D activation and function. *The Journal of the American Osteopathic Association*, 118(3), 181–189.

41. Reddy, P., & Edwards, L. R. (2019). Magnesium supplementation in vitamin D deficiency. *American Journal of Therapeutics*, 26(1), e124–e132.

42. Hussain, S. Z., Belkind-Gerson, J., Chogle, A., Bhuiyan, M. A., Hicks, T., & Misra, S. (2019). Probable neuropsychiatric toxicity of polyethylene glycol: roles of media, internet and the caregivers. *GastroHep*, 1(3), 118–123.

43. Bahgat, K. A., Elhady, M., Aziz, A. A., Youness, E. R., & Zakzok, E. (2019). Omega-6/omega-3 ratio and cognition in children with epilepsy. *Anales de Pediatría (English Edition)*, 91(2), 88–95.

44. Tejada, S., Martorell, M., Capó, X., Tur, J. A., Pons, A., & Sureda, A. (2019). Omega-3 fatty acids and epilepsy. In *The Molecular Nutrition of Fats* (pp. 261-270). Academic Press.

Chapter 26: Autism Spectrum Disorders

1. Baio, J., Wiggins, L., Christensen, D. L., Maenner, M. J., Daniels, J., Warren, Z., Kurzius-Spencer, M., Zahorodny, W., Rosenberg, C. R., White, T., Durkin, M. S., Imm, P., Nikolaou, L., Yeargin-Allsopp, M., Lee, L.-C., Harrington, R., Lopez, M., Fitzgerald, R. T., Hewitt, A., … Dowling, N. F. (2018). Prevalence of autism spectrum disorder among children aged 8 years—Autism and Developmental Disabilities Monitoring Network, 11 Sites, United States, 2014. *Morbidity and Mortality Weekly Report Surveillance Summaries*, 67(SS-6), 1–23. http://dx.doi.org/10.15585/mmwr.ss6706a1external

2. Ozonoff, S., Young, G. S., Carter, A., Messinger, D., Yirmiya, N., Zwaigenbaum, L., … & Hutman, T. (2011). Recurrence risk for autism spectrum disorders: a Baby Siblings Research Consortium study. *Pediatrics*, 128(3), e488-e495.

3. American Psychiatric Association. (2013). *Diagnostic and statistical manual of mental disorders (5th edition)*. American Psychiatric Association.

4. Aran, A., Eylon, M., Harel, M., Polianski, L., Nemirovski, A., Tepper, S., … & Tam, J. (2019). Lower circulating endocannabinoid levels in children with autism spectrum disorder. *Molecular autism*, 10(1), 1–11.

5. Kurz, R., & Blaas, K. (2010). Use of dronabinol (delta-9-THC) in autism: A prospective single-case-study with an early infantile autistic child. *Cannabinoids*, 5(4), 4–6.

6. Kuester, G., Vergara, K., Ahumada, A., & Gazmuri, A. M. (2017). Oral cannabis extracts as a promising treatment for the core symptoms of autism spectrum disorder: preliminary experience in chilean patients. *Journal of the Neurological Sciences*, 381, 932–933.

7. Aran, A., Cassuto, H., Lubotzky, A., Wattad, N., & Hazan, E. (2019). Brief report: Cannabidiol-rich cannabis in children with autism spectrum disorder and severe behavioral problems—A retrospective feasibility study. *Journal of autism and developmental disorders*, 49(3), 1284–1288.

8. Schleider, L. B.-L., Mechoulam, R., Saban, N., Meiri, G., & Novack, V. (2019). Real life experience of medical cannabis treatment in autism: Analysis of safety and efficacy. *Scientific Reports*, 9(1), Article 200.

9. Barchel, D., Stolar, O., De-Haan, T., Ziv-Baran, T., Saban, N., Fuchs, D. O., Koren, G., & Berkovitch, M. (2019) Oral cannabidiol use in children with autism spectrum disorder to treat related symptoms and co-morbidities. *Frontiers in Pharmacology*, 9, 1521.

10. Pretzsch, C. M., Voinescu, B., Mendez, M. A., Wichers, R., Ajram, L., Ivin, G., Heasman, M., Williams, S., Murphy, D. G. M., Daly, E., & McAlonan, G. M. (2019). The effect of cannabidiol (CBD) on low-frequency activity and functional connectivity in the brain of adults with and without autism spectrum disorder (ASD). *Journal of Psychopharmacology*, 33(9), 1141–1148. https://doi.org/10.1177/0269881119858306

11. Caddeo, A., Trampetti, G. M., Porta, E., Di Fede, G., Tartarelli, R., Tartarelli, O., Monzon, A., Porro, G., & Lissoni, P. (2020). A neuroendocrine therapeutic approach with the pineal hormone melatonin, cannabidiol and oxytocin (MCO regimen) in the treatment of the autism spectrum disorders." *Journal of Immunology and Allergy*, 1(2), 1–7.

12. Reviewed in Zamberletti, E., Gabaglio, M., & Parolaro, D. (2017). The endocannabinoid system and autism spectrum disorders: Insights from animal models. *International Journal of Molecular Sciences*, 18(9), 1916.

13. Wei, D., Lee, D., Cox, C. D., Karsten, C. A., Peñagarikano, O., Geschwind, D. H., … & Piomelli, D. (2015). Endocannabinoid signaling mediates oxytocin-driven social reward. *Proceedings of the National Academy of Sciences*, 112(45), 14084-14089.

14. Goldstein, B. (2018, July 29). Personal communication.

Chapter 27: Anorexia and Cachexia

1. Witte, K. K. A., & Clark, A. L. (2002). Nutritional abnormalities contributing to cachexia in chronic illness. *International Journal of Cardiology*, 85(1), 23–31.

2. Fearon, K., Strasser, F., Anker, S. D., Bosaeus, I., Bruera, E., Fainsinger, R. L., … & Davis, M. (2011). Definition and classification of cancer cachexia: an international consensus. *The lancet oncology*, 12(5), 489–495.

3. Zipfel, S., Giel, K. E., Bulik, C. M., Hay, P., & Schmidt, U. (2015). Anorexia nervosa: aetiology, assessment, and treatment. *The lancet psychiatry, 2*(12), 1099–1111.

4. Matias, I., & Di Marzo, V. (2007). Endocannabinoids and the control of energy balance. *Trends in Endocrinology & Metabolism, 18*(1), 27–37.

5. Le Strat, Y., & Le Foll, B. (2011). Obesity and cannabis use: Results from 2 representative national surveys. *American Journal of Epidemiology, 174*(8), 929–933.

6. Vidot, D. C., Prado, G., Hlaing, W. M., Florez, H. J., Arheart, K. L., & Messiah, S. E. (2016). Metabolic syndrome among marijuana users in the United States: an analysis of National Health and Nutrition Examination Survey data. *The American journal of medicine, 129*(2), 173–179.

7. Whiting, P. F., Wolff, R. F., Deshpande, S., Di Nisio, M., Duffy, S., Hernandez, A. V., ... & Schmidlkofer, S. (2015). Cannabinoids for medical use: a systematic review and meta-analysis. *Jama, 313*(24), 2456–2473.

8. Lutge, E. E., Gray, A., & Siegfried, N. (2013). The medical use of cannabis for reducing morbidity and mortality in patients with HIV/AIDS. *Cochrane Database of Systematic Reviews, 4*, Article CD005175. https://doi.org/10.1002/14651858.CD005175.pub3

9. Strasser, F., Luftner, D., Possinger, K., Ernst, G., Ruhstaller, T., Meissner, W., ... & Cerny, T. (2006). Comparison of orally administered cannabis extract and delta-9-tetrahydrocannabinol in treating patients with cancer-related anorexia-cachexia syndrome: a multicenter, phase III, randomized, double-blind, placebo-controlled clinical trial from the Cannabis-In-Cachexia-Study-Group. *Journal of Clinical Oncology, 24*(21), 3394–3400.

10. Jatoi, A., Windschitl, H. E., Loprinzi, C. L., Sloan, J. A., Dakhil, S. R., Mailliard, J. A., ... & Novotny, P. J. (2002). Dronabinol versus megestrol acetate versus combination therapy for cancer-associated anorexia: a North Central Cancer Treatment Group study. *Journal of clinical oncology, 20*(2), 567–573.

11. Gross, H., Ebert, M. H., Faden, V. B., Goldberg, S. C., Kaye, W. H., Caine, E. D., ... & Zinberg, N. (1983). A double-blind trial of Δ9-tetrahydrocannabinol in primary anorexia nervosa. *Journal of Clinical Psychopharmacology, 3*(3), 165–171.

12. Andries, A., Frystyk, J., Flyvbjerg, A., & Støving, R. K. (2014). Dronabinol in severe, enduring anorexia nervosa: a randomized controlled trial. *International Journal of Eating Disorders, 47*(1), 18–23.

13. Monteleone, P., Bifulco, M., Di Filippo, C., Gazzerro, P., Canestrelli, B., Monteleone, F., ... & Maj, M. (2009). Association of CNR1 and FAAH endocannabinoid gene polymorphisms with anorexia nervosa and bulimia nervosa: evidence for synergistic effects. *Genes, Brain and Behavior, 8*(7), 728–732.

14. Ishiguro, H., Carpio, O., Horiuchi, Y., Shu, A., Higuchi, S., Schanz, N., ... & Onaivi, E. S. (2010). A nonsynonymous polymorphism in cannabinoid CB2 receptor gene is associated with eating disorders in humans and food intake is modified in mice by its ligands. *Synapse, 64*(1), 92–96.

15. Monteleone, P., Matias, I., Martiadis, V., De Petrocellis, L., Maj, M., & Di Marzo, V. (2005). Blood levels of the endocannabinoid anandamide are increased in anorexia nervosa and in binge-eating disorder, but not in bulimia nervosa. *Neuropsychopharmacology, 30*, 1216–1221.

16. Frieling, H., Albrecht, H., Jedtberg, S., Gozner, A., Lenz, B., Wilhelm, J., ... & Bleich, S. (2009). Elevated cannabinoid 1 receptor mRNA is linked to eating disorder related behavior and attitudes in females with eating disorders. *Psychoneuroendocrinology, 34*(4), 620–624.

17. Gerard, N., Pieters, G., Goffin, K., Bormans, G., & Van Laere, K. (2011). Brain type 1 cannabinoid receptor availability in patients with anorexia and bulimia nervosa. *Biological Psychiatry, 70*, 777–784.

18. Cristino, L., & Di Marzo, V. (2014). Established and emerging concepts of cannabinoid action on food intake and their potential application to the treatment of anorexia and cachexia. In R. Pertwee (Ed.), *Handbook of Cannabis* (Chapter 24). Oxford University Press. https://doi.org/10.1093/acprof:oso/9780199662685.003.0024

19. Morgan, C. J., Freeman, T. P., Schafer, G. L., & Curran, H. V. (2010). Cannabidiol attenuates the appetitive effects of Δ 9-tetrahydrocannabinol in humans smoking their chosen cannabis. *Neuropsychopharmacology, 35*(9), 1879–1885.

Chapter 28: Drug Substitution and Harm Reduction

1. Reiman, A. (2009). Cannabis as a substitute for alcohol and other drugs. *Harm Reduction Journal, 6*(1), 35.

2. Lucas, P., Walsh, Z., Crosby, K., Callaway, R., Belle-Isle, L., Kay, R., ... & Holtzman, S. (2016). Substituting cannabis for prescription drugs, alcohol and other substances among medical cannabis patients: The impact of contextual factors. *Drug and Alcohol Review, 35*(3), 326–333.

3. Corroon, J. M., Jr., Mischley, L. K., & Sexton, M. (2017). Cannabis as a substitute for prescription drugs—A cross-sectional study. *Journal of Pain Research, 10*, 989.

4. Piper, B. J., DeKeuster, R. M., Beals, M. L., Cobb, C. M., Burchman, C. A., Perkinson, L., ... & Abess, A. T. (2017). Substitution of medical cannabis for pharmaceutical agents for pain, anxiety, and sleep. *Journal of Psychopharmacology, 31*(5), 569–575.

5. Lucas, P., & Walsh, Z. (2017). Medical cannabis access, use, and substitution for prescription opioids and other substances: A survey of authorized medical cannabis patients. *International Journal of Drug Policy*, *42*, 30–35.

6. Mercurio, A., Aston, E. R., Claborn, K. R., Waye, K., & Rosen, R. K. (2019). Marijuana as a Substitute for Prescription Medications: A Qualitative Study. *Substance use & misuse*, *54*(11), 1894–1902.

7. Raby, W. N., Carpenter, K. M., Rothenberg, J., Brooks, A. C., Jiang, H., Sullivan, M., ... & Nunes, E. V. (2009). Intermittent marijuana use is associated with improved retention in naltrexone treatment for opiate-dependence. *American Journal on Addictions*, *18*(4), 301–308.

8. Bisaga, A., Sullivan, M. A., Glass, A., Mishlen, K., Pavlicova, M., Haney, M., ... & Nunes, E. V. (2015). The effects of dronabinol during detoxification and the initiation of treatment with extended release naltrexone. *Drug and alcohol dependence*, *154*, 38–45.

9. Bagra, I., Krishnan, V., Rao, R., & Agrawal, A. (2018). Does cannabis use influence opioid outcomes and quality of life among buprenorphine maintained patients? A cross-sectional, comparative study. *Journal of Addiction Medicine*, *12*(4), 315–320.

10. Hurd, Y. L., Yoon, M., Manini, A. F., Hernandez, S., Olmedo, R., Ostman, M., & Jutras-Aswad, D. (2015). Early phase in the development of cannabidiol as a treatment for addiction: opioid relapse takes initial center stage. *Neurotherapeutics*, *12*(4), 807–815.

11. Hurd, Y. L., Spriggs, S., Alishayev, J., Winkel, G., Gurgov, K., Kudrich, C., ... & Salsitz, E. (2019). Cannabidiol for the reduction of cue-induced craving and anxiety in drug-abstinent individuals with heroin use disorder: a double-blind randomized placebo-controlled trial. *American Journal of Psychiatry*, *176*(11), 911–922.

12. Morgan, C. J., Das, R. K., Joye, A., Curran, H. V., & Kamboj, S. K. (2013). Cannabidiol reduces cigarette consumption in tobacco smokers: preliminary findings. *Addictive behaviors*, *38*(9), 2433–2436.

13. Hindocha, C., Freeman, T. P., Grabski, M., Stroud, J. B., Crudgington, H., Davies, A. C., ... & Curran, H. V. (2018). Cannabidiol reverses attentional bias to cigarette cues in a human experimental model of tobacco withdrawal. *Addiction*, *113*(9), 1696–1705.

14. Labigalini, E., Rodrigues, L. R., & Da Silveira, D. X. (1999). Therapeutic use of cannabis by crack addicts in Brazil. *Journal of Psychoactive Drugs*, *31*(4), 451–455.

15. Dreher, M. (2002). Crack heads and roots daughters: The therapeutic use of cannabis in Jamaica. *Journal of Cannabis Therapeutics*, *2*(3–4), 121–133.

16. Gonçalves, J. R., & Nappo, S. A. (2015). Factors that lead to the use of crack cocaine in combination with marijuana in Brazil: A qualitative study. *BMC Public Health*, *15*(1), 706.

17. Socías, M. E., Kerr, T., Wood, E., Dong, H., Lake, S., Hayashi, K., ... & Milloy, M. J. (2017). Intentional cannabis use to reduce crack cocaine use in a Canadian setting: A longitudinal analysis. *Addictive behaviors*, *72*, 138–143.

18. Aharonovich, E., Liu, X., Samet, S., Nunes, E., Waxman, R., & Hasin, D. (2005). Postdischarge cannabis use and its relationship to cocaine, alcohol, and heroin use: a prospective study. *American Journal of Psychiatry*, *162*(8), 1507–1514.

19. Viola, T. W., Tractenberg, S. G., Wearick-Silva, L. E., de Oliveira Rosa, C. S., Pezzi, J. C., & Grassi-Oliveira, R. (2014). Long-term cannabis abuse and early-onset cannabis use increase the severity of cocaine withdrawal during detoxification and rehospitalization rates due to cocaine dependence. *Drug and Alcohol Dependence*, *144*, 153–159.

20. Gonçalves, J. R., & Nappo, S. A. (2015). Factors that lead to the use of crack cocaine in combination with marijuana in Brazil: A qualitative study. *BMC Public Health*, *15*(1), 706.

21. Edes, R. T. (1887). *Text-book of Therapeutics and Materia Medica*. Lea Brothers.

22. Potter, S. O. L. (1895). *Handbook of materia medica, pharmacy, and therapeutics: Including the physiological action of drugs, the special therapeutics of disease, official and practical pharmacy, and minute directions for prescription writing*. Blakiston.

23. Eli Lilly and Company. (1898). *Hand book of pharmacy & therapeutics* (5th revision). Eli Lilly and Company.

24. *Merck Manual*. (1899). Merck.

25. Mikuriya, T. H. (2004). Cannabis as a substitute for alcohol: A harm-reduction approach. *Journal of Cannabis Therapeutics*, *4*(1), 79–93.

26. Subbaraman, M. S. (2014). Can cannabis be considered a substitute medication for alcohol? *Alcohol and Alcoholism*, *49*(3), 292–298.

27. Reviewed in Chye, Y., Christensen, E., Solowij, N., & Yücel, M. (2019). The endocannabinoid system and cannabidiol's promise for the treatment of substance use disorder. *Frontiers in Psychiatry*, *10*, 63. https://doi.org/10.3389/fpsyt.2019.00063

28. Reviewed in Wenzel, J. M., & Cheer, J. F. (2018). Endocannabinoid regulation of reward and reinforcement through interaction with dopamine and endogenous opioid signaling. *Neuropsychopharmacology*, *43*(1), 103–115.

29. Reviewed in Parsons, L. H., & Hurd, Y. L. (2015). Endocannabinoid signalling in reward and addiction. *Nature Reviews Neuroscience*, *16*(10), 579–594.

30. Reviewed in Parsons, L. H., & Hurd, Y. L. (2015). Endocannabinoid signalling in reward and addiction. *Nature Reviews Neuroscience*, *16*(10), 579–594.

31. Lavie-Ajayi, M., & Shvartzman, P. (2019). Restored self: A phenomenological study of pain relief by cannabis. *Pain Medicine, 20*(11), 2086–2093.

32. Karoly, H. C., Bidwell, L. C., Mueller, R. L., & Hutchison, K. E. (2018). Investigating the relationships between alcohol consumption, cannabis use, and circulating cytokines: a preliminary analysis. *Alcoholism: Clinical and Experimental Research, 42*(3), 531–539.

Chapter 29: Cannabis for Health Promotion and Disease Prevention

1. Buttorff, C., Ruder, T., & Bauman, M. (2017). *Multiple chronic conditions in the United States.* RAND Corporation. https://www.rand.org/content/dam/rand/pubs/tools/TL200/TL221/RAND_TL221.pdf

2. Centers for Disease Control and Prevention (2020, 6 May). *National Center for Chronic Disease Prevention and Health Promotion (NCCDPHP).* Accessed June 18, 2020, at www.cdc.gov/chronicdisease/index.htm

3. Centers for Disease Control and Prevention (2020, 23 Mar). *Health and economic costs of chronic diseases.* Accessed June 18, 2020, at www.cdc.gov/chronicdisease/about/costs/index.htm

4. Liu, Y., Wheaton, A. G., Chapman, D. P., Cunningham, T. J., Lu, H., & Croft, J. B. (2016). Prevalence of healthy sleep duration among adults—United States, 2014. *Morbidity and Mortality Weekly Report, 65*(6), 137–141.

5. Centers for Disease Control and Prevention. (n.d.). *Diabetes and Prediabetes.* https://www.cdc.gov/chronicdisease/pdf/factsheets/diabetes-H.pdf

6. Centers for Disease Control and Prevention. (2020). *National Diabetes Statistics Report, 2020.* https://www.cdc.gov/diabetes/pdfs/data/statistics/national-diabetes-statistics-report.pdf

7. World Health Organization. (2020, April 1). *Obesity and overweight.* https://www.who.int/news-room/fact-sheets/detail/obesity-and-overweight

8. World Health Organization. (2020, June 8). *Diabetes.* https://www.who.int/news-room/fact-sheets/detail/diabetes

9. American Diabetes Association. (2018). Economic costs of diabetes in the US in 2017. *Diabetes Care, 41*(5), 917–928.

10. United Nations. (n.d.). Food. https://www.un.org/en/sections/issues-depth/food/

11. D'Urso, J. (2015, July 10). World's poorest need $160 a year to end hunger: U.N. *Reuters.* https://www.reuters.com/article/us-development-goals-hunger-idUSKCN0PK1K820150710

12. Le Strat, Y., & Le Foll, B. (2011). Obesity and cannabis use: results from 2 representative national surveys. *American Journal of Epidemiology, 174*(8), 929–933.

13. Alshaarawy, O., & Anthony, J. C. (2015). Cannabis smoking and diabetes mellitus: Results from meta-analysis with eight independent replication samples. *Epidemiology (Cambridge, Mass.), 26*(4), 597.

14. Ngueta, G., & Ndjaboue, R. (2020). Lifetime marijuana use in relation to insulin resistance in lean, overweight, and obese US adults. *Journal of Diabetes, 12*(1), 38–47.

15. Meier, M. H., Pardini, D., Beardslee, J., & Matthews, K. A. (2019). Associations between cannabis use and cardiometabolic risk factors: a longitudinal study of men. *Psychosomatic medicine, 81*(3), 281–288.

16. Ross, J. M., Pacheco-Colón, I., Hawes, S. W., & Gonzalez, R. (2020). Bidirectional Longitudinal Associations Between Cannabis Use and Body Mass Index Among Adolescents. *Cannabis and Cannabinoid Research, 5*(1), 81–88.

17. Rodondi, N., Pletcher, M. J., Liu, K., Hulley, S. B., & Sidney, S. (2006). Marijuana use, diet, body mass index, and cardiovascular risk factors (from the CARDIA study). *The American journal of cardiology, 98*(4), 478–484.

18. Smit, E., & Crespo, C. J. (2001). Dietary intake and nutritional status of US adult marijuana users: Results from the Third National Health and Nutrition Examination Survey. *Public Health Nutrition, 4*(3), 781–786.

19. Muccioli, G. G., Naslain, D., Bäckhed, F., Reigstad, C. S., Lambert, D. M., Delzenne, N. M., & Cani, P. D. (2010). The endocannabinoid system links gut microbiota to adipogenesis. *Molecular systems biology, 6*(1), 392.

20. Cluny, N. L., Keenan, C. M., Reimer, R. A., Le Foll, B., & Sharkey, K. A. (2015). Prevention of diet-induced obesity effects on body weight and gut microbiota in mice treated chronically with Δ9-tetrahydrocannabinol. *PLoS One, 10*(12), e0144270.

21. Bermúdez-Silva, F. J., Suárez, J., Baixeras, E., Cobo, N., Bautista, D., Cuesta-Muñoz, A. L., ... & Mechoulam, R. (2008). Presence of functional cannabinoid receptors in human endocrine pancreas. *Diabetologia, 51*(3), 476–487.

22. Jadoon, K. A., Ratcliffe, S. H., Barrett, D. A., Thomas, E. L., Stott, C., Bell, J. D., ... & Tan, G. D. (2016). Efficacy and safety of cannabidiol and tetrahydrocannabivarin on glycemic and lipid parameters in patients with type 2 diabetes: a randomized, double-blind, placebo-controlled, parallel group pilot study. *Diabetes Care, 39*(10), 1777–1786.

23. Benjamin, E. J., Muntner, P., Alonso, A., Bittencourt, M. S., Callaway, C. W., Carson, A. P., ... & Delling, F. N. (2019). Heart disease and stroke Statistics-2019 update a report from the American Heart Association. *Circulation.*

24. Johnson-Sasso, C. P., Tompkins, C., Kao, D. P., & Walker, L. A. (2018). Marijuana use and short-term outcomes in patients hospitalized for acute myocardial infarction. *PLOS ONE, 13*(7), Article e0199705. https://doi.org/10.1371/journal.pone.0199705

25. Desai, R., Patel, U., Sharma, S., Amin, P., Bhuva, R., Patel, M. S., ... & Batra, N. (2017). Recreational marijuana use and acute myocardial infarction: insights from nationwide inpatient sample in the United States. *Cureus, 9*(11).

26. Frost, L., Mostofsky, E., Rosenbloom, J. I., Mukamal, K. J., & Mittleman, M. A. (2013). Marijuana use and long-term mortality among survivors of acute myocardial infarction. *American heart journal*, *165*(2), 170–175.

27. Mukamal, K. J., Maclure, M., Muller, J. E., & Mittleman, M. A. (2008). An exploratory prospective study of marijuana use and mortality following acute myocardial infarction. *American heart journal*, *155*(3), 465–470.

28. Kwok, C. S., Alraies, M. C., Mohamed, M., Rashid, M., Shoaib, A., Nolan, J., ... & Mamas, M. A. (2020). Rates, predictors and the impact of cannabis misuse on in-hospital outcomes among patients undergoing percutaneous coronary intervention (from the National Inpatient Sample). *International Journal of Clinical Practice*, *74*(5), e13477.

29. Richards, J. R., Bing, M. L., Moulin, A. K., Elder, J. W., Rominski, R. T., Summers, P. J., & Laurin, E. G. (2019). Cannabis use and acute coronary syndrome. *Clinical Toxicology*, *57*(10), 831–841.

30. Carbone, F., Mach, F., Vuilleumier, N., & Montecucco, F. (2014). Cannabinoid receptor type 2 activation in atherosclerosis and acute cardiovascular diseases. *Current medicinal chemistry*, *21*(35), 4046–4058.

31. Maslov, L. N., Khaliulin, I., Zhang, Y., Krylatov, A. V., Naryzhnaya, N. V., Mechoulam, R., ... & Downey, J. M. (2016). Prospects for creation of cardioprotective drugs based on cannabinoid receptor agonists. *Journal of cardiovascular pharmacology and therapeutics*, *21*(3), 262–272.

32. Waldman, M., Hochhauser, E., Fishbein, M., Aravot, D., Shainberg, A., & Sarne, Y. (2013). An ultra-low dose of tetrahydrocannabinol provides cardioprotection. *Biochemical pharmacology*, *85*(11), 1626–1633..

33. Steffens, S., Veillard, N. R., Arnaud, C., Pelli, G., Burger, F., Staub, C., ... & Mach, F. (2005). Low dose oral cannabinoid therapy reduces progression of atherosclerosis in mice. *Nature*, *434*(7034), 782–786.

34. Reis, J. P., Auer, R., Bancks, M. P., Goff Jr, D. C., Lewis, C. E., Pletcher, M. J., ... & Sidney, S. (2017). Cumulative lifetime marijuana use and incident cardiovascular disease in middle age: the Coronary Artery Risk Development in Young Adults (CARDIA) study. *American journal of public health*, *107*(4), 601–606.

35. Alshaarawy, O., Sidney, S., Auer, R., Green, D., Soliman, E. Z., Goff Jr, D. C., & Anthony, J. C. (2019). Cannabis Use and Markers of Systemic Inflammation: The Coronary Artery Risk Development in Young Adults Study. *The American journal of medicine*, *132*(11), 1327–1334.

36. Benjamin, E. J., Blaha, M. J., Chiuve, S. E., Cushman, M., Das, S. R., Deo, R., ... & Jiménez, M. C. (2017). Heart Disease and Stroke Statistics-2017 Update: A Report From the American Heart Association. Circulation, 135(10), e146-e603..

37. Heiss, W.-D., & Graf, R. (1994). The ischemic penumbra. *Current Opinion in Neurology*, *7*(1), 11–19.

38. Schmidt-Pogoda, A., Bonberg, N., Koecke, M. H. M., Strecker, J. K., Wellmann, J., Bruckmann, N. M., ... & Minnerup, H. (2020). Why most acute stroke studies are positive in animals but not in patients: a systematic comparison of preclinical, early phase, and phase 3 clinical trials of neuroprotective agents. *Annals of Neurology*, *87*(1), 40–51.

39. England, T. J., Hind, W. H., Rasid, N. A., & O'sullivan, S. E. (2015). Cannabinoids in experimental stroke: a systematic review and meta-analysis. *Journal of Cerebral Blood Flow & Metabolism*, *35*(3), 348–358.

40. Hampson, A. J., Axelrod, J., & Grimaldi, M. (2003, October 7). *Cannabinoids as antioxidants and neuroprotectants* (U.S. Patent No. 6,630,507). U.S. Patent and Trademark Office. http://patft.uspto.gov/netacgi/nph-Parser?Sect1=P-TO1&Sect2=HITOFF&d=PALL&p=1&u=%2Fnetahtml%2FPTO%2Fsrchnum.htm&r=1&f=G&l=50&s1=6630507.PN.&OS=PN/6630507&RS=PN/6630507

41. Maas, A. I., Murray, G., Henney III, H., Kassem, N., Legrand, V., Mangelus, M., ... & Knoller, N. (2006). Efficacy and safety of dexanabinol in severe traumatic brain injury: results of a phase III randomised, placebo-controlled, clinical trial. *The Lancet Neurology*, *5*(1), 38–45.

42. Nguyen, B. M., Kim, D., Bricker, S., Bongard, F., Neville, A., Putnam, B., ... & Plurad, D. (2014). Effect of marijuana use on outcomes in traumatic brain injury. *The American Surgeon*, *80*(10), 979–983.

43. Di Napoli, M., Zha, A. M., Godoy, D. A., Masotti, L., Schreuder, F. H., Popa-Wagner, A., & Behrouz, R. (2016). Prior cannabis use is associated with outcome after intracerebral hemorrhage. *Cerebrovascular Diseases*, *41*(5-6), 248–255.

44. Malhotra, K., Rumalla, K., & Mittal, M. K. (2018). Association and clinical outcomes of marijuana in patients with intracerebral hemorrhage. *Journal of Stroke and Cerebrovascular Diseases*, *27*(12), 3479–3486.

45. National Toxicology Program. (1996). *NTP toxicology and carcinogenesis studies of 1-trans-delta9-tetrahydrocannabinol (CAS no. 1972-08-3) in F344 rats and B6C3F1 mice (gavage studies).* (National Toxicology Program Technical Report Series 446). U.S. Department of Health and Human Services, Public Health Service, National Institutes of Health. https://ntp.niehs.nih.gov/ntp/htdocs/lt_rpts/tr446.pdf

46. Hashibe, M., Morgenstern, H., Cui, Y., Tashkin, D. P., Zhang, Z. F., Cozen, W., ... & Greenland, S. (2006). Marijuana use and the risk of lung and upper aerodigestive tract cancers: results of a population-based case-control study. *Cancer Epidemiology and Prevention Biomarkers*, *15*(10), 1829–1834.

47. Zhang, L. R., Morgenstern, H., Greenland, S., Chang, S. C., Lazarus, P., Teare, M. D., ... & Brhane, Y. (2015). Cannabis smoking and lung cancer risk: Pooled analysis in the International Lung Cancer Consortium. *International journal of cancer*, *136*(4), 894–903.

48. Thomas, A. A., Wallner, L. P., Quinn, V. P., Slezak, J., Van Den Eeden, S. K., Chien, G. W., & Jacobsen, S. J. (2015).

Association between cannabis use and the risk of bladder cancer: results from the California Men's Health Study. *Urology*, *85*(2), 388–393.

49. Gurney, J., Shaw, C., Stanley, J., Signal, V., & Sarfati, D. (2015). Cannabis exposure and risk of testicular cancer: a systematic review and meta-analysis. *BMC cancer*, *15*(1), 897.

50. Reviewed in Huang, Y. H. J., Zhang, Z. F., Tashkin, D. P., Feng, B., Straif, K., & Hashibe, M. (2015). An epidemiologic review of marijuana and cancer: an update. *Cancer Epidemiology and Prevention Biomarkers*, *24*(1), 15–31.

51. Reviewed in Huang, Y. H. J., Zhang, Z. F., Tashkin, D. P., Feng, B., Straif, K., & Hashibe, M. (2015). An epidemiologic review of marijuana and cancer: an update. *Cancer Epidemiology and Prevention Biomarkers*, *24*(1), 15–31.

52. Veligati, S., Howdeshell, S., Beeler-Stinn, S., Lingam, D., Allen, P. C., Chen, L. S., & Grucza, R. A. (2020). Changes in alcohol and cigarette consumption in response to medical and recreational cannabis legalization: Evidence from US state tax receipt data. *International Journal of Drug Policy*, *75*, 102585.

53. Weil, A. (1972). *The natural mind: A new way of looking at drugs and the higher consciousness*. Houghton Mifflin Company.

54. Santini, Z. I., Jose, P. E., Cornwell, E. Y., Koyanagi, A., Nielsen, L., Hinrichsen, C., ... & Koushede, V. (2020). Social disconnectedness, perceived isolation, and symptoms of depression and anxiety among older Americans (NSHAP): a longitudinal mediation analysis. *The Lancet Public Health*, *5*(1), e62-e70.

55. Steptoe, A., Shankar, A., Demakakos, P., & Wardle, J. (2013). Social isolation, loneliness, and all-cause mortality in older men and women. Proceedings of the National Academy of Sciences, 110(15), 5797–5801.

56. Cohen, S., Doyle, W. J., Skoner, D. P., Rabin, B. S., & Gwaltney, J. M. (1997). Social ties and susceptibility to the common cold. *Jama*, *277*(24), 1940–1944.

57. Knox, S. S., & Uvnäs-Moberg, K. (1998). Social isolation and cardiovascular disease: An atherosclerotic pathway? *Psychoneuroendocrinology*, *23*(8), 877–890.

58. Caspi, A., Harrington, H., Moffitt, T. E., Milne, B. J., & Poulton, R. (2006). Socially isolated children 20 years later: risk of cardiovascular disease. *Archives of pediatrics & adolescent medicine*, *160*(8), 805–811.

59. Knox, S. S., & Uvnäs-Moberg, K. (1998). Social isolation and cardiovascular disease: An atherosclerotic pathway? *Psychoneuroendocrinology*, *23*(8), 877–890.

60. Soueif, M. I. (1975). Chronic cannabis takers: Some temperamental characteristics. *Drug and Alcohol Dependence*, *1*(2), 125–154.

61. Feldman, H. W., & Mandel, J. (1998). Providing medical marijuana: The importance of cannabis clubs. *Journal of Psychoactive Drugs*, *30*(2), 179–186.

62. Lavie-Ajayi, M., & Shvartzman, P. (2019). Restored self: A phenomenological study of pain relief by cannabis. *Pain Medicine*, *20*(11), 2086–2093. https://doi.org/10.1093/pm/pny176.

63. Dewals, P. (2015, September 25). Marijuana, reconsidered: Dr. Lester Grinspoon on 45 years of cannabis science. *MyMPN*. www.mintpressnews.com/MyMPN/marijuana-reconsidered-an-interview-with-doctor-lester-grinspoon/

64. Grinspoon, L. (1971). *Marihuana Reconsidered*. Harvard University Press.

About the Author: My Path to Cannabis Medicine

1. Zimmer, L. E., & Morgan, J. P. (1997). *Marijuana myths, marijuana facts: A review of the scientific evidence*. Lindesmith Center.

2. Watson, S. J., Benson, J. A., & Joy, J. E. (2000). Marijuana and medicine: Assessing the science base: A summary of the 1999 Institute of Medicine report. *Archives of General Psychiatry*, *57*(6), 547–552.

3. Feuer, B., Sulak, D., Christ, W. J., Lapenta, R. J., & Feuer, M. (2018). *Process for the production of a concentrated cannabinoid product* (U.S. Patent No. 10155176). U.S. Patent and Trademark Office. http://patft.uspto.gov/netacgi/nph-Parser?Sect1=PTO2&Sect2=HITOFF&p=1&u=%2Fnetahtml%2FPTO%2Fsearch-bool.html&r=1&f=G&l=50&co1=AND&d=PTXT&s1=10155176.PN.&OS=PN/10155176&RS=PN/10155176

Index

In this index, *f* denotes figure, *n* denotes footnote, and *t* denotes table.